Promoting a Good Death
for cancer patients of Asian culture:
An evidence-based approach

Promoting a Good Death for cancer patients of Asian culture: An evidence-based approach

Mui Hing June Mak

Whiting & Birch
MMVII

© Mui Hing June Mak 2007
Published by Whiting & Birch Ltd,
Forest Hill, London SE23 3HZ

EAN 9781861771001
ISBN 1861771002
Printed in England and the United States by Lightning Source

Promoting a good death for cancer patients of Asian culture

Contents

List of Figures

Foreword

THERE IS A popular view, even among academic researchers, that the study of dying is now quite advanced. This is a highly exaggerated view but supported by casual observations such as the world-wide spread of hospice and palliative care services, by the impressive and enduring sales of books such as Kubler-Ross's 'On Death and Dying' (1969), or the regular publicity that people with cancer or HIV attract when lobbying for new treatments or services.

Sadly, these book sales and services are no measure of our far more modest advances in the study of dying people and their needs. Rather, the popularity of hospice often reflect a region-specific growth of a new health service under the pressure of its aging population or the growing curiosity and openness towards death and loss – and more particularly in the Western world. Elizabeth Kubler-Ross's work represents - even today - only one of a precious handful of actual empirical work examining the needs and conduct of dying people. Empirical work, theoretical development and interpretation of dying people's needs, or a more than passing understanding of the role of culture on dying conduct remains in its infancy. Furthermore, of those few studies that pioneer our understanding of these end-of-life needs and behaviours little of this research employs non-Western samples.

Dr Mui-Hing June Mak's present work is both exceptional and pioneering in just this way. Most of our current understanding about Asian dying remains locked away from the Western gaze in non-English publications or in unpublished theses scattered around different university libraries around the world. In presenting her insights, Dr Mak not only provides us with fresh insights into how a Good Death expresses itself in Hong Kong, but also how this ideal varies and is modified in other Asian societies as this is observed in the their own, often inaccessible literature.

We have, in this important book, both a review of the literature on dying conduct and needs from several Asian points of experience but also an in-depth study of one example of this experience from an author who is both a nurse clinician and a social scientist. Dr Mak brings to her words not only the disciplined eye of a hospice clinician and academic but also the empathy – what the famous European sociologist Max Weber called 'Verstehen' (a sense of personal connection) - from her direct personal experiences. Her close, personal relationship with three dying people – her grandmother, her professional medical mentor, and one of her own students - was not only formative of her current research and professional interests but also the driving concern in ensuring that all the voices of her study participants are heard clearly, sympathetically, and poignantly.

Dr Mak's book is hallmark study of the dying experience that brings together compassion, academic insight and an inclusive view of Asia that consolidates and advances our understanding of the needs of dying in this part of world. It is essential reading for all of us who wish to deepen a trans-cultural understanding of our common fate.

Allan Kellehear, PhD
Professor of Sociology & Head of Department
Department of Social & Policy Sciences
Centre for Death and Society (CDAS)
University of Bath
UK

Preface

MY MOTIVATIONS FOR researching this area and writing this book were two-fold. First, I wanted to help improve the care of those dying of cancer, particularly in Chinese communities, which was what prompted me into an exploration of the meaning of Good Death from a cultural perspective. Second, this would be an important element in my personal and professional development. In Hong Kong, cancer has been the leading cause of death since 1971 and accounts for one-third of total deaths. Therefore, caring for cancer patients has long been an everyday task for many healthcare professionals.

However, adequate attention has not been paid to the complexity of health problems that were experienced by such patients in Hong Kong. For example, as a student nurse, I was assigned to look after patients with terminal cancer in a chronic medical ward. It was apparent that most cancer patients suffered more intensely than people with other illnesses. One patient had cancer of both breasts. She experienced a lot of pain every time she had her wound cleansed. Quite often, these patients did not receive adequate pain control, and made constant requests for analgesics. Unfortunately, some nurses who did not seem to understand the complex health problems of the dying gave them 'placebo' injections because they did not want their patients to become addicted to analgesics. Consequently, the patients' pain was not relieved. Many also did not receive sufficient support as the number of nursing staff on this ward was relatively small.

Meanwhile, three significant persons in my life had inspired my investigation of the meaning of death and dying. The first was my grandmother, who had died of thyroid cancer in her seventies, and with whom I had a close personal relationship. After a tracheotomy, my grandmother could neither eat nor speak properly. I observed that the nurses were too busy to attend adequately to my grandmother's needs as she was not able to communicate verbally. I saw that she felt distressed in her last few days.

The second was Dr M. Aquinas, medical director of Ruttonjee Hospital and visiting consultant at Grantham Hospital where I was a nurse educator. I saw Dr Aquinas as a role model, who greatly encouraged me in my research. Unfortunately, she was diagnosed with cancer, and she suffered greatly from oedema of the legs. Thus, she refused to receive any visitors before she died.

The third person to inspire me was Yip Kwok Chuen, one of my students, who shortly after his graduation, was diagnosed with cancer of the liver. He subsequently became very depressed and refused to talk to me when I visited him in hospital. At his funeral, Yip's father said that his son had appreciated my visit although he did not speak to me. From my personal and professional experiences, I became aware that many people died poorly with inadequate care.

The book will be of interest to all those with concerns in the area of health, illness, life, death and care for the dying. This includes students and teachers across the medical, health, behavioural and social sciences, anthropology, philosophy, thanatology, not to mention the humanities. Readers with interest in the topic of Good death and palliative care should also find this book of interest, as indeed they might have with previous scholarly treatments of this subject in sociology (Kellehear, 1990), community studies (Young and Cullen, 1996), medicine (Lee, 1995 and Webb, 1997). This book will be the first monograph to approach the subject from a cultural perspective. It is suitable for use as a student text on cancer/ palliative nursing, social work, medicine, counselling, gerontology, sociology and qualitative research programmes.

In addition to this, I expect particular interest from healthcare professionals who work in palliative/ hospice settings in multi-cultural countries. The book is based on research done on Chinese patients; however, it is also relevant to those working with other Asian patients, particularly those whose beliefs are founded in Confucianism, Taoism or Buddhism, and also those from other parts of the world with these beliefs. The book suggests a system of more culturally-appropriate palliative care interventions and demonstrates the importance of considering culture when designing methods for measuring the quality of life among dying persons.

Acknowledgements

Many people deserve my special thanks for their help in the completion of this book. Most noteworthy, of course, are the people who participated in the interviews. Because the participants in this research were dying people, most of them felt unwell at the time of interview. My gratitude to them is profound. I hope I have adequately represented the stories that I was privileged to hear. I am particular grateful to my academic supervisor and mentor, Professor Allan Kellehear for his excellent intellectual support, continuous encouragement and many insightful suggestions.

I am also grateful to Mr David Whiting, Director of Whiting and Birch Ltd for his encouragement and keen interest in the project. I would like to thank several scholars for their expertise and thoughtful suggestions at different stages during my preparation of this research: Dr Derek Doyle, Professor Renee Fox, Professor Daniel Overmyer, Professor Clive Seale, Dr Bruce Rumbold and Dr Peter Kok Wan Tan. My gratitude also goes to several staff in the hospice units: Dr Chak Wah Lam and Ms Ellen Yeung of Ruttonjee Hospital and Dr Helen Tinsley Dr Doris Tse and Ms Catherine Ho of Caritas Medical Centre.

To my family, I owe a special debt. I thank all of them for their patience, understanding and unfailing support, a support that comes from an intimate family connectedness.

*

I am grateful to Baywood Publishing for granting me permission to reprint extracts from the following articles.

Mak, MHJ. Death awareness: An experience of Chinese patients with terminal cancer. *Omega. Journal of Death and Dying.* 2001; 43 (3): 259-279.
Mak, MHJ. Accepting one's death: An experience of Chinese hospice patients. *Omega. Journal of Death and Dying.* 2002; 45 (3): 229-244.

Mui Hing June Mak
Hong Kong
November 2007

1
Introduction

FROM A REVIEW of the literature, it appears that a Good Death is an uncommon phenomenon. The findings of some pioneer studies [1-5] have stimulated a closer examination of the needs of the dying. An individual's perception of death and a Good Death are clearly associated with his or her cultural and religious beliefs. 'Death itself is not only a state but a complex symbol, the significance of which will vary from one person to another and from one culture to another, and is also profoundly dependent upon the nature and vicissitudes of the developmental process'. While there are a few existing studies on Good Death based on first-person accounts by dying individuals in Western countries,[7,8] limited studies have been conducted in the East.[9] Three main broad questions emerged from this review of the literature. How did people with terminal cancer become aware of their impending death? I asked this question to identify their ideas and personal experiences of the awareness of approaching death. The next question to emerge from the first was what were the needs and concerns of these people? In other words, what did it mean to die a Good Death from the dying person's perspective? I sought to understand and document the experiences of dying people and what they preferred to encounter, and if any discrepancy existed. Such documentation would allow me to identify implications, which would facilitate people's achievement of their desirable Good Death.

There was little to draw on from the existing literature to provide an understanding of the ideal of dying a Good Death, due to the limitations and perspective of existing research and the lack of a systematic review of what could be inferred about Good Death. In reality, there was scarce evidence of the effectiveness of interventions aimed at helping hospice patients to attain a Good Death. Efforts to examine the experiences of patients receiving hospice care in Hong Kong were limited,[11] and patient-desired outcomes were seldom identified. Therefore, it was logical to assume that healthcare professionals needed more information about patients' desires before they could be helped to achieve the outcomes they preferred. Accordingly I decided to focus on the area of palliative care, having earlier investigated psychological responses towards dying and death of terminally ill cancer patients in a Chinese community.[12]

My motivation for conducting my research was further inspired by the current hospice movement in Chinese communities such as Hong Kong, Taiwan, and mainland China. In the West, the introduction of hospice care has provided an alternative way of dying.[13, 14] It has been a major force in deepening understanding of the phenomenology of illness, in helping human relationships and health care, and in advancing the rights of the dying[15]. More importantly, the awareness of death has strengthened people's appreciation of the uniqueness of life. In Hong Kong, the idea of hospice care was first introduced in 1982.[16] Since then, awareness of the need for hospice care has grown steadily. At present, three types of service are offered: hospital-based, hospice-based, and home-based hospice care.[17]

In Taiwan, Dr. David Chung, the Medical Director of Mackay Hospital, set up the first hospice in 1990 after a visit to Japan in 1982.[18] Compared with Hong Kong and Taiwan, however, the demand for developing hospice service, teaching, and research in China is even greater. 'Although hospice care in this country is a new branch of science and a new concept for most Chinese people, the source of the spirit of revolutionary humanitarianism and the glorious moral faith of human beings embodied by the modern hospice movement can also be traced back to traditional Chinese culture'.[19] The first Hospice Research Centre was set up in Tianjin in 1988. Today, hospice services are provided in hospitals, hospices, at home, and in nursing homes. The development of hospice services in China is growing relatively fast. By 2002, there were said to be hundreds of palliative care services in urban areas.[34] Hospice services are available or are being developed in more than two-thirds of China's provinces, autonomous regions, and municipalities.[20] The hospice services are offered to cancer, cardiac, and chest patients.

The introduction and development of hospice care may have been motivated by a desire to improve the quality of care for the dying.[21]

The practice has expanded from the West to the East. Thus the need for, and further development of, hospice care in China is important. Of equal importance, 'the development of a Chinese model of hospice care which is applicable to Chinese people is suggested...'[22] The authors recommend that China should develop models that are suited to its particular needs, culture, and customs rather than imitate models developed in other countries. The operationalisation of the concept of Good Death from the patient's point of view is essential.

This book is important for several reasons. First, it makes an important contribution to building knowledge about thanatology by describing the perceptions of death of the hospice patients. The lack of sound research to study the phenomenon of death and dying was identified by Kastenbaum and Costa.[24] and further substantiated in a search of international theses and dissertations between 1988 and 2000. Furthermore, there is a significant difference between responses of patients and primary caregivers in their views on quality of life.[25, 26] This difference in attitudes to death has important clinical implications because effective communication is best achieved when care receivers and caregivers share a common understanding of the patients' experiences.

Second, it provides further understanding of what Chinese hospice patients believe it means to die a Good Death. It will help provide the necessary culturally-based practical guidelines to achieve it. An important role of healthcare professionals is to interpret the patient's concerns to the family.[27] This role is clearly difficult to fulfil when the patient and healthcare professionals do not share the same culture. Methods of care are largely derived from culture and therefore require culturally-based knowledge and skills to be effective, legitimate, and relevant to people of diverse culture.[28-30] In her theory of transcultural care, diversity and universality, Leininger [28] offers assumptions derived from an anthropological base. She maintains that care has been an essential feature of human survival, development, and confrontation with such life events as illness, disability, and death. Human care is therefore universal although it has diverse expressions, that are patterns and methods of action in care giving, care expressions, patterns, and styles which take on different meanings in different cultural contexts.

I have built on the work already done on thanatology in Asian cultures. 'Asian' refers to people with ancestral origins in East Asia (China, Japan, Korea, Mongolia and Taiwan), Southeast Asia (Brunei, Cambodia, East Timor, Indonesia, Laos, Myanmar, Malaysia,

Philippines, Singapore, Thailand and Vietnam), South Asia (India, Bangladesh, Pakistan, Sri Lanka, Maldives, Nepal) and Middle East. 'Asian' accounts for about four billion people or more than 57 percent of the world's population. The People's Republic of China is the most populated country in the world. The Han Chinese, make up about 20 percent of the world population. Meanwhile, there are approximately thirty-four million 'overseas Chinese' who live mostly in Southeast Asia.[36] Many, however, live in other parts of the world, where they may still retain their Chinese culture.

The research on which this book is based, is largely a case study of one Asian cultural form of Good Death from Chinese hospice patients in Hong Kong. Chinese culture is one of the two key influences on beliefs and behaviour in death, dying and bereavement in Asian cultures. The other influence is Indian culture.[36] Chinese culture expresses the different configurations of Confucianism, Buddhism and Taoism. Taoism and Buddhism, along with an underlying Confucian morality, have been the dominant religions of Chinese society for almost two millennia and the neighbouring countries when these religions are spread to them. On the other hand, Buddhism, Hinduism, Sikhism and Jainism all have their origins in India.

Confucianism is a complex system of social, political, moral and religious thought.[36-38] The cultures most strongly influenced by Confucianism include those of China, Korea, Japan, Singapore and Vietnam.[36] Buddhism originated in India and was transferred to China during the first century and later spread throughout East Asia. Today, India, China (including Tibet), Korea, Japan, Vietnam and Taiwan all practise Buddhism. It is estimated that about six percent of the six billion world population practise Buddhism. Only within the past century, Western cultures have reached out to embrace Buddhist wisdom to awaken and to serve. Meanwhile, Taoism, one of the Chinese philosophical works of the Warring States era, enjoys a wide following in the West. There are some movements in the West that claim this point of view as well, but most do not maintain traditional ritual practice. Today, Taoist churches still survive in Taiwan, Hong Kong, other Chinese communities and have been re-established in China.[36-37]

Third, this book offers suggestions on improving the quality of palliative care. Some significant statistics that highlight the importance of studying the dying are reported.[31, 32] These authors concluded that about 70 per cent of all deaths in adults were associated with diseases. This, together with the phenomenon of an ageing population, means that a majority of the world's adult population will have to cope with the prospect of their own impending death. For example, cancer has been the major killer in Hong Kong for many years.[17] The situations in Taiwan and mainland China are similar. In the developed countries, diseases of the circulatory system and cancer (both associated with advanced age) are the chief takers-of-life, accounting for approximately two-thirds of all deaths.[37] '...the war against cancer is one in which the foe's order of battle changes constantly'.[33] It is found that many patients associate their diagnosis of cancer with death, as cancer is a life-threatening disease. Dying, as a prolonged social and physical process, has been under-researched, and the focus of previous literature has been on the caregivers of the dying patients rather than the patients themselves.

About this book

This book is a comprehensive description of the needs and concerns of the people dying with cancer through face-to-face interview. Seven important outcomes of the patients to facilitate a Harmonious Good Death are identified. These seven elements include death awareness, hope, comfort, connectedness, control, preparations, and completion. These elements constructively unite the dying person and his or her caregivers (health care professionals and family) and the universe (ancestors, heaven/gods), in a beneficial hierarchical and socio-cultural relationship. The aim of the book is to present these seven elements and their relationships for dying a good death. It also gives health care professionals insights to the implications to promote better quality of life for the dying and their caregivers based on the evidence of the research findings.

This book has been organised in the following manner. Chapter One introduces my inspiration in writing about death and dying, which is considered a subject of contemporary social taboo in most Asian societies. The chapter also presents the organisation of the book. Chapter Two provides a detailed critical review of death, dying, and Good Death from a global overview. The review begins with a close scrutiny and examination of death and dying from the Western perspective. The historical development; meaning of death and dying; factors that influence the dying process; theories of death and dying and Good Death, from different disciplinary discourses such as philosophy, psychology, sociology, and health sciences are explored. Then Chinese views on death, dying, and Good death from a cultural perspective, and discuss traditional Chinese beliefs, Chinese popular beliefs, and contemporary studies are examined. The review summarises the main studies of death and dying from different cultures and highlights that while some theories of death and dying exist in the West, limited studies have been conducted in the East, and notes the scarcity of related works in Chinese culture.

Chapter Three describes the Grounded Theory approach, which is the research method used in this research. The need and benefits of using Grounded Theory approach are justified. It presents a detailed discussion of the research process, which includes preparations, ethical considerations, sample description, data collection and data analysis. Interviewing is the key method of data collection and constant comparison is used for data analysis. Then, the chapter comments on the reliability and validity of the research process and limitations of the methodology.

The next seven chapters of the book deal separately with the seven elements of Harmonious Death. The seven elements are death awareness, hope, comfort, connectedness, control, preparations, and completion. Each chapter discusses one main element of Harmonious Death as they emerged from the findings of the research and its clinical implications. 'Today, the integration of palliative care into the main stream health system, and the development of an 'evidence-based' model of practice and organisation are crucial to long-term viability.'[35]

Large sections of direct quotes from the patients are woven into the style of these accounts, which reproduced to provide useful and accurate illustrations of the issues.

Chapter Four describes awareness of dying (Death Awareness), which is an essential first step of dying a Good Death. The discussion stresses the importance of awareness. Three main issues are identified: being informed; receiving 'bad news'; being aware of the diagnosis of cancer and being aware of dying. I emphasise that the taboo on death remains in most contemporary Chinese societies, which might add to the complexity of death awareness issues. Chinese people may have different exhibit diverse presentations of death awareness but they may have similar experiences of dying.

Chapter Five focuses on the second element: maintaining hope

(Hope). Two main sources of hope for dying persons are identified: receiving treatment and making adjustments. Many of the dying persons I interviewed continued to strive for new hope after they developed an awareness of dying. Traditional Chinese medical treatment emerges as a popular alternative therapy. In addition, the chapter discusses the three major strategies of adjustments: adjusting to hospice environment, changing lifestyles, and making psychological adjustments, and examines the nature of hope during the course of illness.

Being free from pain and suffering (Comfort) is the third element of Harmonious Death, and is discussed in Chapter Six. The chapter is divided into two sections. The first section reveals my findings related to the dying persons' perceptions of being free from pain and their existential experiences of pain. Correspondingly, the second part of the chapter discusses the patients' perceptions and experiences of suffering. These human experiences are subjective, emotional, and often multi-dimensional in nature. The chapter further explores the phenomenon of unresolved pain and suffering, with a focus on the issues of euthanasia and suicide.

The fourth element, maintaining social relations (Connectedness), is discussed in Chapter Seven. Dying people are concerned with two main social relationships: with the hospice staff, and with the family. As death becomes an institutional event, hospice staffs have replaced the family as the primary caregivers for dying persons. Nevertheless, many Chinese, such as the patients in this study, believed that the living and the dying continue their relationships through the practice of filial piety and ancestor worship. The function of family connectedness is clear as it may also offer spiritual comfort to dying persons. The chapter further examines the factors affecting connectedness with both hospice staff and the family.

Chapter Eight describes my findings on experiencing personal control (Control). The chapter begins with an exploration of the concepts of personal control, and examines the dying persons' views on where and with whom they would like to die. The chapter also discusses several factors affecting a person's ability to effect control, which include the person's psycho-social, physical, and spiritual status, are discussed.

Chapter Nine discusses the element of preparing to depart and bidding farewells (Preparations). The chapter focuses on the issues of personal preparations for death: organising material affairs, leaving instructions, and giving gifts. The discussion then deals with public preparations — preparing funerals. Funeral arrangements may give social and spiritual meaning to the dying and their families. Examples of cultural preparations and bidding farewells are also presented.

Accepting the timing of one's death (Completion) is the last element of Harmonious Death, and is the focus of Chapter Ten. The patients may first guess the timing of death. They either choose to accept or reject the timing of their death. The chapter identifies four circumstances in which the patients may have better acceptance of the timing of death: completing social obligations, dying in old age, accepting death as a natural part of life, and experiencing meaningful lives.

Chapter Eleven presents the theoretical framework of Harmonious Death that unites the above elements. The chapter summarises the findings of the research, and explores the association of these seven elements and the dying person's harmonious relationships with heaven, medical practitioners, and the family respectively. It then examines the extent of the influence of Chinese moral traditions, such as Confucianism, on Harmonious Death. Lastly, the chapter compares the present theory with some existing models of Good Death in order to highlight the significance of the present framework.

In conclusion, Chapter Twelve provides a short summary of the findings and outlines future implications of the research. Several broad suggestions are made to translate the theoretical concepts into practical guidance for future policy and research directions.

2
Literature review

Introduction

THIS LITERATURE REVIEW on death and dying serves as a detailed background to the study. The review explores Western views of death and dying, because studies and research in these areas were initiated in Western countries in the 1940s.[1] The pioneer studies of dying and death have shown that many people died rather poorly. They experienced significant emotional turmoil on learning of their imminent death. This has further stimulated consideration of the needs of the dying person – particularly what each individual meant by dying a Good Death. Thus this chapter explores and analyses the concept of Good Death and the elements that constitute a Good Death. Since views on dying and death are essentially cultural phenomena, I then consider the Chinese perspective on death and dying with the aim of identifying cultural influences thereon.

Death and dying:
The Western perspective

Historical development

One of humanity's most distinguishing characteristics is its capacity
to grasp the concept of a future and inevitable event – death. 'The
place of death in psychology was practically *terra incognita* and an
off-limits enterprise until the mid-20th century'.[2] Psychology's initial
organised approach to death was a symposium, 'The concept of death
and its relation to behaviour' in 1956.[3] In the succeeding years, there
was an increase in the number of activities in the field.

Death is manifestly too complex to be the special sphere of any
one discipline'.[2] Death-related research in sociology, psychology,
and psychiatry emerged between 1940 and 1960. Feifel, [4-5] Becker,[6]
Kastenbaum and Aisenberg [7] studied attitudes towards death, fear
of death, and bereavement. Psychologists also made significant
contributions to the study of suicide and suicide prevention, developing
guidelines for suicide prevention work.[8, 174] Between 1960 and 1970,
there were significant contributions to knowledge about the personal,
interpersonal, and social meanings of dying and death. Understanding
derived from investigations by sociologists such as Fulton, [9-11] Glaser
and Strauss, [12-15] Sudnow,[16-17] nurse sociologist Benoliel, [18-20] and
psychiatrists Hinton,[21] Kubler-Ross,[22] Parkes, [23] and Weisman.[24] Other
pioneering works include Choron,[25] and Gorer.[26] Meanwhile, Saunders
[27] was concerned with the clinical problem of intractable pain when
she began her work in hospice care. Further, Moody's studies, [28-29],
which focus on near-death experiences have drawn attention to the
issue of life after death. Near-death experiences are real phenomena,
which have attracted the interest of psychologists, psychiatrists,
sociologists, and philosophers.[30-31, 175-176]

What do death and dying mean?

Dying is an integral part of life, as natural as being born. Weisman
describes it in the following poetic way: 'Dying is a great way of
going to sleep, you can't help it if you're tired enough, and can't think

of anything else'.[32] Death and dying are mysterious and complex processes. When does dying begin? When does death occur? There is still no consensus on these questions. The label of dying is commonly applied to terminally ill patients.[33] The traditional view in Western culture is that a person dies at the moment the soul leaves the body.[34] This view is religiously oriented and emphasises the spiritual aspect of life. The third view is that dying begins when a fatal condition is recognised by a medical practitioner.[35] Kellehear [36] argues that dying is no longer a self-detected matter. Today, people gain an awareness of dying from other people, either through medical (announced by the medical practitioner) or social means (informed by relatives). In other words, the patient begins to be aware of the possibility of his or her death when the medical practitioner breaks the bad news.

The medical practitioner certifies a person's death when death signs are present on examination. This is called clinical death. Sweeting and Gilhooly [37] identify two other categories of death: biological and social death. Biological death is the cessation of cellular activity; in other words, brain death occurs, [37] when the brain is not functioning although the heart is still beating. In this case, the relatives often experience a sense of hopelessness, as the patient has no chance of recovering. Once the definition of death is applied to an individual, the behaviour of others towards that person can be expected to change.[38] The individual is said to be socially dead when he or she is treated as though already dead by another person or a group of people, before actual clinical death.[17, 36, 37, 178] Social death is a phenomenon that may occur in institutions such as hospitals, and may have a great impact upon many people. It can be the end of an individual's social identity as a result of dehumanisation and depersonalisation. Furthermore, Kalish [39] and Kastenbaum [40, 41] suggest a new category, psychological death, which is said to occur when a person ceases to be aware of his or her own existence.

Researchers have highlighted that death is not solely associated with clinical evidence. It may exist in other circumstances. Therefore other categories of death – biological death, psychological death, and social death – are suggested. Clinical death may be good or bad. In biological death, the dying process is unpredictable and prolonged. The dying person often suffers from a lingering death until his or her vital organs cease to function. His or her relatives also suffer from seeing their loved one dying helplessly. Similarly, people who are in the state of psychological death cannot communicate their needs to others, and may also become a burden on the family. For the dying person who experiences social death, he or she is isolated or receives depersonalised care. This person's needs may not be met, subsequently, he or she may be emotionally disturbed. Therefore, people generally do not consider a 'premature death' which results from disease, suicide, disaster, murder, war, or accident as a Good Death.[42] Instead, such deaths are considered bad. Bad deaths are uncontrolled: they happen in the wrong place at the wrong time.[43] In conclusion, a Good Death does not appear to be a common occurrence in health care institutions.

Factors that influence the dying process

Many factors contribute to the experience of the dying process. The following factors will be examined accordingly: age, gender, social values regarding death, the nature of disease, religion and culture.[44]

Age

Attitudes towards death are related to developmental level, extent of life experiences, and chronological age. The dying process of a mature adult with a well-developed cognitive structure and diverse life experiences will differ considerably from that of a young child, who may not comprehend the nature of death. A dying person's ascribed social value also influences the kind and quality of care received. For example, age influences the dying process in terms of the degree of control the patient has over the situation. Age also affects how relatives, health care professionals and others respond to the dying person. For example, some Chinese believe that dying in old age is a blessing from heaven, while a premature or young death is a curse.[45]

Glaser and Strauss [12] suggest that patients attributed with high social value tend to receive more than routine care whereas those carrying low social value might not. The latter may also suffer a reduction in their social network due to residential mobility or death among friends or family. Death of a spouse further represents the loss of another social role. As a result of the above factors, old people are more likely to die in an institution.[46] Hospice staff sometimes complain that they are unable to fulfil hospice ideals because elderly patients are too passive and do not want to participate actively in the care plan. Therefore, institution staff will make most of the patients' decisions for them [47] and in this way, elderly people may experience premature social death.

Gender

Kastenbaum [48] suggests that gender affects the dying experience because of the difference in life roles for men and women and the resulting difference in values. A man may have more concern with financial provisions for his family, whereas a woman may be more concerned with family integrity. Cultural values may play their part, too. The death of a man was traditionally seen as more important than the death of a woman in China.[49, 50] Nevertheless, changing contemporary gender-role patterns and lifestyles have reduced the influence of gender on the dying experience.[44]

Social values regarding death

An individual's attitudes towards and experiences of death are largely created by society. In the past, the whole family witnessed and was involved in the two most important family events: the birth of a baby and the death of a family member.[51] The dying person would die at home and the family accepted the event of death and their responsibility to participate. The family often surrounded the dying person at the moment of death. Therefore, people maintained a social connectedness with their families until they died.

In recent times the industrialisation and urbanisation of some countries has led to the disintegration of the multi-generation family living in close proximity. As a result, elderly people are often sent to a nursing home or hospital to be cared for until they die.[51] Thus, health care professionals have replaced the family as witnesses of death and in the responsibility for caring for the dying person.[51-53] Fewer people have any immediate contact with dying and death. People may even avoid the sight of a dead person.[54] His Royal Highness, The Prince of Wales[55] (p.5) describes the situation precisely. 'I have been living my life up to now in a society that has tended to push death away, no longer to see it as a natural part of life, but to make it a thing apart, something to be spoken about only in hushed voices, something to be dreaded and shunned.' As the patterns of social values change, a relatively higher number of people experience a biological, psychological, or social death rather than a Good Death.

The nature of disease

Death from cancer is often perceived as a 'bad death'. The diagnosis (of cancer) and the names and descriptions of the disease are as invasive and damaging as the disease itself.[56-57] Thus, the equation of cancer with death has been well documented in literature.[58-60] The perceived relationship between cancer and death profoundly affects the person who has cancer and those who share their experiences, such as the person's primary caregivers.[61] Essentially, all cancers are treatable and many can be cured. Unfortunately, the outcome is seldom certain at the time of diagnosis and for most patients, relapses, recurrences, or secondary tumours are possible. Cancer patients have to face such frightening possibilities as debilitating illness, pain, disfigurement, loss of physiological function, and death.[62] Consequently, psychological morbidity can be expected.

Health care professionals have also been observed to be overly pessimistic about the prognosis for cancer patients. Corner [63] reports that registered nurses often associate cancer with death, pain, and suffering. This association of cancer with death means that it is difficult for both the care receivers (patients and relatives) and caregivers (health care professionals, friends, and volunteers) to see the value of the active treatment of cancer. People therefore tend to avoid having contact with dying patients, eventually contributing to a social death.

Religion and culture

The deepest hopes and fears are expressed in religious beliefs and activities.[64] A person's religious background is an essential element that affects his or her dying experience. Cancer patients who are church attendees can cope better and have lower levels of stress.[65] They may also have a higher level of life satisfaction. Although many Chinese practise Chinese popular religions, Christianity is also common. For example, about 300,000 Protestant Christian and 242,500 Catholics live in Hong Kong.[66]

Christians believe in and hope for eternal life. One way to

understand Jesus's experience of suffering and dying is reflected in the last words that Jesus spoke before He was crucified: 'My God, My God, why hast thou forsaken me?' (The Holy Bible: Matthew 27: 46, Matthew 15: 34) and 'Father, forgive them, they do not know what they are doing' (The Holy Bible: Luke 23: 34). The first sentence reflects His human suffering of confusion and abandonment before His death, while the latter sentence reflects His unbelievable compassion.[67] The strength of Christian attitudes towards death and dying and the impact of Christianity's claims, stands or falls on the reality of Christ's resurrection. Paul stated that if 'Christ has not risen, then one's faith is in vain'. Christ also prayed both in Gethsemane and from the cross just before he died. Christians pray their way into death, too. The believer cultivates a prayerful attitude of heart and mind in order to keep Christ's presence alive throughout the dying process.

Theories of death and dying

In order to understand the universal phenomena of death and dying more fully, the following section examines some of the pioneer theories, including: contexts of awareness, [12] Kubler-Ross's stage theory, [22] Weisman's four phases, [65] Pattison's living-dying model, [68] and Shneidman's personality approach.[69]

Contexts of awareness

Glaser and Strauss [12-15] have contributed extensively to the study of death and dying. Their field study on 'awareness concepts' has provided one of the most influential contributions to the understanding of the social contexts of dying.[70] The authors identify four basic types of awareness: closed awareness, suspected awareness, mutual pretence, and open awareness. In closed awareness, the patient does not recognise that he or she is dying, but everyone else does. Family and health care professionals jointly keep the secret by preventing communication to the patient of information that may lead to a realisation that death is a prospect. In suspected awareness, the patient suspects what others know and attempts to prove the suspicion that he or she is dying by tricking family members and staff into admitting the truth. In this situation, health care professionals prefer to allow the patient to realise their condition for themselves, rather than tell the patient directly. Although the patient, family, and staff are aware that the patient is dying, they continue to act as if this is not the case. Mutual pretence is also said to occur, and is useful in helping staff to keep a safe emotional distance from the dying patient and in giving some patients more privacy, dignity, and control. Open awareness exists when everyone involved knows the patient is dying and acknowledges the fact in interactions.[12] This allows the patient to complete the necessary tasks associated with dying.

Nevertheless, some patients, families, or health care professionals do not prepare to function in an open awareness context because of the highly anxious nature of the situation or their limited communication abilities. These people may use denial as a compromise with death.[71] It must be acknowledged that people, including the patient and family members, have different capacities for handling difficult situations.[72]

Kubler-Ross's five stages

Kubler-Ross[22] was the first psychiatrist to draw attention to dying patients' neglected needs. She reports the five ways her patients coped when they were confronted with terminal illness: denial, anger, bargaining, depression, and acceptance. However, there has been some controversy surrounding Kubler-Ross's stage theory. For example, sadness increases from the early to the later phase of illness but no systematic pattern was found for anger and happiness (acceptance) among a sample of terminally ill patients.[73] In addition, there has been no confirmation of the validity of Kubler-Ross's stages or their reliability more than thirty years later. Some clinicians who have worked with dying people have criticised the stage theory as inadequate, superficial, and misleading.[36, 68, 69, 74]

Kastenbaum[75] makes several criticisms of Kubler-Ross's theory. First, there may be many more than five ways in which human beings cope with anything as fundamental as dying. Second, there is no evidence that people actually move from stage one through to stage five. Corr[76] asserts that one should not speak of 'stages' unless one intends to speak about elements in a linear standard of measurement. Third, the theory makes an insufficient distinction between description and prescription. Fourth, the totality of a person's life is neglected in favour of the supposed stages of dying. Lastly, the resources, pressures, and characteristics of the immediate environment can also make a tremendous difference. Clearly, a stage-based model may risk stereotyping vulnerable dying individuals. Kubler-Ross has neither responded to these criticisms nor offered any evidence or additional arguments to support her stage theory.[76] Nevertheless, her efforts to draw wide attention from health care professionals and the general public, to the needs of the dying, are undeniable. As a psychiatrist, she is sensitive to the most basic ways in which human beings react to the challenges of dying. Kubler-Ross[77] also claims that death should not be perceived as an event that brings about negative experiences, and that dying may be the final stage of growth when acceptance evolves with peace and dignity. This insight has provided inspiration for future studies, such as the exploration of the features of a Good Death in this book.

Weisman's four phases

Based on experience of working with terminal cancer patients, Weisman[65] constructed the theory of 'psychostaging' in the life of a patient, which includes existential plight, mitigation, and accommodation, decline and deterioration, preterminality and terminality. Existential plight is the initial shock of an abrupt confrontation with unquestionable evidence of one's vulnerability and mortality. Mitigation and accommodation reactions often follow initial treatment while the possibility of relapse or recurrence remains real. Subsequently the patients' energy for living begins to wane. This third phase is called decline and deterioration. The last phase of preterminality and terminality follows in which everyone involved begins to realise that the focus must shift to the palliation of symptoms and assurance of as much comfort as possible. Weisman's psychostaging hypothesis, which is continuously sequential, does not seem to have any empirical support.[78]

Pattison's living-dying process

The dying process can be viewed as a transition. Taking into account both the subjective views of the dying person and objective observations of the person's coping mechanism, Pattison[68] describes three phases of dying transition. These phases are the acute crisis phase, the chronic living-dying process, and the terminal phase. The acute crisis phase that immediately follows the discovery of impending death generally consists of a stage of intense anxiety. The patient may experience immobilisation, alterations in consciousness, and feelings of inadequacy, anxiety, and fear, and may exhibit pathological defence. It is during the acute crisis phase that peak anxiety is experienced. The chronic living-dying phase represents an adaptive process when the patient and the family learn to live with the knowledge of impending death on a daily basis. This is the phase of longest duration and may be experienced through integration or disintegration. In this phase, the patient may experience progressive fears associated with dying. The terminal phase is the period when the dying patient begins to withdraw. Some subsequent studies supported the concepts of this theory.[79, 80] These authors have described their theories in a linear way, implying that people move from one phase to another sequentially when they die.

Shneidman's personality approach

Shneidman's[69] approach to dying and death seems to be more objective and acceptable to the holistic concept of care, as he does not adopt a set framework of dying. This view is quite different from the theories of Kubler-Ross, Weisman, and Pattison. Shneidman maintains that it is imperative to understand the ways in which dying persons have lived through and experienced previous stressful life events. Thus, the ways they respond to the challenges inherent in the dying process can be understood.[44] Shneidman leans quite heavily on the general personality theory and the detailed long-term approach to the study of individual behaviour. He believes that individuals tend to die as they have previously reacted in periods of threat, stress, failure, challenge, shock, and loss. In other words, one dies as one has lived in the terrible moments of one's life. Hinton's[81] findings are valuable in that he studies the relationship between each patient's personality and state of mind before and during terminal cancer. He identifies the need for detailed knowledge of the individual's previous patterns of handling life's demands. Shneidman's individual personality theory also appears practical and workable and its overall reliability would appear to be higher than that of other approaches.[78] Nevertheless, the over-emphasis of a person's individuality and personality may overlook the importance of the social and cultural influences that affect the dying process.

Dying and death as a special stream of study has attracted scholars and researchers from various disciplines since the 1950s. All of the findings indicate that most people die poorly and experience a wide range of emotions upon learning of their life-threatening illness. More importantly, these theories of dying and death have stimulated thought on the needs of dying persons – what they mean by dying a Good Death.

Good Death

Development of the concept of Good Death

Regardless of their cultural background, people come to death with a variety of beliefs, attitudes, superstitions, fears, and hopes.[69] Most of the studies on dying persons present a negative and dismal picture of the process.[82-84] It is only recently that researchers have shown an increasing, though insufficient, interest in describing the elements of a Good Death.[36, 85-88] and that dying people themselves have been encouraged to influence the process.

From the Græco-Roman world, the early Christians inherited an attitude towards death, which they accepted as a universal phenomenon and as something not to be feared.[89] Death is seen as a collective destiny, therefore, not to be feared. People with religious faith believe that a Good Death signals entry into heaven.[43] More explicit notions of what it means to die a Good Death have arisen from the work of psychologists, sociologists, and anthropologists.[90] For example, Glaser and Strauss [12, 14-15] have conducted well-known studies on the behaviour of dying patients and have developed ideas about levels of awareness of impending death and about dying trajectories more generally. Although Glaser and Strauss were careful not to privilege one form of dying trajectory over others, many health care professionals have assumed it is better to die in full awareness that one is dying, rather than to die in a closed awareness context in which impending death is not openly acknowledged. Similarly, the theory of death and dying developed by Kubler-Ross [22] has become very widely accepted and valued by many health care professionals. Kubler-Ross's description of the stage of acceptance is regarded as an important element in dying a Good Death. Weisman [24] has further encouraged belief in the possibility of a Good Death with notions of a very good or an appropriate death. More recently, Kellehear[36] has pointed out that despite its development, and influence on health care professionals, the concept of Good Death is inadequately defined. Consequently, several studies were undertaken on what it means to die a Good Death from the perspective of different health care professionals, such as hospice coordinators [71] and nurses.[87,90-96] At the same time, there is little doubt that the work, which has been done on death and dying, has largely ignored social and cultural responses to dying.[90] Insufficient attention has been paid to the possibility that ideas about a Good Death may be different in Chinese communities from those known from studies of death and dying in the West.

Terms of Good Death

In Western culture, a Good Death has been variously defined. The simplest definition is a death in which the patient's wants and needs are met.[87] Other descriptive terms and labels also have been proposed. For example, Blauner, [52] Hinton, [21] Shneidman [69, 97] and Weisman [24, 98] have used the concept of 'Appropriate Death', others have used the terms 'Healthy Death' [71, 99, 100], 'Correct Death' [71, 101] "Tame Death', [89] 'Happy Death',[102] 'Peaceful Death' [103-108] while the use of the term 'Good Dying,' [35, 109] 'Dying Well' [110, 111] and 'Good Death' has continued.[36, 90, 91, 92, 99, 112-123] In Chinese, there is a colloquial saying to the effect that 'a good birth is not as good as a good death'. I will present a detailed discussion of Chinese views of Good Death in the last section of this chapter. Despite the variation in adjectives, all of the above phrases point to a common possibility – that it is possible to die in a way that is consistent with one's principles. However, it is important to identify what this means, and I will consider some possibilities.

Elements of Good Death

Rather than relating to an assisted and timely death, a Good Death may be viewed as involving a more complex set of relations and preparations. On this view, a Good Death is not a single event, but a series of social events.[90] From the perspective of hospice staff, a death may be perceived as 'good' if it goes well overall.[88] Recently, a number of studies have focused on caregivers' perceptions of Good Death.[87, 90-96] Nurses as health care workers have been seen as integral to palliative care. They 'have a definite role when a patient is dying and therefore their perceptions of Good Death will play a significant role in how they provide care to the dying patient'.[124] Smith and Maher[100] survey the opinions of the hospice coordinators, while some studies have preferred to obtain patients' ideas of Good Death directly.[35,36,122,125] What, then, does the literature imply are the characteristics of this broader concept of Good Death? The following section will review the literature, and seek to ascertain what it means to die a Good Death from both the caregivers' and the dying persons' perspective.

Controlling pain and symptoms

Nurses often see a Good Death as one where the patient is comfortable;[126] i.e. the patient is pain- and symptom-free.[90-96] Some hospice coordinators also strongly maintain this view.[100] Just as important, alertness must be considered in any notion of Good Death.[92] Although technology has developed rapidly, some nurses have expressed concern about the way it might be used.[124] They emphasise that dying people should not receive any active or aggressive medical treatment, because over-treatment and over-medication during palliative care are seen as detrimental to Good Death.[90, 93, 94] Therefore, a Good Death should neither be sudden nor prolonged.[92, 95]

From the patients' perspective, freedom from pain is also one of the most commonly cited elements of a Good Death.[24, 86, 98, 122, 126] The state of freedom from pain emphasises that the patient's suffering should be reduced, and his or her emotional impoverishment should be kept to a minimum.[24, 98] 'Without adequate pain relief, quiescence of nausea, and other debilitating symptoms, the remaining quality of life is drastically damaged, and an appropriate (good) death rendered impossible' (p.71).[98] The World Health Organisation [117] also connects the concepts of freedom from pain and alertness by stating that 'one of the essential elements of a Good Death is freedom from [the] pain that dominates consciousness and may leave the patient physically and mentally capable of reaching whatever goals he or she may want to achieve before death'.

At the same time, the concept of natural death can be considered as a form of freedom from pain. There are two kinds of natural death. The first kind is death that occurs in good health and old age.[45, 64, 127] Such a death is desirable because it is assumed to be free from fear and pain. The second kind is one in which medical intervention is kept to a minimum. As mentioned earlier, some people actively reject the idea of medical intervention to prolong life.[90, 93, 94, 124] For them, a Good Death is one where the only medical interventions that take place are those of pain and symptom relief, highlighting once again the importance of being comfortable.

Accepting death

Many nurses have associated dying a Good Death with a sense of acceptance. They agree that dying people should have an acceptance of their impending death.[90, 96] Hunt[91] specifies that relatives need to accept the reality of death as well. What, then, are the possible predisposing factors for people to accept a death? Some commonly cited answers from interviewees are dying in old age as one form of natural death[45] and knowing the truth of their condition.[100]

Likewise, dying people assert that a Good Death is allied with a sense of acceptance[65, 86] and of appreciation for having lived according to the best standards possible.[24, 98, 138] Acceptance begins when a patient becomes aware of impending death and accepts that nothing more can be done. The literature stresses that once patients have accepted that death is approaching, they might need help to give meaning to their lives.[32] Therefore, a Good Death is one in which a patient dies with an acceptance of the timing of his or her death. There is a sense in which death is essentially good only when it occurs 'on time'.[86, 115] 'To die at the right time in the right way those are the hallmarks of a sterling death' (p.29).[97] When is the appropriate time to die? A common view is that a timely death is one that occurs 'when a person has completed his span of life, his powers wane, and the eventual increasing decline suggests that it is time for the individual to depart this life' (p.43).[21] Correspondingly, a Good Death occurs when a person is about to die in old age,[21, 37, 45, 115, 116, 128, 129] when he or she has completed his or her life, and all unfinished business.[24, 97, 112, 126]

Maslow[112] has described his personal feelings towards a meaningful (timely) death following a serious heart attack that occurred soon after he completed writing a book that was important to him. He states, 'I had really spent myself. This was the best I could do, and here was not only a good time to die but I was even willing to die. It is what David Levy called the "completion of the act". It is like a good ending, a good close. I think actors and dramatists have that sense of the right moment for a good ending, with a phenomenological sense of good completion – that there is nothing more that you could add' (p.16). Furthermore, as an individual approaches death, he or she may possess a sense of readiness which is related to his or her style of living, situation in life, and mission (aspiration, goals, wishes) in life.[97] Kearl [115] points out that factors such as the time at which death normally occurs in the life span and how long it typically takes for people to die shape both cultural beliefs about death and individual fears.

Making decisions

In most situations, dying determines the kind of behaviour exhibited by the dying person; in Good Death, the dying person's behaviour determines the kind of death.[124] Thus, dying people experience a certain degree of personal control over their end-of-life journey. Personal control is defined as the feeling that one can make decisions and take effective action to produce desirable outcomes and avoid undesirable ones.[130]

Some caregivers argue that dying persons should have the right to define their needs and choices.[87, 100] They may have a sense of participation in physical care [96, 100] or a sense of having control, [100] which is essential for dying a Good Death. They 'preferred to have as much control as possible in making decisions concerning care rather than its opposite of having others make decisions' (p.26).[100] In this way, the autonomy of the dying person is respected.[90, 94] For example, the person may have a peaceful death at home[91] and may have significant others (family and/or friends) around him/ her[100] when he or she dies. For the hospice patient, the nature of the setting and the experiences of fellow patients are also relevant to achieving a Good Death.[92]

For some people such as college students, the hospice movement appears to provide a more acceptable option for dying patients than typical institutional settings. In their view, hospice services delivered in the home seem to be particularly suitable for supporting a person in their passage towards a Good Death.[128] However, within the hospice, a positive experience of a fellow patient's death was typically helpful. Johnston and his colleagues [131] point out that hospice patients who have witnessed a death are found to be significantly less depressed in standardised measures of emotional distress.

Dying people maintain a similar view of having personal control. Weisman [24, 98] stresses repeatedly that the dying individual must not lose control. The dying person does not completely eliminate the effects of death, but he or she does, as much as possible, choose to set conditions on what kind of death is wanted. The imperative for the person to retain a sense of control until the very end is implicit.[24, 31, 35, 98, 132, 133]

People live with the consequences of where they choose to die.[172] Those who choose a hospice face a different set of challenges from those who choose to die at home, although neither route is easy. There can be no easy road to death. Patients prefer to stay in a restful and quiet environment [35, 113, 173] which the hospice can provide. In his study of Hindu villagers (Pandits), Madan [133] demonstrates the importance of the place of death and of culture in a stronger sense. He points out that a Good Death is a great 'passing on', which does not just happen, but is achieved if one can let go of the life-breath in full consciousness, at a time and place of one's choosing. When one achieves 'these things', one will die in a state of dignity. In general, Pandits prefer to die at home, in the house in which they have lived, because they regard their house as a microcosm of the universe.

Death in an environment of emotional care and support relieves the individual's discomfort and isolation.[126] The presence of the family is particularly relevant. Some patients may have the chance to choose where to die but they may also wish to avoid dying in a lonely way. Therefore, they ask significant others to listen, share, understand, accept, and pray.[35] Several authors emphasise that dying persons consider being surrounded by people they love when they die as a Good Death [92, 134] Thus, the quality of connectedness between the dying person and the family is an important element in Good Death [122] because death is a dual process that simultaneously involves the dying and the surviving.[115] Respect for the patients' personal control and good communication among patients, families, and health care professionals complement this element of Good Death. Therefore, health care professionals are exhorted to acknowledge patients' autonomy and to accommodate their wishes by allowing them more control over the dying trajectory and establishing a partnership in decision making .[135]

Maintaining hope

Hope can be defined as a feeling of the possible, inner readiness, and an unused resource.[136] The sense of hope is a belief that the present situation can be modified and that there is a way out of difficulties. A desire to live, a sense of enjoyment of life, and a determination to keep 'mobile' and to 'fight back' are all related to one's sense of hope.[91] Thus, maintaining hope is another element in a Good Death from the nurses' perspective. Nurses have a predominant perception that death must be peaceful.[92,93,124] Some dying persons might explore the idea of an afterlife as yet another source of hope. This interest in an afterlife seems to have occurred independently of patients' involvement in organised religion. In this way, they may wait actively rather than passively.[100]

The ways in which people live through their final days may reflect their personal philosophy, maturity, and sense of self-realisation.[97] The dying person needs to have a sense of hope.[21,97] It has become self-evident in the West that Good Deaths are those that demonstrate control over events and can be seen to equate to a kind of victory over nature. For people with religious faith, their concepts of Good Death appear to follow the more religiously oriented belief of hope in entry into heaven.[43] At the same time, hospice patients require social and emotional support. These elements play a crucial role in what might be regarded as a form of sharing in the present, [137] in which mutual emotional and social support sustains the hopes of the person and the family. It is the absence of what might be called such mutuality that renders people hopeless, because the experience of supporting and being supported transforms the dread of abandonment and the terrors of isolation into hope, [98] and later acceptance and spiritual contentment.

Receiving social and family support

Several studies report the need for family and social support in order to die a Good Death.[90,92,94,95,96,100] The presence, love, and encouragement of family members are significant. Both the dying persons and their families and caregivers should have the opportunity to experience 'self-worth, dignity, and freedom of choice during the natural passage from life to death'.[138]

Consistent with the ideas of caregivers, dying patients perceive the family as an important source of support and care for them. Relationships of terminal cancer patients with their spouses often remain the same or become closer. The patients' social experience with their children is often positive. For example, most adult children pay more visits and help around the house.[36] According to Young and Cullen,[122] in a Good Death, a person has a generally harmonious relationship with his or her kin.

Preparing for death

Smith and Maher[71] maintain Kellehear's [36] beliefs about a Good Death in their emphasis on the importance of personal preparations for death, noting that bidding farewells to staff, friends, and family is an essential element in an individual's quest for a final resolution. Patients need to have time to prepare themselves emotionally for dying.[93, 100] They need to fulfil their wishes, say good-bye and give messages, and organise their funerals in preparation for farewells.[96] Some dying persons are concerned with their personal cleanliness and appearance.[35, 100]

When cancer patients are aware of their impending death, they also have an awareness of the limitation of time. The patients' personal and public preparation for their own deaths can be regarded as evidence that they are able to regain some types of control over their future. In this context, Kellehear[36] has identified preparation for a person's death as an element of Good Death. The dying persons' preparations for their impending death include personal completion of their significant role, bidding farewells and giving instructions, and public preparations such as funeral arrangements.

Weisman [24] notes the importance of being able to resolve residual conflicts and to satisfy any remaining wishes. To achieve a Good Death, a person completes his or her unfinished business and makes all the necessary preparations. Other main activities include informal willing; talks about death and dying and talks about role reorganisations for illness.[36] Kellehear also observes that more women conduct informal willing than men do. Other personal preparations include simply talking, and making arrangements for their pets. Apart from personal preparation, public preparation for death is also identified as an essential element of a Good Death.[36, 122] It has been an important part of dying according to some studies in the United States in the 1960s and 1970s. Examples include studies by Lipman and Marden, [139] Glaser and Strauss, [14] and Kalish and Reynolds.[140] In Australia, Kellehear's [36] study has elaborated two forms of public preparation: material preparation and religious preparation for death. He also compares his findings before and after awareness of dying. He perceives that people tended to make most of their material preparations before they became aware of dying. A large part of the material preparations made after awareness of dying was ratifying and redrafting intentions. Religious preparation occurred mostly after the person had gained an awareness of dying. People's main concerns were talking with their clergyman and praying. Similar to the findings of two previous American studies, [140, 141] the people in the Australian sample had made wills, had taken out life insurance, and had made funeral preparations. However, the percentage of people who made these preparations was different from that in the USA. The pattern of public preparation has suggested a pattern of social priorities, which puts the welfare of survivors above one's own. Factors such as sex, age, usual work status, and occupational prestige were also found to influence patterns of public preparation.[36]

There have been no similar surveys of public preparation in Chinese communities. Nevertheless, Chao[35] indicates that planning for one's remains and funeral is important for some Taiwan Chinese patients and indifferent for others. Some families would comply with the patients' will but some would not. Some were concerned about the performance of religious rites of passage.

Some hospice coordinators believe that dying people tend to review 'past pleasures and pains, accomplishments and regrets' (p.28).[100] This is what Aries [89] calls a dying person's farewells to the world. These farewells can be completed in several ways: a family conference chaired by the dying person, individual conferences between the dying person and his or her significant others, letters, journals, audiocassettes or videotapes.[100]

Similarly, some dying persons will bid farewell formally or informally in their last days. According to Kellehear, [36] farewells can have four mutual components: affection, regard, reassurance, and acceptance, which will often be interspersed in conversations about other things. Therefore, it may be hard to determine if any farewells take place at all. Nevertheless, earlier studies reported that such an event was not uncommon [140, 142] but has not been reported by researchers in more recent studies.[35, 122, 125]

Awareness of dying

From the point of view of people with terminal cancer, awareness of dying is the foremost essential element of a Good Death.[36] Theories of awareness of dying stem from the important work of Glaser and Strauss, [12, 14-15] which suggests that dying patients should know the truth about their illness, including diagnosis and prognosis so that they will gradually accept their impending death and make preparations for a definite departure. According to Smith and Maher (p.28),[100] a healthy death is characterised by the dying person wanting 'to hear the truth, even when painful' as opposed to wanting 'to be protected from painful truths'. Patients will then need time to fulfil whatever they want to complete. Open discussion between patients and caregivers is essential.

Kellehear [36] modifies Glaser and Strauss's [12] theory of death expectation and suggests a further division, relating to certainty of dying, in the fourth category of death expectation. This means the dying person may experience five sets of death expectations: '1) uncertain about death, with unknown time when this will be resolved; 2) uncertain about death, but time known when this will be resolved; 3) certain about death but uncertain about when this will occur...4a) certain about death and certain when to generally expect it. Most terminal cancer patients expect to have such certainty; 4b) certain about death and certain when to precisely expect it' [36] (p.75–76). The latter death expectation can apply to most people who are about to commit suicide. The above researchers studied the behaviour of dying patients, developed ideas that related to the awareness or otherwise of impending death, and conceived of the process of dying as a social trajectory. Their work has led others to believe that a Good Death is a form of passage in which everyone involved is aware of and accepts the imminence of death, and in which the dying person has resolved socio-emotional and material concerns.[24]

Authors seem to agree that having an awareness of dying is an essential first step in achieving a Good Death.[24, 36, 65, 114, 122]. The 'death awareness movement' has introduced the notion of 'openness' as an element of Good Death.[143] With the recent advocation of patients' rights, the 'resulting openness has made possible a new kind of Good Death for more people' (p.175).[122]

There seems to be a growing concern over whether dying people must tolerate a terminal situation over which they have minimal control. It is believed that the circumstances of dying can be made more compatible with the person's needs and wishes. Several studies have explored the meaning of Good Death according to people who have confronted death and to the caregivers.

Both caregivers and patients are in general agreement on several elements contributing to a Good Death. These elements are: controlling pain and symptoms; accepting death; making one's own decisions; maintaining hope; receiving family and social support; preparing for death; and bidding farewells. First, the dying person should be comfortable and free from pain and symptoms. Acceptance of one's mortality is the next prerequisite for final departure if one is to die with a sense of inner freedom and without narcissism.[114] Therefore, a person usually refers to having a Good Death when he or she is about to die in old age, and when he or she has completed his or her unfinished business. Death should occur on time. Third, the patient needs to experience a sense of personal control until the end of their life. He or she is allowed to make his or her own decisions regarding care in the remaining part of life. Fourth, the dying person needs to be hopeful, so that he or she can wait actively instead of passively. The nature of hope varies depending on a patient's social, emotional, and religious support. Fifth, both caregivers and patients maintain that family and social support are significant for a Good Death in that it can provide emotional comfort, hope to live, and a better chance of accepting their death. On the other hand, relatively fewer studies from the caregivers' perspective have identified preparation for death and farewells as essential in dying a Good Death.[93, 96, 100] Nevertheless, Kellehear [36] has made a detailed description of patients' personal and public preparations, while other studies identify funeral arrangements as common preparations before a person's death.[35, 122, 125] In several studies, dying individuals agree that having an awareness of dying is an essential first step of achieving a Good Death, although this issue has not been well considered by caregivers. Most of these elements are social and emotional in nature. Nevertheless, the state of being comfortable and free from pain and symptoms relates more closely to the physical needs of dying persons, while accepting death and maintaining hope have more to do with their spiritual needs.

Table 2.1
Studies relating to elements of Good Death

Elements of Good Death	Studies
Controlling pain and symptoms	Nimocks, Webb, and Connell, 1987, Hunt, 1992; Wilkes, 1993; White, 1994; McNamara, Waddell, and Colvin, 1994 and 1995; McNamara, 1996; Taylor, 1995; Smith and Maher, 1993; Weisman, 1972, 1988; Nimocks, Webb, and Connell, 1987; Wilson, 1989; McCracken and Gersen, 1991; Young and Cullen, 1996.
Accepting death	Hunt, 1992; Wilkes, 1993; White, 1994; McNamara, Waddell, and Colvin, 1994 and 1995; McNamara, 1996; Taylor, 1995; McDonald and Carroll, 1981; Smith and Maher, 1993; Wilson, 1989; Weisman, 1972; 1988; Hull, 1989.
Making one's own decisions	Weisman, 1972 and 1988; McDonald and Carroll, 1981; Nimock et al., 1987; Smith and Maher, 1991; Madan, 1992; Chao, 1993; McNamara et al., 1994, 1995; Hunt, 1992; Kalish, 1981; D'Angelo, 1986; Chao, 1993; Young and Cullen, 1996; Jennings, 1997.
Maintaining hope	Hunt, 1992; Smith and Maher, 1993; Hinton, 1967; Shneidman, 1973; Bradbury, 1993; Anderson, 1989; Weisman, 1988; Chao, 1993.
Receiving family and social support	Wilkes, 1993; Smith and Maher, 1993; McNamara et al., 1994, 1995; Taylor, 1995; Hull, 1989; Kellehear, 1990, Young and Cullen, 1996.
Preparations for death	Kellehear, 1990; Chao, 1993; Young and Cullen, 1996; Webb, 1997; Smith and Maher, 1993; White, 1994.
Awareness of dying	Glaser and Strauss, 1965, 1968, 1971; Alizade, 1988; Kellehear, 1990; Smith and Maher, 1991; Young and Cullen, 1996.
Farewells	Kellehear, 1990; Smith and Maher, 1993.

Death and dying
The Chinese perspective

Hong Kong is a cosmopolitan city with a population of 6.3 million people, of whom some 98% are Chinese. Many of Hong Kong's older residents came to Hong Kong after World War II. Because they were born and raised in China, they maintain strong Chinese traditions although Hong Kong was a British Colony until June 1997. Many traditional Chinese ideas and behaviours are still observed in contemporary social life, [144] including attitudes towards death.

However, aspects of other cultures, mostly Western culture, have now become incorporated into mainstream thinking. While there have been several studies on death and dying in the West, few have been conducted in the East.[35, 145] Whether the findings of such studies in Western societies can be applied to Asian countries such as Hong Kong is a topic for future research. There are a number of ethnic and cultural groups in Hong Kong, with differing religious beliefs and practices. The following section examines the three most common Chinese religions – Confucianism, Taoism, and Buddhism.[146]

Traditional Chinese beliefs

According to Li's [45] commentary on *The Book of History* (*Shang Shu*), long before Confucius, during the Zha, Zhang, and Zhou Dynasties the Chinese recognised the infinite nature of the universe. They believed in the supernatural power of heaven and they worshipped it accordingly. It should be noted that the ancient Chinese understanding of heaven was not equivalent to that of the Christians point of view in Western countries. *The Book of History* is an historical official document which describes how Chinese emperors should rule the country. It stresses that if an emperor governs the country by moral principles, his people will be blessed by heaven with the Five Blessings – longevity, wealth, serenity, the love of virtue, and Good Death. The latter means dying naturally of old age, without pain and suffering, 'as if they are asleep'.[45, 116]

These teachings have had an important impact on Chinese beliefs.

Conversely, if an Emperor did not fulfil his role properly according to the will of the heaven, his people would be persecuted with the Six Sufferings – bad death, illness, apprehension, poverty, unkindness, and weakness.[45]

Confucianism:
Emphasis on this life and care until the end

Confucius (551-479 BC) was one of several intellectuals who started questioning the meaning of life, and the role of the gods and the spirits. He was born during the Warring States Period and developed a system of ethics and politics that stressed five virtues – charity, justice, propriety, wisdom, and loyalty. His teachings were recorded by his followers in a book called the *Analects*, and formed the code of ethics called Confucianism which has been the cornerstone of Chinese thought for many centuries.[147]

Confucius' guiding belief was that of 'Tien Ming' or the influences of fate and mission. 'Tien Ming' states that all things are under the control of the regulatory mechanism of heaven. This includes life and death, wealth and poverty, health and illness. Confucius believed that understanding 'Tien Ming' was his life's mission.[147, 148] He encouraged people to accept whatever happened to them, including death.

The following statement made by the Master to his Disciple Tzu Lu can best illustrate the dominant Confucian attitude toward death. Confucius affirmed that 'if we do not yet know about life, how can we know about death?'.[149] Without a knowledge of how to live, a person would not know about death and dying. However, Confucius was criticised for avoiding discussion of death. He did not encourage his followers to seek eternal life, [150] nor did he discuss death, gods, ghosts, and the unknown future or afterlife in detail.[148] He maintained that ghosts were spirits and were not easy to understand. Confucius concluded that these issues were complicated and abstract, and that it was better to spend time solving the problems of the present life than to look into the unknown world of death and afterlife. He wanted to convey the importance of valuing the existing life and of leading a morally correct life according to one's mission from heaven.[151]

The virtues of goodness and righteousness are the essence of Confucian teaching. Confucius considered righteousness to be a basic requirement of a good person, stating that such a person 'would not seek to stay alive at the expense of injuring virtue'. He encouraged people to uphold these moral principles and care for each other until death.[150] His followers were exhorted to be loyal and dutiful towards family, kin, and neighbours, and to respect their superiors and the elderly. Filial piety to parents and ancestors are fundamental to these beliefs. The Confucian view of death is that of continuous remembrance and affection. 'Death does not sever the relationship of the departed with the living, but merely changes it to a different level. Far from being characterised by fear, the attitudes of the living towards the departed members of the family or clan are one of continuous remembrance and affection' (p.198).[64]

These beliefs may go some way to explaining why people such as Qu Yuen, and those who died in the 'June 4th massacre' in 1989, are prepared to give up their lives to advocate the values of justice and goodness for their country. Those who follow such beliefs would have no regret when confronted with their own death and would accept death readily. This is regarded as a high level of moral behaviour of family or social virtue.[151] Although Confucius did not express it explicitly, to die for righteousness is an example of a Good Death for the individual as well as the nation.

Taoism:
The notion of mutual interpenetration of life and death

Between the fourth and third centuries BC, some thinkers tried a non-interference approach – letting things be in their natural state. For the Taoists, non-action refers to contentment with one's lot: to preserve the principles of nature and to live out one's allotted span of life.[35] The person united with the Tao shares its creativity and harmony.

Similar to the Confucian view, Taoists believe that everything in the world is produced by the cosmic Way (Tao), which provides harmony and balance. Since creation occurs at the moment of the separation of being into Yin and Yang, at the beginning of the universe, there existed a unity of Yin-Yang (light-darkness, heat-cold, dry-moist). Lao Tzu further teaches that:

The Tao engenders one
One engenders two
Two engenders three
And three engenders the myriad things

> *The myriad things engender the Yin vapours and embrace the Yang*
> *And through the coalescing of these vapours*
> *They attain a state of harmony.*[177]

The process of death was a natural transition from a conscious state to an unconscious one, from a life-body to a death-body.[152] According to Lao Tzu and Chuang Tzu (399–295 BC), the eternal way of the universe is much wiser than any person can possibly be. Most people assert their egos and try to substitute their own limited knowledge for the wisdom of the universe. Such action would create fear and suffering.[148] 'Life is the companion of death [and] death is the beginning of life. Who understands their workings? Man's life is a coming together of breath. If it comes together, there is life, if it scatters, there is death. And if life and death are companions to each other, then what is there for us to be anxious about?' [153]

Unlike other philosophers of the time, Chuang Tzu openly discussed his views on death. People often experience sadness and depression when their relatives die but Chuang Tzu did not feel the same.[148] He argued that he could not reject or escape the natural law of the universe. For example, he did not feel joyful or upset when he was confronted with his wife's death. When Chuang Tzu lost his wife, Hui Tzu found Chuang Tzu sitting with his legs sprawled out, pounding on a tub and singing. The following conversation has been frequently cited to illustrate Chuang Tzu's point of view on death and dying.

> *Hui Tzu said, 'You lived with her, she brought up your children and grew old'. It should be enough simply not to weep at her death. But pounding on a tub and singing – this is going too far, is it not?' Chuang Tzu replied, 'You are wrong. When she first died, do you think I didn't grieve like anyone else? But I looked back to her beginning and the time before she was born. Not only the time before she was born, but the time before she had a body. Not only the time before she had a body, but the time before she had a spirit. In the midst of the jumble of wonder and mystery, a change took place and she is dead. It's just like the progression of the four seasons, spring, summer, fall, winter. Now she is going to lie down peacefully in a vast room. If I were to follow after her bawling and sobbing, it would show that I do not understand anything about fate. So I stopped. (Translated from Chuang Tzu)* [154]

Likewise, when Chuang Tzu was dying, his disciples suggested that he had an elaborate burial with an expensive coffin. He replied that he was just part of the universe and would not require any extravagant funeral.

> *I will have heaven and earth for my coffin and coffin shell, the sun and moon for my pair of jade discs, the stars and constellations for my pearls and beads, and the ten thousand things for my parting gifts. The furnishings for my funeral are already prepared. What is there to add? Above ground, I'll be eaten by crows and kites, below ground I will be eaten by ants. Wouldn't it be rather bigoted to deprive one group in order to supply the other?* (Translated from *The Complete Works of Chuang Tzu*) [155]

Chuang Tzu was able to face his own death with such apparent nonchalance. Meanwhile, Lao Tzu and Chuang Tzu have said very little about gods or rituals, although they had a strong sense of the mystery and power of the universal Tao, which was present everywhere.

Unlike the Christian God, the Tao has no consciousness or will.[64,155] By the fourth century BC, a set of beliefs had emerged in which there were ways for human beings to escape death, either by living for a very long time, or by being reborn in a new form after what only appeared to be death. The Taoist priests, who had a real knowledge of Taoist beliefs and techniques, had the power to drive away demons, heal illnesses, and renew the forces of life and fertility in the community. At the same time, most Chinese may not have been sure of what happened after death[152] and if they could escape death. They also believed in the effect of Feng Shui (geomancy) when they buried the dead. An incorrectly performed funeral may cause illness and accidents.[155]

Buddhism:
The emphasis of reincarnation and reward or punishment

Buddhism, which has exerted tremendous influence on traditional Chinese beliefs, was introduced to China in about the first century AD. Buddhism originated in India in about 500 BC with Gautama Siddhartha. Because of the richness of its teaching and of its well-organised rituals and monastic life, Buddhism has exerted a deep influence on all classes and nationalities of Chinese society.

Buddhists believe that life moves according to regular patterns of cause, which the human mind can understand. There is a cause or reason for everything that happens. Every result or effect of one cause in turn becomes the cause of something else. That is, people's feelings and actions operate according to the Law of Cause and Effect. This concept is called 'karma' (an Indian word meaning 'act' or 'deed'). Buddhism encourages people to have sufficient self-control to reach a point where the old sense of ego disappears. One simply acts in response to situations as they arise, without any concern for gain. In other words, it is the intentions behind an action that cause its effects.[64, 150]

The Buddhist teachings instruct people to accept that life is basically impermanent and full of suffering. Most religions teach that there is something eternal behind the changes of life, something they call God. For Buddhists, such solidity is an illusion. They believe that most people are anxious and fearful because they are egocentric, and that one should develop compassion and fairness in order to build up good karma for a better rebirth. Buddhists believe that all humans live for many lifetimes, not just one, with the form of each life shaped by how one has lived in the previous life. Good living will lead to a happy rebirth (that is, a Good Death) as a person or even a god. Evil deeds lead to rebirth as a beggar or an animal. This is the concept of reincarnation.[150,] If one meditates long enough, one can reach a level at which one's actions cause no reactions. In such a case, one need no longer continue on the cycle of birth and rebirth, but instead enter a state of perfect peace, known as Nirvana. Nirvana is what remains when illusion and ignorance have passed, and when desire and attachments have fallen away. 'As the profound antidote to death and dying, nirvana is liberation from suffering, extinction of desires, elimination of ignorance, absence of self, the abolition of all concepts including of nirvana itself, and the cessation of all desires to enter nirvana'.[67] Buddhism teaches acceptance of the inevitable, ever-changing character of life and death. Such acceptance will eventually bring about a new peace of mind and a new sense of compassion for other living things.

For almost 2,000 years, Taoism, Confucianism, and Buddhism have coexisted as China's three dominant religious systems. Their mutual tolerance may be explained, in part, by the fact that each emphasises one aspect of three important concerns of religious consciousness: a person's relation to nature (Taoism), to society (Confucianism), and to the absolute (Buddhism).[146] People in Hong Kong are free to choose their religion. Buddhist and Taoist believers are most prevalent. Baker

[50] observes that most Chinese people do not adhere to one particular faith. Instead, they amalgamate and choose from various religious practices. Therefore, Buddhist and Taoist deities are often honoured together in the same temple. Though differing in many respects, the three traditional Chinese religions and belief systems have many similarities.

All three believe in the fundamental goodness of human nature. Both Confucianism and Buddhism encourage people to keep moral principles and self-control, but each emphasises different intentions. They teach people to live a morally good life and have faith in self-improvement, which will eventually lead to a state of spiritual contentment. According to Confucianism and Taoism, the individual has little control over one's life and death. Buddhism, on the other hand, believes that people need to control their ego if they want to reach a state of spiritual contentment.

All three Chinese religions believe in the law of the universe that is people should not work against heaven because they can never win. Although Buddhism does not use the word heaven, its belief in the Cause and Effect as a regulating mechanism of human behaviour is quite similar to that of Confucianism and Taoism. Therefore, many Chinese people accept dying in old age as a natural life event, but mourn for a premature death.

The traditional Chinese religions have not identified the meanings of Good Death explicitly. In Confucianism, to die for the sake of righteousness and/or to complete one's social roles would be a form of Good Death. Meanwhile, the view of Buddhism is that a Good Death is one in which a person reaches a state of perfect peace or has a better rebirth. Similarly, Taoism encourages people to maintain a harmonious relationship with the universe, that is, to live and die with peace of mind according to the natural order. Although both Confucianism and Buddhism stress achievement and social moral behaviour, they support Taoism in the view that all people should work according to the good will of heaven. They agree that a Good Death emerges from a good life.

Chinese popular beliefs

Chinese religious thought can be seen as a philosophical distillation essentially rooted in folk traditions older than Confucianism and

Taoism. Chinese religions never discard earlier beliefs and practices when adopting new ones.[152, 156] Today, some Chinese people might not be sure of the traditional beliefs of the Chinese philosophies and religions. However, the majority seems to practise one or more popular belief systems, such as fate, ancestor worship, god worshipping, and Feng Shui, which have their origins in Taoism, Buddhism, or Confucianism.

Fate:
The divine decides all things, including the direction of life and death

Most traditional Chinese people believe in the divine direction of life. Since the Zhou Dynasty, people have offered sacrifices to heaven. Every ruler was given a mandate to rule by heaven, but only while he remained compassionate and just. If he failed to practise morally, the divine right to rule could be transferred to someone else. Such ideas, which comprise the concept of 'Tien Ming', have become important in Chinese history because they impose an ethical and religious monitoring on the king's behaviour. Confucius has emphasised the importance of following the mission of heaven – 'Tien Ming'. According to 'Tien Ming', fate decides all things and hence exerts a great deal of power. Heavenly fate decides the time of birth, the hour of death, the manner of death, and the experiences between birth and death, as well as who will rule the country. Therefore, one should learn the will of fate and conform to the highest possible degree.[152] This may explain why Chinese people are often viewed as obedient and passive, because their belief system decrees they have to endure and accept whatever happens in their lives, including pain, suffering, and death.

Ancestor worship: The continuation of a 'social tie'

Ancestor worship is said to be the universal religion of China.[157] It is considered as the most important element of the Chinese belief system, operating on the basis of male relationships. As early as prehistoric times, the Chinese honoured their ancestors. They attempted to discover their will through divination and made offerings to the powers of nature.[64] They also believed that most illness or misfortune was caused by demons or angry ancestral spirits. Such events would result from neglecting to take care of their ancestors' graves or the fact that ancestral spirit(s) have not received enough sacrificial offerings to sustain them in the next world.

The Chinese make three general assumptions about ancestor worship. First, all living persons owe their fortunes or misfortunes to their ancestors. Second, the departed ancestors have needs similar to those of the living. Lastly, the departed ancestors continue to help their relatives in this world, just as their living descendants can help them. The strength of such belief is demonstrated by the continuation of a 'social tie' and a family's obligation to their ancestors. Ancestors are remembered and honoured through regular acts of worship, such as daily offerings of burial incense before wooden tablets inscribed with the ancestors' names, on the family altar. By their actions at the home altar, the Chinese indicate that they are both offering their oblations to the departed and receiving benefits from the family's spiritual resources.[67]

Feng Shui

In Chinese society, the preparation of a good funeral is essentially the obligation of the descendants. A Good Death should include a good Feng Shui (geomancy) reading of the grave. When a person dies, his or her family may ask a Feng Shui master to locate an appropriate spot to bury the dead body so that the spirit can rest in peace. Geomancy implies that if people take proper care of the way they place themselves or their ancestors in the environment, they will be able to benefit their own interests. Accordingly, the major reason for economic success would be that the rich have succeeded in locating their ancestors in a more appropriate setting than that of the poor. It is evident that older Chinese value and believe in Feng Shui more than the younger generation.[158]

God-worshipping

According to historical writings, five types of god were commonly worshipped in ancient China, and continue to be worshipped even today. They are known as the gods of the door, gods of the household, gods of the well, gods of the stove, and gods of the land. People worship many deities in Chinese communities. Chinese popular deities are very often former human beings. They might be moral exemplars who attained a spiritual appointment after death or locals whose lives were prematurely cut short.[156]

Today, many Chinese maintain popular beliefs about fate, ancestor worship, Feng Shui, or god-worshipping which have their origins in the traditional religions of Confucianism, Taoism, or Buddhism. Chinese who believe in fate will respect the divine rights of the universe and may accept death more readily. Meanwhile, they worship different gods and hope for good health and a good death. Most Chinese feel that they are obliged to practise filial piety while their parents are alive, and that they should continue to respect them through the practice of ancestor worship when their parents die. These beliefs have their origins in Confucianism. To bury one's parents properly is one way of respecting one's ancestors. This aspect of cultural beliefs and practice reinforces the Chinese values of hope, family, and spiritual connectedness.

Contemporary studies

Although 'the past decades have seen much learning of psychological, social and spiritual, as well as physical needs', [159] denial of death and death anxiety are not uncommon responses to a poor prognosis.[161, 162] Peck[162] observed that, 'I found that I had to push at least half of my patients to face the reality of their death. Indeed, their reluctance to do so seems to be a part of their illnesses' (p.50). Patients have indicated in several studies that they had unmet spiritual needs.[162-164] In a recent study in Hong Kong, Chinese hospice patients rank strategies for spiritual care the lowest while the priorities on the effectiveness of hospice care also ranked low.[165] Therefore, greater sensitivity is required to help patients to fulfil their needs to worship according to their faith, or to cope with a lack of faith. Studies that relate to spiritual issues have been constrained by a variety of factors, including discomfort among nurses. They believe that spirituality and spiritual needs are patients' private matters; they exhibit difficulty in distinguishing psychosocial needs from spiritual needs, a lack of valid and reliable measurement tools that address spiritual concerns, and confusion about differences between spiritual concerns and religiosity.

At the same time, an increasing number of research studies have focused on Chinese views on dying and death. Hwang[171] concludes that cultural differences exist concerning attitudes towards death and dying: American college students have less fear of their own death and dying and that of their loved ones than Chinese students do. However, his study was limited to college students. Hwang [155] summarises sixteen other studies conducted in Taiwan between 1984 and 1991, half of which are post-graduate theses.[155] From the findings, religious background, self-identity, family, gender, and age are identified as factors contributing to death anxiety among Chinese. Correspondingly, people with a religious background, positive self-identity, and family achievements were more accepting of death. Furthermore, people began to develop their attitudes on death as children. In Hong Kong, some studies have been conducted with the spouses of terminally ill patients. For example, Choy [166] explores anticipatory grieving in spouses of terminally ill patients. Ng [167] and Tsang [168] examine approaches to working with these spouses. Wong [169] investigates communication between health care professionals and hospice patients. These authors conclude that social welfare services for dying patients in Hong Kong were inadequate.

Chao[35] studied the meaning of Good Dying for terminally ill Chinese cancer patients in Taiwan. She identifies three patterns of Good Dying: peace of body, peace of mind, and peace of thought. The first pattern, peace of body, has four themes. These four themes are: minimising the agony of physical symptoms, a short dying process without a lingering death, cleanliness, neatness, and integrity of the body, and mobility. The second pattern is peace of mind. This pattern consists of five themes: yielding, non-attachment, not being lonely, settling all one's affairs, being in a preferred environment, and enjoying nature. The third pattern is peace of thought. The three themes in the pattern are getting through each day without thinking, having a meaningful life, expectation that the suffering would end. Rather unexpectedly, Chao [35] concludes that her findings of good dying were similar to those of studies in Western countries.

The findings of Chao's [35] study have laid the groundwork for future research related to death and dying among the Chinese population. However, her study has some limitations. First, the difference between the second theme of peace of mind and the theme of peace of thought is rather unclear. 'Mind' and 'thought' connote quite similar ideas. Second, Chao mentions that she performed some 'humanistic nursing interventions' while she was interviewing her patients. Such actions may have an influence on the interviewees' responses to the research questions.

Summary and statement of the problem

The theme of dying and death as a special stream of study has attracted scholars and researchers from various disciplines in Western countries since the 1950s. Several pioneer researchers have made attempts to investigate how patients responded to dying. Among them, Kubler-Ross [22] reports five stages, Weisman [24] identifies four phases, Shneidman[69] emphasises the patient's personality, while Pattison [68] establishes the living-dying model. Their findings tentatively conclude that a Good Death is an uncommon phenomenon. These have stimulated a closer examination of the needs of the dying. Thus, the death awareness movement has emerged in the ensuing decades. Individual perceptions of death and dying are clearly associated with one's cultural and religious beliefs. While there are some existing theories of death and dying in the West, limited studies have been conducted in the East. It is noted that little work is known to have been conducted on death and dying in the Chinese culture. Today, many Chinese maintain the popular beliefs of fate, ancestor worship, Feng Shui, and god-worshipping, which have some relationship with the traditional philosophies and beliefs of Confucianism, Taoism, and Buddhism. They agree that a Good Death emerges from a good moral life. A good moral life includes practice of ancestor worship, proper funeral arrangements for the family member, and god-worshipping. Further, the tenet of the Five Blessings includes dying a Good Death, signifying a natural painless death in old age.

A number of studies have looked at the perception of Good Death from the point of view of health care professionals such as nurses and hospice coordinators. Few have obtained data directly from patients themselves. As health care professionals may well hold a different idea of what death should be like than the patients themselves, [69, 120] more research is required to ensure that the preferences of patients are taken into account in the development of measures to evaluate their quality of life. Of equal importance, the need to identify cultural differences in perceptions of Good Death, especially from the perspective of people in Eastern cultures such as the Chinese, becomes significant. By such attempts, it may be possible to provide more culturally appropriate care to Chinese dying people and to demonstrate the importance of considering culture when designing methods for measuring the quality of life among dying people.

On reviewing the research studies that related to dying over the past twenty years, I found that given the significance of this problem, there was very little information about dying persons and their experiences before death on which to make a generalisation.[170] The research literature focused on viewpoints of the relatives and caregivers of the dying people, omitting first-hand information from the patients themselves. Subsequently, several researchers have attempted to explore the notion of Good Death, choosing dying persons as their respondents.[35, 36, 120, 122] Following this line of thought, I decided to obtain information directly from Chinese hospice patients.

Current research on death and dying follows two general directions. One direction focuses on the process of an individual's death in order to learn more about the human experience. The other direction focuses on the epidemiological aspect of death in order to estimate the use of health services towards the end of a person's life.[102] This book aims to cover the former aspect.

3
Methodology

Introduction

THIS CHAPTER PRESENTS the research methodology used to conduct the research. First, I review the need for a qualitative approach, and explain the benefits and rationale of choosing the Grounded Theory method for the present research. The discussion is presented in three main phases: preparation; method and data collection; analysis and theory generation. Finally, I consider the study's reliability, validity, limitations, and ethics.

The need for a qualitative approach

In selecting the appropriate design for a research, it is generally agreed that the approach should be determined by the research question and the state of existing knowledge.[1] The purpose of this research was to understand what is meant to die a Good Death from the perspective of Chinese hospice patients. I considered the use of a qualitative research method more appropriate than a quantitative method for the following reasons. Qualitative methods allow one to discover 'meanings, concepts, definitions, characteristics, metaphors, symbols, and descriptions of things rather than the counts and measures of things which are emphasised in classical quantitative method'.[2]

Qualitative inquiry is an interpretative science.[3] The word 'qualitative' implies an emphasis on process and meanings that are not rigorously examined, or measured, in terms of quantity, amount, intensity, and frequency.[4] 'Qualitative methods can be used to uncover the nature of people's actions and experiences and perspective which are yet little known in the world of research products'.[5] Therefore, qualitative methods are commonly used to explore problems about which relatively little is known. The literature review presented in Chapter Two as a background to the research confirms the need for more research into the experiences of dying people. Therefore, I use hospice patients' viewpoints, such as their verbatim statements, thoughts, feelings, and actions, as the data for this research. This focus allows the exploration and identification of patterns and themes relevant to Chinese hospice patients' perceptions of what it means to die a Good Death.

Central to quantitative methods are underlying modes of inquiry. Therefore, quantitative researchers usually study concrete phenomena. 'Quantitative research focuses upon the empirical and objective analysis of discrete and pre-selected variables that have been derived *a priori* as theoretical statements in order to determine causal and measurable relationships among the variables under study'.[6] In addition, in quantitative research, every attempt is made to reduce the effects of the researcher by developing an explicit, standardised set of experimental or interview procedures. In this way, an assessment of the reliability of the findings is possible by replication of the research procedure.

The main difference between the qualitative and quantitative approaches to research is the way in which the phenomenon under study is identified. Human beings are conscious of their unique continuous behaviour and intentions. Therefore, qualitative research aims to explore their thoughts, perceptions, and experiences. Qualitative researchers are interested to learn how people attach meanings to their lives and how this affects their actions. They stress the socially constructed nature of reality, the intimate relationship between 'me' and what is studied.[4] Consequently, they use research methods, such as in-depth interviewing and/or participant observation, which allows them to gain access to the perceptions, meanings, actions, and reactions of people in the context of their daily lives. This approach does not rely on the predetermined and rigid application of the predictive and prescriptive requirements of quantitative methods to understand people and their perceptions. The goal of qualitative research is not to reveal causal relationships, but to discover the nature of experienced phenomena.[7]

In an attempt to investigate what it meant to die a Good Death from the perspective of hospice patients, I hoped to gain first-hand information of the experiences of dying people and how they perceived the meaning of dying well.

I had neither the intention to impose a preconceived hypothesis on the patients, nor to attempt to fit the patients' answers into preconceived categories. On the contrary, I hoped to listen to what the patients had to say, using their own terms and frames of reference about their experiences and what they perceived as dying a Good Death. Thus, I chose a qualitative research method because it permitted an inductive approach to the study of the experience of hospice patients. It also allowed me to understand the patients' frames of reference sensitively so that I could stay close to the reality of the hospice unit. This qualitative approach further allowed me to establish a rapport with the people I interviewed, and enhanced natural and spontaneous conversations with few barriers. In sum, the qualitative approach fitted well with the nature and purpose of the research and facilitated greater cultural and human sensitivity.

The benefits of Grounded Theory

Relatively little is known about what it means to die a Good Death in an Asian context. Chao's [8] study of the meanings of good dying among terminally ill Taiwan Chinese cancer patients pioneered work of this kind in the Chinese context. In the present research I proposed to explore what it meant to die a Good Death from Chinese hospice patients' perspective. There were two main reasons. First, Chao[8] concludes that her results are similar to findings in Western studies. Although Chinese is the major ethnic group in both Hong Kong and Taiwan, the cultural context of these communities has some differences. For example, moral education based on the teachings of Confucius is emphasised more in formal education in Taiwan than in Hong Kong.[9] Confucian beliefs may have an impact on perceptions and meanings of life and death in Taiwan. Therefore, the perceptions of dying or Good Death may not be the same among Taiwan Chinese and Hong Kong Chinese.

Second, Chao[8] chose as her patients the terminally ill cancer patients in oncology wards. Some of these patients may not have known that they had cancer and therefore may have had different reactions towards dying from those who were aware of their impending death. Some researchers report that more hospice patients accept their death than do conventional care patients.[10]

Furthermore, knowledge about what it means to die a Good Death from the Chinese perspective is relatively unexplored. I selected the Grounded Theory approach from among the existing qualitative methods, in order to formulate an indigenous theory about the phenomenon. Several researchers have pointed to the need to formulate such a theory. For example, they pointed out that the range of human responses to terminal illness and dying should be explored and described so as to build a culturally sensitive base for hospice care. Feifel [11] and Corr [12] have made similar observations.

Grounded Theory derives from the study of phenomena. It is discovered, developed, and provisionally verified through systematic data collection and analysis of data pertaining to specific phenomena. Therefore, data collection, analysis, and theory stand in a reciprocal relationship. Using this approach, I begin with an area of study and allow what is relevant to that area to emerge. The identified codes and categories are then constantly compared for their similarities and differences in order to increase the precision and consistency of the theory discovered. This method is called the constant comparative method of analysis and is used throughout this research. Consequently, concepts and a theory of Good Death would be grounded in observations of the social world rather than generated in the abstract.[13]

Compared with other qualitative research methods, Grounded Theory emphasises theory development rather than mere description of phenomena. It aims to evolve new theories grounded from data, whatever the level of analysis. Numerous definitions of theory exist in the literature. For example, theory is 'logically interconnected sets of propositions from which empirical uniformities can be derived' (p.39).[14] Maxwell[15] extends the definition as 'a set of concepts and proposed relationships among these, a structure that is intended to represent or model something about the world'. Theories may be complex, providing a means for description, explanation, prediction, or a more explicit representation of reality.[16] There are two levels of theory: a higher general theory and a substantive theory. My research is concerned with generating a substantive theory of what it means to die a Good Death. According to Strauss,[17] a substantive or empirical theory differs from formal theory in levels of generality. Formal theory is developed for a conceptual theory. As 'substantive theory is grounded in research on one particular substantive area (work, juvenile delinquency, medical education), it might be taken to apply only to that specific area'. [18] However, it may have important general implications and relevance, and become a stepping stone to the development of a formal theory. In terms of the research process, Grounded Theory studies share some similarities with other modes of qualitative research. First, all qualitative methods emphasise the interpretative roles of researchers in making judgements about the data collected.[19] Second, similar to other qualitative approaches, the data for Grounded Theory can be obtained from various sources such as interviews, observation, and reviews of documents. Correspondingly, the data from each of these sources can be coded in the same way as other qualitative interviews or observations. I have applied these principles in conducting my interviews and field work. Most important of all, I have set out to secure the trustworthiness of the research findings. [20]

Therefore, 'a "good theory" must be readily applicable to the data under study, it must be meaningfully relevant to and be able to explain the behaviour under study' (p.3).[21] It is hoped that, the discovery of a substantive theory of Good Death will be derived from the clinical settings appropriate to Chinese and other Asian communities. Second, the theory, which will be inductively generated, will be grounded in the actual experiences of the people under study.

The research process

The following paragraphs will describe the procedures of the research process. I was interested to know both what people experienced as they approached death, and their views on what it meant to die a Good Death. Since operationalisation of the concept of Good Death from the patients' points of view was essential, and given the poor state of the understanding of a Good Death within the local context, a legitimate first step was to apply a qualitative analysis to patients' viewpoints, in order to achieve greater conceptual clarification. The Grounded Theory is a non-linear process that is difficult to describe.[22] The research process, which includes data collection, sampling, and analysis, occurs simultaneously as the research progresses.[21] I will present the following description of the research process according to the three major phases of Grounded Theory: preparatory, data collection and data analysis, and theory generation.

Preparations

During this initial phase, my main task was to gain access to the research setting, to recruit people for the research, and to build a relationship with hospice staff. When I had decided on the focus for the research, I worked to gain access to a hospice unit. I did not approach the independent hospice because I had recently completed a preliminary study of the relationship between pain and the mood of the patients in this hospice.[23] Therefore, I had acquired experiences in interviewing dying people, who could serve as the target patients for the present research. Nevertheless, I had no intention of making a comparison between the two types of hospice service.

The research setting

I chose a hospital situated in the town centre of Hong Kong Island as the research setting. This hospital has provided hospice services since 1986. The hospice unit is a ten-bed unit, which is situated next to a medical unit and is under the care of a medical consultant. There are also two single rooms, and each room has two beds. Male and female patients stay in the cubicle or in the single rooms depending on the number of patients in each group. The hospice team consists of a medical practitioner, a hospice nurse specialist, and two other hospice nurses. The patients also receive care from other disciplines, namely medical social workers, physiotherapists, and occupational therapists. Hospital volunteers and some charitable agencies also visit the patients. The medical practitioner visits the patients every morning. At night, the ward nurses look after the patients. Patients can be discharged home or to a nursing home if their condition improves. They can then be followed up at the outpatient clinics that run one afternoon per week. Hospice nurses also make home visits to discharged patients.

The second clinical setting, a hospice unit in Kowloon, is similar in nature, except it is a bigger unit with 16 beds. There is also one single room, which is designed for patients who want to avoid the busy main ward. Some patients and/or relatives may prefer a quiet and private environment for their remaining days. The duration of my field work for the first phase in the first hospice unit in Hong Kong was 13 months while that of the second phase in the second hospice unit in Kowloon was three months. Thus, the total time spent on field work was sixteen months.

Ethical considerations

I had to obtain the formal approval of the hospice unit before I started data collection. Since no ethical committee had been set up for the purpose of approving studies in the hospital, I wrote to the medical practitioner in charge of the hospice unit to apply for formal ethical approval to conduct my research. The medical practitioner in charge consented to my conducting my research in his palliative unit. I undertook the same procedure before I conducted my research in the second hospice unit. The Hospital Chief Executive gave me consent to carry out my research.

Confidentiality and anonymity were established and maintained in documentation. During the research process, I did not carry out the practice of written consent, as the patients did not feel comfortable signing a consent form. Another reason was that cognitive failure is extremely prevalent during the last weeks of life. Consequently, the reliability of informed consent for participating in a research during the final stages of life may be questioned.[24] Verbal consent was, however, obtained prior to the interviews, when the hospice staff approached the patients individually. In addition, at the beginning of the interview, I explained the objectives and purposes of the research to the patients. They also had opportunities to ask questions and were free to withdraw from the research at any time. To ensure that consent was ongoing in the research (during the second or third interview), assurance was repeated that patients were free to withdraw from the research at any time. For example, one patient requested to end the interview when questions on preparation for departure were raised. To some patients, preparation before one's death was a private matter. Confidentiality was assured. Moreover, trust and mutual respect were established through honesty and openness as I hoped that the patients would see the value of the interviews I conducted.

The Participants

The Chinese hospice patients who stayed in the hospital-based hospice unit were recruited. They were either admitted from their homes or transferred from nursing homes. Staying in the hospice unit is quite different from staying at home or in a nursing home. Before the patients were admitted to the hospice unit, they were interviewed and assessed by hospice nursing staff. They were informed of their condition and diagnosis before admission to the unit.

As the aim of the research was to find out what it meant to die a Good Death, all hospice patients were potential participants for the research. Nevertheless, four criteria were set to guide the recruiting process. The criteria for the sample were that they were:

1. adult (over 21 year olds), male or female, receiving hospice care;
2. diagnosed as having cancer with a life expectancy of 6 to 12 months. These criteria were the same as for admission to the hospice unit;
3. aware of their diagnoses and prognosis which made them consider the matter of death and dying;
4. conscious, able to communicate clearly, and willing to be interviewed. Therefore, patients with communication difficulties such as those who spoke less common Chinese dialects were excluded from the research.

As the patients were aware of their diagnoses and prognosis, it was expected that they had a sense of dying psychologically and interpersonally.[25] Nevertheless, I did not mention the word 'death'. Instead, I attended to and observed patients' conversations carefully. Some patients used the word 'death' explicitly but some used alternative words or terms to describe the notion of death and dying. Examples of alternative terms included: 'passing away', 'going to sleep', and 'returning to my old home'.

For the purpose of theoretical sampling, I recruited five hospice patients, who were relatively young and who had different types of cancer, from the second hospice unit. Glaser and Strauss[21] stated that, 'the sociologist trying to discover theory cannot state at the outset of this research how many groups he will sample during the entire research; he can only count up the groups at the end' (p. 61). The researcher may collect data from a single group, and return to the group when needed, while simultaneously seeking new groups. In total, 33 Chinese hospice patients participated in the research and 64 interviews were conducted. This fits well with the estimate that between 20 and 50 interviews is necessary to elicit major, repetitive themes of a topic under research.[26] Therefore the number of interviews conducted in this research was within the suggested range and was considered appropriate.

During this preparatory phase, I was able to gain a general, yet deeper understanding of the characteristics of hospice patients and hospice care in Hong Kong. Based on my previous research experiences with the hospice patients in the independent hospice, I was prepared to interview patients with some broad questions in mind.

Of the patients in this research, 17 were men and 16 were women. As has been the case in some previous studies[25, 27] there was a high representation of older people and 70 per cent of the patients were over 60 years old. The age range was from 34 to 86 with a mean age of 67. Among the patients, 49 per cent were married, 27 per cent were widowed, 15 per cent were divorced, and 9 per cent were single. Regarding educational background, 24 per cent of the patients had had no formal education, 61 per cent had received primary education, and only 15 per cent had had secondary education. Fifty-two percent of the patients were retired, 18 per cent were in employment, 15 per cent were senior citizens, 9 per cent were unemployed because of their illness and 6 per cent were housewives. None of the patients had any financial support, such as a retirement fund or pension, and most had to rely on their children for financial support. Some received social assistance for disability from the government.

Sixty-nine percent of patients had cancer of the lungs and 9 per cent had cancer of the colon. These cancers are common in Hong Kong.[28] Other types of cancer included: rectum, palate, kidney, pancreas, cervix, ovary, and the parotid glands. In addition, 63 per cent of patients had developed metastases. The average duration of the cancer trajectory for this sample was 14.5 months, ranging between 5 and 53 months. Eighteen per cent of the patients were Christians, 15 per

Table 3.1
Demographic characteristics of the sample (*N*= 33)

Characteristics	no.	%
Gender		
Male	16	51
Female	17	49
Age		
30–39	1	3
40–49	3	9
50–59	6	18
60–69	6	18
70–79	12	37
80 and over	5	15
Marital status		
Single	3	9
Married	16	49
Widowed	9	27
Divorced	5	15
Occupational Status		
Employed	6	18
Unemployed	3	9
Senior citizen	5	15
Retired	17	52
Others	2	6
Education		
No schooling	8	24
Primary	20	61
Secondary	5	15
Religious background		
No religion	10	30
Christian	6	18
Ancestor worship	6	18
Buddhist	5	15
Fate	5	15
Others	1	3

Type of cancer		
Lung	23	70
Colon	3	9
Cervix/ ovary	2	6
Kidney	1	3
Palate	1	3
Pancreas	1	3
Parotid glands	1	3
Rectum	1	3

Time since diagnosis		
Less than 6 months	8	24
6–12 months	14	43
1 year	4	12
2 year	4	12
3–5 years	2	6
6–10 years	1	3

Time before death		
Less than 1 month	12	36
1–2 months	9	27
3–4 months	8	24
5–6 months		
7–8 months		
9–10 months		
Over 10 months	1	3
Unknown	1	3
Still alive at time of writing	2	6

cent were Buddhists; 15 per cent believed in Fate, while 18 per cent of the patients practised ancestor worship. That is, about half of the patients followed Chinese popular beliefs. At the same time, 30 per cent of the patients had no religious affiliation.

Other information such as the time when the interview took place was considered important. The life expectancy of the hospice patients was 6 to 12 months. The median time from diagnosis to the time of interview was 15 months. In other words, a majority of patients had already undergone 15 months of adjustment. However, the range of duration of illness from cancer was wide. One patient was interviewed in the same month as 'receiving the bad news' while one was interviewed seven years after the diagnosis. Two-thirds were interviewed within 12 months of diagnosis: 24 per cent were interviewed within six months and 42 per cent of the patients were interviewed 6 to 12 months after they were diagnosed.

I calculated the interval between the date of the first interview and date of death retrospectively. This provided information about the context of the dying experiences that the patients underwent. The range was large: one patient was interviewed five days before her death, while another was interviewed one year before his death.

In total, 33 hospice patients were recruited for this research, of whom 16 took part in one interview and 17 in more than one. The number of interviews depended on the saturation of data gathered during the first interview. I conducted 64 interviews, which I taped and transcribed. The data were then coded and categorised. I wove quotations from the patients into this account to reflect the true voices and experiences of the patients. During the dying process, the patients expressed feelings of pain, suffering, and emotional stress, which were described as 'bad' experiences. On the other hand, some patients experienced something beneficial from their illness experiences. These were referred to as elements of Good Death. The findings of this research indicate that individual patients often had a mixture of 'good' and 'bad' experiences. The proportion of 'bad' experiences and 'good' experiences varied from individual to individual.

Data collection

This section will present the details of data collection: how theoretical sampling was performed, the processes of interviewing and observation, and information on desirable data sources. At the beginning of my research, I had prepared some broad questions. As the research process continued, I gradually gained deeper insights and engaged simultaneously in data collection and analysis. The concepts and insights that emerged from the data guided the whole research process.

Like ethnography, the Grounded Theory approach relies primarily on less structured interviews and observations from data. In this research, interviewing was used as the primary research method. The principles of theoretical sampling were used to guide the interview phase.[21] Regarding the number of patients, the principle was that it was the quality of data that counted rather than the size of the sample. 'Adequacy of sample size in qualitative research is relative, a matter of judging a sample neither small nor large *per se*, but rather too small or too large for the intended purposes of sampling and for the intended qualitative product' (p.179).[29] For example, Morse[30] recommends the phenomenologies to include about six participants, ethnographers, and grounded theorists, about 30 to 50 interviews and/or observations. More important, the depth and quality of interviews must be considered.

Theoretical sampling

I employed the theoretical sampling procedure developed by Glaser and Strauss. 'Theoretical sampling in the Grounded Theory approach is the process of data collection for generating theory whereby the analyst jointly collects, codes, and analyses the data and decides what data to collect next and where to find them, in order to develop the (grounded) theory as it emerges'[21] (p.45). The entire process of data collection is guided by the theory as it gradually emerges. Initial decisions for theoretical collection of data are based on a general understanding of the problem area instead of a pre-conceptualised theoretical framework. Therefore, the procedures of data collection cannot be planned in advance. The research process is controlled by the emerging theory which gives direction to the types of data collected. I began and continued my field research following these principles. Examples of the broad questions I used at the beginning of the interview: What is the nature of your current illness? Where would you like to be in your final days and with whom? What would you like to prepare for the end when the time comes?

Theoretical sampling involves gradually enlarging a population description through the selection of elements, such as the background to the patients' illnesses, and their age. Each phase is different from the preceding one. The method involves active sampling of new patients as the analysis proceeds. Therefore, patients were chosen as needed and not before the research began.[22] I continually adjusted my data collection to ensure both its relevance and the nature of my emerging theory.

Therefore, it was essential to have a diverse sample of participants. During the initial phase of data collection, I required the support of hospice nurses, who would obtain initial consent from potential patients. Moreover, it was necessary to recruit patients who represented an adequate range of experiences and backgrounds so that their perceptions and meanings of Good Death could become data from which to generate theory.[22] Therefore I included all hospice patients and not just those who were perceived by the nurses to have 'problems'.

During data collection, I had to be theoretically sensitive so that I could conceptualise and formulate a theory as it emerged from the data.[21] Theoretical sensitivity is the ability needed to develop continuously, which would help me to conceptualise the categories and sensitising questions relating to the research.

As the hospice unit was attached to a chest medical unit, the majority of the patients suffered from lung cancer. After interviewing twenty patients, I found that only three patients presented with dyspnoea, which affected the progress of interviews. The remaining 17 patients had a wide range of symptoms. They had different sites of metastasis, such as the pleura, liver, bone, brain, and spinal cord. Nevertheless, I felt that the suffering of these people might not be unique, and purposefully looked for patients with other types of cancer. As a result, seven patients with cancer of other sites were recruited. The cancers they had included cancer of the palate (1), cancer of the cervix (1), cancer of the parotid glands (1), cancer of the kidney (1), cancer of the pancreas (1), and cancer of the colon (2).

After interviewing 10 patients, it was found that most of the patients were about 60 years of age, so I began to look for both older and younger patients. At the end of data collection, I managed to recruit four patients below 50 years of age and five patients aged about 80, in order to facilitate the constant comparative method used in the research. In comparing the data, I found that people of all ages have similar experiences and dying processes. For example, most of the dying people presented with anxiety as they approached death. In addition, the assumption that older patients were more 'ready to die' was found to be untrue. The even ratio of female and male patients was maintained approximately.

I then looked for patients who presented with intensified experiences, such as patients with altered body image or poor social support, and patients who experienced anger or abandonment. For example, I interviewed two female patients who suffered from facial disfigurement. One of them had cancer of the palate and the other had cancer of the parotid glands (The parotid glands are in the face behind the cheeks). Both patients had undergone surgery on the oral cavity, producing marked facial disfigurement.

I recruited my patients through a gradual and developmental process in which I allowed the insights and concepts generated from my interviews to guide my sample selection. Through this theoretical sampling process, I was able to increase the size of my sample according to my theoretical purposes. Eventually I felt that the data had reached a stage of saturation.[21] Theoretical sampling was achieved when additional analyses yielded neither further directions for purposeful sampling nor anything new.[31]

Interviewing

I chose interviewing as the major method of data collection, since this approach is the most flexible method to use.[25] The interview method allows for the collection of a mass of heterogeneous data. Interviews were conducted 'face-to-face', thus allowing the observation of a full range of non-verbal behaviour. This method also facilitated a closer rapport with the patients. Thus, my approach reflected the statement that: 'the fullest condition of participating in the mind of another human being is face to face interaction' (p.2).[32]

The hospice staff may have had concerns that the interviews would create emotions such as anxiety, and allow for the revelation of the patients' intimate secrets. This is because psychosocial research involves some risks.[42] Therefore, I closely followed the guidelines for the ethical conduct of research throughout the research process. At the beginning of the interview, I introduced the aims of the research. The patients were reminded that they were under no obligation to participate and they could withdraw from the research at any time.

I developed a semi-structured interview guide (Appendix 1) to facilitate data collection. The interview guide was helpful because it enabled me to explore, probe, and ask questions that would elucidate and illuminate the experience of the particular patient. Depending on the current situation and the willingness of the patient, I carried out the interview more formally, following the semi-structured interview guide to yield the data. The focused interview was thought to collect the maximum amount of information in the most useable form. The interviews elicited patients' views and feeling about their conditions and their needs. I did not use the words 'cancer' and 'death' when I asked the patients for their opinions because I did not want to induce any strong emotional feelings. Bryant and Payne[33] point out that anyone researching into cancer is entering into a very sensitive and complicated area of human concern. I had to bear in mind that a proportion of people preferred not to reflect on their experience of their illness or talk about cancer *per se*, a concern that, of course, needed to be respected within a flexible research approach. [34]

The patients often started the interview by describing the onset of their illnesses. Some of them then went on to talk about how the medical practitioner had announced their diagnoses. Some patients talked about their feelings on hearing their diagnoses. Many went on to describe what types of treatment they received and the level of symptom control they had. Most patients expressed their feelings freely and naturally. Several expressed feelings of helplessness and hopelessness. Occasionally, these interviews elicited disclosures that the patients had not shared with their families.[35] At the end of the interview, I asked the patients how they felt about the interview process. I wanted to ensure that I had not caused the patient any distress. Most of the patients felt that the experience of being interviewed was beneficial in several respects. For example, one patient thanked me for listening to him. One older man felt more relaxed having somebody with whom to share his views on death.

I followed an open-ended conversational style in interviewing, allowing the patients to raise the issues about death that were important to him or her. It is essential to be aware that the process of dying may be the most individual thing that happens in life. I assessed this by asking how the patient felt during and at the end of the process, and attempted to maintain an open mind so as to remain sensitive to data which I had not foreseen. Because I was also the person deciding on the purpose of the research, this facilitated much greater flexibility during the interview itself. Sue Jones has described the advantages of using this approach.

> *In qualitative research the notion of some kind of impersonal, machine-like investigator is recognised as a chimera. An interview is a complicated, shifting, social process occurring between two individual human beings, which can never be exactly replicated... There cannot be definitive rules about the use of open-ended questions, leading and loaded questions, and disagreements with patients and so on. Such choices must depend on the understanding researchers have of the person they are with and the kind of relationship they have developed in the encounter. Some relationships may allow, without destroying trust or comfort, much more of the to-and-fro debate between two human beings than others. What is crucial is that researchers choose their actions with self-conscious awareness of why they are making them.* [36]

Observations

I used my observation of non-verbal cues to supplement the verbal information provided by the patients. I followed the four features that Lofland[32] highlights are to be observed when a researcher conducts field work. Firstly, I established closeness with the patients in both a physical and social sense. It is desirable that this involvement is on a long-term basis so as to enhance understanding and to reduce reactivity due to my presence. I made weekly visits to the patients, and my contact with the hospice lasted for more than one year. Therefore, the hospice staff and the patients gradually became familiar with my presence and because of this, several patients agreed more readily to be interviewed. I also greeted those patients who had already participated in the research when I saw them during my visits. Secondly, the report had to be authentic. I had to learn to be sensitive, yet as objective as possible, when I collected and interpreted the data I obtained. Thirdly, the data contained a large amount of 'pure description of action, people, activities and the like. The reality of the place was conveyed through representation of its mundane aspects in a straightforward manner' (p.4).[32] Fourthly, my observation notes and memos contained direct quotations from the patients. Note-taking and audio recordings were appropriate for conveying the reality of the situation. Observation offered a unique opportunity to examine the dying persons' experiences and their interactions.

Other methods

Qualitative data do not emerge only from interviews. The collection of other data directly from the field was also important. In addition to in-depth interviews and field notes of observations, the patients' notes on some critical incidents, published texts, transcripts of conversations,[37] and their photographs were useful sources of data for analysis. One patient recorded his past medical history, while two patients noted down their symptoms, the drugs used, and the effects of their medication, in their notebooks. Others wrote down their critical incidents because they were dyspnoeic and wanted to find a way to communicate with their medical practitioners.

Two patients were keen to show me their photographs, which were taken before their illnesses. This was considered a sign of trust and mutuality. The photographs provided me with some visual insights and knowledge of the events that had occurred, leading to richer data and greater understanding of the events. Photographs can serve as a powerful agent of memory. In these cases, both patients recalled the happy times they had had in the past in order to keep up their morale. They shared with me their experiences of losing their past identities after they acquired cancer. Another advantage was that the photographs helped the patients to tell their stories more spontaneously, especially when the research focused on the compassionate dimension of the experience of dying.

To minimise the problem of over-reliance on the verbal presentation and perceptions of the patients, I sought to understand the 'ethnographic context' of the patients through observation at the hospice units and informal discussion with hospice staff and patients' relatives. I talked to relatives, hospice staff including hospice nurses, medical practitioners, medical social workers, health care assistants, and volunteers such as those from Comfort Care Concern Group, which aimed to promote hospice care and bereavement care. In order to obtain a more comprehensive picture of ongoing hospice care, I spent one afternoon as an observer at the out-patient clinic. It was noted that the hospice patients who came for follow-up, were in reasonably good physical condition. Most of them had good social support and were accompanied by their relatives. In addition to visiting the out-patient clinic of the hospice unit, I visited other hospice units so as to cultivate my sensitivity in interpreting the needs of Chinese hospice patients.

During the phase of data collection, I taped interviews whenever the patients gave their consent. The first four exploratory interviews were not taped. Other data, such as observations and untaped interviews, were written in the form of memos, since the writing of memos is seen to be the foundation of theory generation;[17, 38] Immediately after each interview, I wrote memos on my impressions to describe the interview context. These were used to select the focus of the subsequent analysis. For example, the questions I recorded in one memo were: Were the hospice patients aware of their impending death? Who was responsible for letting them know that they would die? How was the 'breaking the bad news' performed? Did the hospice patients know they had cancer? How would they relate the diagnosis of cancer with death? What were their (and their relatives') reactions on hearing the bad news? Did it have an impact on the hospice patients throughout the dying trajectory?

Data analysis

The first task in data analysis is to be extremely familiar with the data.[22] After the completion of a tape-recorded interview, I replayed and checked the tape. I listened carefully to the content, as well as to the questions asked and the responses. It was crucial that the tape was transcribed exactly (word for word) from the interview and not paraphrased. Pauses were shown by using brackets with the duration inserted. All expressions, including laughter, crying, and sighing, were included in the text and separated from the verbal text. I then recognised persistent symbolic words, phrases, or themes within the data. One example of symbolic words was the word(s) the medical practitioners used to substitute for the word 'cancer' when they announced the 'bad news'. Thus, I labelled the theme and identified the characteristics that were indicative of the process.

The frequencies of the codes and categories were counted. Counting in qualitative research is important to ensure that the researcher has not simply trawled through a mass of data and selected anecdotes to report that support his or her particular bias. This is an aspect of validity, [13] which helps generate confidence in the report.

Since I conducted the interviews in Chinese, all tapes were first transcribed to Chinese. Typical examples of 'conversation' would be quoted in the sections of results and discussion. A few samples of the Chinese transcripts were translated into English. The translated transcripts were then cross-checked by another researcher for accuracy. In addition, a non-Chinese-speaking person with relevant expertise further validated the translated transcripts. A great amount of material was collected during the research process; therefore, the less relevant material was reduced.

Constant comparative method

As mentioned previously in this chapter, I use the constant comparative method of data analysis in this research to generate a Grounded Theory from the data. The constant comparative method is an inductive method of qualitative analysis and theory development, and is concerned with generating and suggesting many categories, properties, and hypotheses about the research problem. These properties may be causes, conditions, consequences, dimensions, types, and processes, and will generate a theory through the process of constant comparison and vigorous analysis of data. This method enhanced the ability of my analysis to explore the diversity of the data. By diversity, it is meant that each incident is compared with other incidents, with the properties of each consistent category, in terms of as many similarities and differences as possible. As a result, a tentative theory was developed. While comparing the incidents, I learnt to see my categories in terms of both their internal development and their changing relations to other categories. In this way, I was able to bring out underlying uniformities and diversities, and began to use more abstract concepts to account for differences in the data. [21]

Coding and categorising

Based on the interview transcripts, sets of notes describing observations, and some other qualitative materials, my first task was to develop a set of codes that reflected the initial aim of the research. I had to take into account any unexpected issues that emerged during data collection. Unlike the classical social survey, where the aims of the research stay relatively fixed from beginning to end, qualitative research can often be more exploratory in nature, and can end up addressing issues that were not imagined before the research began.[37] For example, the initial aim of this research was to make an ethnographic study of Chinese hospice patients on death and dying. After my interview with the second patient, who discussed his viewpoints on Good Death with his fellow drug addicts, I decided to focus my research on the meaning of dying a Good Death rather than dying and death *per se.*

In the first stage of coding, I coded each incident in the data into as many codes of analysis as possible. Coding involves placing like with like, so that patterns can be formulated. Coding was therefore the first step of data analysis. This process was later structured, and I coded the data diversity into my emerging categories. Codes are subdivided so that a category begins to develop branches. Categorisation of the qualitative replies to open-ended questions in the semi-structured interview is one way of turning quality into quantity so that patterns can be detected in data analysis.[37]

As my knowledge of the categories gradually accumulated, I integrated the diverse properties and categories into a unified whole and gradually developed the theory. The third stage was the delimiting stage, in which I reduced the properties I considered to be irrelevant or overlapping. More effort was paid at this stage to developing those properties which are central to the theory. The final stage was the writing up of the theory. At this stage, I transformed the coded data and memos into major themes and then developed a theory which was genuinely grounded in the data collected.

For this process, I followed the constant comparative method closely to analyse my data. I first coded the transcribed data using the 'open-coding' method (p.27-29).[17] I thoroughly examined all the interviews and memos, in an attempt to produce preliminary concepts and meanings of Good Death from the data. Open-coding helped me to open up my analysis and to begin making tentative interpretations of the data. It further allowed me to develop initial theoretical understanding and theories about what it meant to die a Good Death from the perspective of Chinese hospice patients. These steps formed the initial process of conceptualising theory from the data.

During the process of open-coding, I became aware of the different elements that contributed to dying a Good Death, such as, being aware of death, experiencing minimal pain and suffering, maintaining hope, and so forth. I had gained a preliminary understanding of the condition, dynamics, and consequences of achieving a Good Death from hospice patients' perspective. I was also aware of some strategies the patients used to adjust their lifestyles while they underwent the dying process and of the cultural factors that had influenced the achievement of a Good Death.

The second method I used for coding was 'axial coding', carried out after generating some initial codes from my data.[17] During the process of axial coding, I attempted to analyse the data intensively, revolving around an 'axis' of one category at a time. I considered axial coding around the categories that I had determined during the previous stage of open coding. For example, the categories around the axis of 'being aware of dying' included: being informed; receiving bad news; being aware of cancer and being aware of dying. At this stage, some fundamental properties started to define themselves, as 'certain differences between incidents create boundaries and relationships between categories are clarified'. [39]

Some concepts appeared more prominent than others and the inter-relationship between the categories began to emerge. Certain patterns and linkages were also identified.

In the process of axial coding, I began to note that my data offered an initial conceptualisation of what Chinese hospice patients meant by dying a Good Death. I also pinpointed some core categories that were central to the emerging Grounded Theory. I proceeded to work on 'selective coding' (p.69-74),[17] continuing to code systematically for the core categories. I delimited coding by categorising, re-categorising and condensing all first-level codes, only to those codes that related to the core codes of emerging theory which were related to dying a Good Death from the Chinese hospice patient's perspective. Therefore, I focused only on coding categories of Good Death experience. The coding of the core categories helped me to integrate and generate the Grounded Theory and rendered the theory theoretically dense and saturated. At the end of the coding stage, I derived seven core categories as elements of Good Death. These seven elements were: being aware of dying (death awareness), maintaining hope (hope), being free from pain and suffering (comfort), experiencing personal control (control), maintaining social relationships (connectedness), preparing to depart (preparations) and accepting the timing of one's death (completion).

Developing theory

The process of open-coding, axial-coding and selective coding is thought-provoking; though monotonous. I gradually discovered how Chinese dying people perceived dying a Good Death, through the eyes of the hospice patients I interviewed. The constant comparative method and the coding paradigm were particularly useful in facilitating a systematic, yet rigorous data analysis.

The process of analysis helped me to generate the conceptions of theory truly grounded from the collected data. Therefore, the theory reflected well the perspective and perception of dying a Good Death for Chinese hospice patients. The gradual evolution of conceptualisation moved systematically to higher levels of abstraction. Initially, I explored and formulated some basic categories that reflected the experience of dying Chinese hospice patients. Next, I conceptualised two core categories of dying experiences – the good experience and the bad experience – through vigorous constant comparative method. Subsequently, using the constant comparative method of analysis, I identified the seven major elements which the Chinese hospice patients viewed as constituting a Good Death. I further grouped the seven elements into three relationships with which the patients were concerned. These three relationships thus formed the theoretical framework of the theory of Harmonious Death. This theory emerged from an inductive method of theory development through a joint process of data collection, coding, and data analysis.

Reliability and validity
of the research process

Reliability is concerned with whether a test or way of taking measurements will tend to produce the same result upon repeated administrations. Validity is generally concerned with the accuracy of measurement. The whole philosophy of qualitative research is founded upon an explicit move towards increased validity. In Glaser and Strauss's work, [21] this was demonstrated by the notion that the grounded theories should work, fit, and be recognisable and of relevance to those studied. Therefore, it implied that some forms of validity criteria could be employed.

Appropriateness of the sample

In Grounded Theory, reliability is established by ensuring the appropriateness of the sample and the adequacy of the data. [40] The selection of the sample is considered as one essential step to maintaining reliability and validity in qualitative research. The use of a purposeful sample ensured appropriateness. I selected the sample according to the theoretical needs of the research, the willingness of the patients to participate, and the ability of the patients to describe their experiences and needs.[40, 41] The selection of Chinese hospice patients as the sample led to a challenge: patients did not usually survive for very long after the interview. Consequently, I had no opportunity to return to some patients to validate data as they were either too ill to receive my visit or had died. As Davies et al.[42] have suggested, validation had to be addressed in other ways, such as talking with other patients in similar situations. In addition, I verified data with secondary patients from the second hospice unit, and sought negative cases or exceptions. Thus, I obtained a sample representative of the population according to the knowledge domain, rather than according to demographic characteristics. [22]

Comparative analysis and systematic coding

To sustain the reliability, validity, and objectivity of research study, the interviews and observational notes were monitored throughout the process of comparative analysis. The process of systematic coding also helped in improving the validity of reports of qualitative data. This was achieved chiefly by 'presenting counts of how many times, and in which circumstances, a thing happens, and by using coding categories to search for negative instances that may contradict, or help to develop, an emerging theory' (p.153).[37]

Combination of methods

I also used several methods to compare different kinds of data from different sources to see whether they corroborated one another, thus comparing data relating to the same phenomenon. Data was derived from different phases of fieldwork, different points in time and accounts of different patients, or using different methods of data collection. [37]

Lincoln and Guba [20] recommend several strategies to ensure the credibility or trustworthy of the data and findings. The four standards for assessing rigour in qualitative research are credibility, transferability, dependability, and confirmability, which define these criteria and describe the individual strategies used to establish trustworthiness in this research.

Limitations of the study

The research has several limitations as it used a purposeful sampling method. First, the patients of this research were all cancer patients. Cancer is not the only life-threatening illness in Hong Kong today, although it has the highest mortality in Hong Kong, mainland China, and Taiwan. AIDS has become the most high-profile life-threatening illness. Patients with other illnesses, such as cardiac failure, renal failure, and neurological disorders, are also confronted with their imminent death. Therefore, the findings of this research may not be generalised to people who die from illnesses other than cancer.

Second, as cancer has commonly occurred in the elderly population, a majority of the patients selected for this research were older people. Age has been a predominant factor affecting Chinese people's perception of dying a Good Death. Therefore, the findings of this research may be more applicable to the elderly population.

Third, most of the patients in this research were in the terminal stages of their illness. The research is limited in that it does not provide understanding of what it means to die a Good Death for people in the different stages of the cancer after diagnosis. Since less than half of the patients were interviewed once, the data may be confined to one particular stage of the dying trajectory. Even when patients agreed to a second interview in the following week, his or her condition did not always allow him or her to do so. For example, one patient did not feel free to disclose his opinions on death issues with me because he felt the hospice staff did not like him. He was also a demanding patient. Nevertheless, I managed to gain his trust during the first interview, and he promised to discuss it in the next interview. When I returned again the following week, the patient was dying and could not communicate with me. Therefore, a future longitudinal study is suggested to identify the meaning of dying a Good Death throughout the different stages of illness. More data relating to interactions between the patients and their caregivers would be collected.

Fourth, there were several uncontrollable factors. First, the amount of time with each patient was uncontrollable. The first interview could also be the last interview due to uncontrolled changes in the patients' condition. Therefore, I tried to discuss the major issues with the patient in the first interview. I would follow up if the patient was still in the hospice unit in the following week.

Fifth, as death is a taboo subject for many Chinese people, several patients were not prepared to disclose their opinions to an outsider such as myself. For example, one patient told me that she considered the discussion of death-related issues as a private matter which she would share only with her family.

Summary

In summary, on reviewing studies which related to dying, first-person information from dying individuals has been omitted. Consequently, several recent research studies have attempted to explore the notion of Good Death and chose dying persons as their patients. Nevertheless, a scarcity of knowledge existed about what it meant to die a Good Death in Chinese culture. Thus, I chose a qualitative approach to explore what Chinese hospice patients meant by dying a Good Death. I selected a Grounded Theory approach so as to formulate an indigenous theory about the phenomenon. Grounded Theory emphasises development of theory rather than description of phenomena, and aims to evolve new theories grounded from data. It is hoped that the discovery of a substantive theory of Good Death will be fitted to the clinical settings appropriate to Hong Kong and other Asian countries.

The research process consisted of three phases: the preparatory phase, data collection and data analysis. In the preparatory phase, I prepared the research setting and respected ethical considerations. Confidentiality was assured. Theoretical sampling was used. In total, thirty-three Chinese hospice patients were interviewed, all of whom were terminally ill cancer patients. Data was collected and analysed using the constant comparative method. Through the process of open-coding, axial-coding, and selective coding, I derived the theory of Harmonious Death from the perspective of Chinese hospice patients. Meanwhile, I addressed the reliability and validity of the research process, with special attention to the appropriateness of the sample and research process.

The next seven chapters of the book discuss the main results of the data analysis and the seven major themes that emerged from the analysis. These themes consequently comprise the seven elements of Harmonious Death from the Chinese patients' perspective. Chapter Four describes awareness of dying (Death Awareness) which is an essential first step of dying a Good Death. Death remains a social taboo in most contemporary Chinese societies, which might add to the complexity of death awareness issues in Asian patients. Chapter Five focuses on the element of maintaining hope (Hope). Receiving treatment and making adjustments are identified as the main sources of hope for the dying persons. Therefore, the nature of treatment and strategies of adjustments are further examined. Chapter Six examines the third element of being free from pain and suffering (Comfort). These human experiences are often subjective and multi-dimensional. The topics of euthanasia and suicide are explored as people with unresolved pain and suffering have raised these issues. The fourth element is maintaining social relations (Connectedness) and is discussed in Chapter Seven. Dying people are mainly concerned with their connectedness with the hospice staff and their families. Factors affecting connectedness are therefore examined. Chapter Eight describes the findings of experiencing personal control (Control). The nature of personal control and factors affecting a person's ability to control are discussed. Chapter Nine examines the element of preparing to depart and bidding farewells (Preparations), and explores both personal and public preparations. Chapter Ten describes the last element of accepting the timing of one's death (Completion). In this chapter, the four circumstances in which patients may have a better acceptance of the timing of death are discussed. Chapter Eleven presents the final theoretical framework of Harmonious Death which unites the above elements. In addition, I compare the present theory with some existing models of Good Death in order to highlight the significance of the present framework.

4
Being aware
of dying
(Death awareness)

Importance of awareness

IT IS IMPORTANT for patients to know their condition so that
they can develop an awareness of dying, and are able to adjust to
changes that occur as a result of the illness and or to prepare for their
death. However, since some individuals have complex psychological
defences, one can never be absolutely sure of this awareness.[2] In
this research, nineteen patients mentioned the word 'death' during
the interviews, which may be considered quite specific evidence of
awareness of dying. The evidence of death awareness was specific in
the book because death has been a subject of social taboo, and death
is a forbidden word in most Chinese communities.[3] Among these
patients, fourteen of them made adjustments to maintain their hope
and thirteen of them made preparations for death. These preparations
include personal preparations such as arranging properties, leaving
instructions, giving gifts and funeral arrangements after becoming
aware of dying. It was apparent that these people, who knew that
they were dying, were ready to fulfil the dying person's social role by

preparing for their death and adjusting to changes that occurred as a result of having cancer. This is the beginning of Good Death.

This chapter will discuss the nature of death awareness in terms of three issues:

1. being informed: receiving 'bad news',
2. being aware of the diagnosis of cancer; and
3. being aware of dying.

In order to obtain a precise picture of the dying persons' views, the frequencies of their responses were recorded and counted. These procedures enhance the validity and reliability of the research. It also enables an analysis of the depth and the breath of their viewpoints. Therefore, the file numbers of the patients are marked as numbers in parentheses to allow reference to the appropriate sources if necessary. For example, (1, 2, 3) indicates that Patient 1, Patient 2, and Patient 3 made this response. The page number (p.) indicates the reference page in the patient's file. Due to the nature of a qualitative study, the number of the patients' responses will give a general impression of the data, but I do not intend to quantify the data.

Being informed: Receiving 'bad news'

Consistent with some previous studies in Western cultures, [2, 4-6] a majority of hospice patients in this research preferred to know that they had cancer. The patients' knowledge about their conditions depended largely on the process of receiving 'bad news'. During the interviews, I asked the patients how much they knew about their conditions and from whom they obtained the information. Other details included the place and people who were present when the medical practitioner delivered the 'bad news'. Thus I assessed the patients' understandings about their conditions and their level of awareness of dying. I did not mention two words 'cancer' and 'death' when I conducted the interviews for the following reasons: first, I did not know what information the patient had received. Second, I did not want to lead the topic of discussion by introducing the words of cancer and death. Third, I was cautious not to induce adverse emotions in the patients for ethical reasons.

A majority of patients reported that they received the 'bad news' at the out-patient clinic. Five patients consulted private medical practitioners, with the remainder attended public sector clinics. Only one patient had learnt about his condition after admission to the hospice. His ignorance about his condition was probably a result of his dementia.

The process of receiving 'bad news' can consist of three phases. These phases are perception, communicating, and accepting 'bad news'. Each phase will be examined in relation to the findings of this research.

Perceptions of the 'bad news'

Cultural beliefs about death have certainly made the event of receiving 'bad news' a critical one. Despite current advancements in cancer treatment, some patients felt bad because they were given a 'death sentence' once they heard the 'bad news' that they had cancer. This finding supports the findings of a recent local research on Chinese cancer patients[7] and Galanti's observation.[8] Galanti observes that 'Asians have a tremendous fear of cancer, perceiving it as a death sentence, although many forms can be successfully treated'[8] (p.87).

Accordingly, six patients considered receiving 'bad news' most distressing. Receiving a diagnosis of cancer has been perceived as one of the significant points of psychological distress in the course of an illness.[9] This result also parallels work by Kubler-Ross[10] and Weisman[11] that highlights the initial emotional turmoil experienced by a patient upon hearing the diagnosis of a terminal illness such as cancer. According to Pattison,[12] receiving 'bad news' initiates the acute crisis phase in his living-dying model. Several patients experienced immobilisation, alterations in consciousness (that their minds were empty), feelings of inadequacy, anxiety and fear. Consequently, the message (a death sentence) could be so traumatic to the patients that they became agitated and wanted to commit suicide.

Medical practitioners are always responsible for disclosing the 'bad news'. Therefore, the consequences of this particular event rely on their attitudes towards death and dying and their communication skills. While the patients may take the word 'cancer' as a death sentence [7-8] medical practitioners may consider cancer and/or death a medical failure. It is possible that both practitioners and patients perceive cancer in a negative way. Further, disclosing 'bad news' requires a commitment to truth-telling, which means a responsibility to be honest; such honesty does not come painlessly [13] Therefore, some medical practitioners admit that 'breaking bad news' has been an unpleasant and complicated task. To tell a patient that he has a fatal illness is one of their most difficult dilemmas. [14]

Communicating the 'bad news'

Receiving 'bad news' often hits an individual very hard emotionally. From the present findings, all patients responded to the news that they had cancer with intense and mixed emotions. Consistent with Cheng's [7] study, several patients recalled that they were shocked and depressed after the announcement of 'bad news'. Some patients reported that the disclosure of their diagnosis was the most difficult time of their illness. Two illustrated their feelings by stating that it was as if they had been hit by a thunderstorm. Many patients developed an awareness of dying when the 'bad news' was announced. Therefore, the episode of receiving 'bad news' was a significant reference point in cancer patients' illness. This episode also had an enormous impact on the quality of their lives, as they went through their unique dying processes. Many of them remembered the details of the episode clearly, such as the tone of the medical practitioner's voice, the place, time, date, and subsequent events.

Further, the patients reported that some medical practitioners withheld information and that some of them also appeared frightened. The medical professional is generally considered an authority, which is in contrast with the obedient and passive role of the patients. 'In China and Japan, where medical practitioners are often seen as authority figures in a hierarchical and patriarchal society, patients are told little about their conditions. If the patient has cancer, the family might be told, but the patient rarely given the diagnosis' (p.87). [8] Galanti's description also reflects the situation in some Asian countries. The medical practitioners of general wards and out-patient clinics often discuss the patients' conditions with their families. Likewise, some medical practitioners' accounts from Western cultures show that they control the information through their management of the information-giving process.[15] They may adopt a paternalistic attitude when they carry out their duties. The families will decide what to tell and what not to tell the patients. If the family members and other professionals were absent when the 'bad news' was delivered, the patients may be more vulnerable to the medical practitioner's control of information.

As medical practitioners are dominant in the health care team, patients may be unable to establish a mutual relationship with them. This is particularly true for elderly patients. Despite the introduction of the Patient's Charter in Hong Kong in 1994, many patients do not consider that they have the right to be informed about their condition. They feel 'safe' playing the 'sick role' of reacting passively and obediently. [16-17] Patients in the present research seldom raised questions about their condition, in this way, hoping to receive the best possible health care.

After the announcement of the 'bad news', most medical practitioners left the patient alone and thought they had completed their tasks. They may not be aware of the extent of the emotional impact that the patients had after the disclosure of the information. The medical practitioners who work in general wards or who maintain private practice may not consider supporting the patients after receiving the 'bad news' as their obligation. The patients needed immediate psychosocial support but that was not always available.

Accepting the 'bad news'

From the findings of this research and some previous ones, awareness of dying used to be self-detected but has now mostly been replaced by medical detection. [2] Awareness of dying seems to be controlled largely by medical professionals and sometimes relatives, when they deliver the 'bad news' of a life-threatening illness such as cancer. The patients had little or no control over the information the medical practitioner would tell them. Further, the procedure of disclosing 'bad news' was found to be inconsistent. [18] Therefore, it was not surprising that one-third of cancer patients in Hong Kong may die without discussing their diagnoses with their medical practitioners. [19]

Even when the patients had an open awareness, the degree of acceptance may vary. The psychological acceptance of death or dying and establishing awareness is not necessarily a logical association. Being aware of dying may not become the 'dominant social expression of a person' (p.74).[2] Consequently, health care professionals may be unsure as to whether their patients have accepted the 'bad news'. No patient in the present research accepted the 'bad news' immediately. Some patients may demonstrate acceptance of impending death by preparing for death or fighting against it (or making adjustments).[4] Some patients were aware of the truth but were unable to deal with it, and some experienced many emotions that lasted until they died. Some of them could not take in even the most basic part of the message because they were in shock. Meanwhile, some patients did not seek further information about themselves and refused to express to others that they could not cope with the 'bad news'. Most of these patients were likely to avoid an open discussion of death. This was especially difficult for them if their relatives were not with them when they 'received the bad news'. Most patients attended the clinic on their own and only three patients reported that their relatives accompanied them when the medical practitioner disclosed the 'bad news'. Likewise, the spouses of the patients also reacted to 'the bad news'.

> My wife (who was with me) reacted more intensely. The disease is almost like a family disease, isn't it? She cried immediately. I did not have the same strong feeling. She has more intense feelings. Yet, I did not have much feeling. I am not helping myself. I just feel that this is not serious. This is life that (we) must walk along. It (life span) can be long or short. If I do not have this illness, I may have other illness in the next year or so.

The following is a typical example of receiving 'bad news'. A fifty-year-old patient was found to have cancer of the ovary. Coincidentally, her husband had also died of cancer. Her medical practitioner disclosed the 'bad news' to her in an out-patient clinic when she was unaccompanied. From her professional experience as a nurse and personal experience as the spouse of a cancer patient, she immediately associated cancer with a life-threatening illness. She was shocked and found it very difficult to accept that she had cancer. She complained to the medical practitioner for not supporting her. Her relationship with her family was reasonable. Understandably, she was very upset about the 'bad news'.

> In April 1993, I detected a small, hard lump in my lower abdomen. I also developed polyuria. I thought I had urinary tract infection and I could improve the situation by drinking more water and taking antibiotics.

Later, I guessed there must be something wrong (with my body) as my condition was getting worse. Then I went to see the medical practitioner at the casualty unit (of Tang Siu Kin Hospital). I used to be very careful with money, so I did not go to a private practitioner, who may palpate my abdomen and give me Buscopan on a routine basis. At Tang Siu Kin Hospital, the medical practitioner (at the casualty unit) told me that I had cancer when he palpated my abdomen. He told me that I had cancer... I was shocked (because he had not done any examination). He was serious. I needed to be hospitalised immediately and he did not allow me to leave the casualty ward. I had prepared nothing (for my hospitalisation!). I had not brought my face towel, tooth brush, or tissue paper. I wanted to go home and get some of these things, but he would not let me. He asked me to be admitted to Queen Mary Hospital. At that moment, I found it very difficult to accept (repeated three times). I did not phone my family because my elder daughter was having a dinner party and my younger daughter was in her (nurses') residence.

The medical practitioner performed an ultrasound examination later. He said that there was a tumour in my ovary, around 14x7cm. After a series of investigations, my operation was scheduled for 13th June 1993. They confirmed that the tumour was cancer. The staging was stage 3 grade 3.

The patient was a nurse who had worked in this hospital previously. She felt excited when she found a new job in a nursing home in her fifties. She started her new job in 1991 when the Hospital Authority took over this hospital.

Being aware of the diagnosis of cancer

Knowing the diagnosis

In Hong Kong, all hospice patients are informed about their condition before they gain access to hospice services. Therefore, all patients in this research were expected to be aware that they had cancer. About half of the patients reported that they had cancer and sixteen of them did not mention the word 'cancer'. According to the patients, even some of the medical practitioners had avoided using the word 'cancer'. They used other terms such as toxic boil(s), a lump, tumours, weak lungs, and shadows in the lung to describe the patients' conditions (Table 4.1). They also told them that their illness was inoperable, incurable or serious, and that their prognoses were poor. Some patients were angry to hear that they had cancer. No matter what terms the medical practitioners had substituted for the word 'cancer', the patients' emotions were likely to be intensely disturbed by such 'bad news'. In other words, they realised that their illness could not be cured and they also lost the hope to live.

Table 4.1
Examples of terms used by medical practitioners to explain 'cancer' in this research

You have *toxic boils.*

There were *tumours.*

The medical practitioner said I have a *toxic tumour* and it has many complications.

Your x-ray has lung *shadows.*

The medical practitioner said there were several *shadows* on the lung.

I know nothing about my diagnosis. The medical practitioner said there is a *lump* in my lung. He asked me to have an operation.

Your lungs are very *weak.*

Understanding cancer

Although not every medical practitioner informed the patients that they had 'cancer', and patients may not have understood the biological nature of the illness, the patients often associated cancer with death. [5, 20] They believed that cancer was incurable and that they would die soon. Some of them had acquired this knowledge from previous contact with family members or friends who had cancer. Some learnt about cancer from public media such as newspapers and television. However, some patients had misconceptions about cancer, its symptoms, and treatment. Their misconceptions may have resulted from their age or educational background. A majority of them had little knowledge about cancer, which indicated a demand for further attention in patient education in the future. The following are some examples.

A fifty-two-year-old housewife, who had received little formal education, knew very little about cancer. She knew that cancer was a tumour and her life was threatened. However, she did not understand what cancer was.

> Cancer is a tumour. I do not know exactly what a tumour is. I know it is cancer but I do not understand what cancer is. [I know] cancer is inoperable and death is coming.

A forty-six-year-old man, who also had little schooling, explained that his knowledge of cancer came from his previous contact with cancer patients. He recalled that his friend had died with a lot of suffering after receiving radiotherapy. Therefore, he associated radiotherapy with dying a 'bad death'. He was anxious when his medical practitioner suggested that he have radiotherapy.

> I have come across six or seven people who died of cancer. They died soon after they knew their diagnoses. I do not know which types of cancer they had. I have not just heard about it, I have also seen them... I do not know what cancer is. What do you mean by having a tumour or cancer? Is it incurable?

Another seventy-year-old man had cancer of the lungs. He described his cancer as a 'bag of water' because he had recurrent pleural effusion. The invasive power of the cancer cells was strong and he predicted that he would be 'eaten up' by these cancer cells.

> My medical practitioner told me that I have cancer and it is incurable. Yes, he said it this way. It is incurable. Even [I] want to have an operation, it is inoperable. If it is operable, it will be curable and it offers me a hope. Now it is inoperable. It is not just a lump... Yes, it is not a lump. If it is a lump, it is operable. [I think] you understand this. There is so much water in it and the whole lung is like that... Yes, it is a different type of cell. Now I am waiting to be 'eaten up' by the cancer cells. If it (his lung) is eaten up, then I will finish (die) too. Yes, they are like evil, they eat me up.

Responses to cancer

Some patients reacted to the 'bad news' of having cancer by complaining about the medical practitioners who withheld the truth of their diagnoses. They could be in a state of denial or shock, or be frightened, anxious, and/or angry. The following are some examples.

Denial

According to Glaser and Strauss, [4] a patient may respond to the announcement by choosing either to accept or to deny the imminence of his or her death. Mrs. L had difficulty in accepting the 'bad news' that she had cancer and wanted to commit suicide. At the beginning of the interview, she insisted that she did not know about her diagnosis. However, she described her emotions towards cancer at a later stage of the interview.

> No, I do not know my diagnosis. My daughter talked to the medical practitioner because she understood English. At the beginning, he (the medical practitioner) said I had a terminal illness, my God, it was incurable ... (the medical practitioner was) crazy! He said I had a terminal illness. I asked if this was cancer. Then, I could not eat for three months. I just drank water. I cried... (She began to cry...) No, I could not accept it but I didn't have the courage to jump from my flat.

Shock and fear

The initial response of a patient to disclosure is often depression or shock.[10] Six patients feared the unknown and uncertainty. They were uncertain about how long they would live and what would happen tomorrow.

> I have worried for my life... the medical practitioner has not mentioned what happened to me, I cannot talk to my family because I do not want them to worry.

Eight patients were frightened and anxious about death. For example, an elderly woman with lung cancer, experienced fear of dying.

I am afraid that my condition would deteriorate, I'm afraid of death... (It is) incurable...I cannot find a good medical practitioner, that (I won't receive) good treatment. I have to experience death myself.

Mr. W, a drug addict, had cancer of the lung. He felt anxious because the medical practitioner appeared frightened when he disclosed the 'bad news'.

The medical practitioner said that I had five to six shadows (from the X-ray report). Yes, I was shocked. He (the medical practitioner) seemed frightened too! (The patient raised his voice). I looked at the medical practitioner, who was frightened. He was frightened; of course, I was frightened, too, for this (tumour) was with me! His facial colour changed and looked fearful. I felt immediately that my life would end (after 8.6 minutes of interview). The medical practitioner was very frightened and I was frightened too, even though it was none of his business. My life may end. It was possible that my life will end. Yes, I thought, my life will end and I have to leave soon...

Ms N, a young clerk with cancer of the pancreas, felt shocked, frightened, confused, and angry when she knew that she had cancer.

The medical practitioner said I have a toxic tumour and many complications. My family was not with me. When I heard this, I was shocked, confused, and frightened. My whole body was still. I did not want to see anybody and I just could not help crying. Why was I chosen? Why me? I have a lot of unfinished business.

Anger

Mrs. M described her frustration when the medical practitioner withheld the information on her diagnosis. She had to confront him instead.

It was not the medical practitioner who informed me of the diagnosis. I said it myself. I said to the medical practitioner that I had cancer. I guessed I had cancer because the symptoms had not been relieved for some time. I knew that it was cancer because no medical practitioner could treat me well. I am very angry... Why should I have cancer?

One common reaction of a patient to cancer is to see it as an enemy or as a competitor, in which either the patient wins (and lives) or loses (and dies) the battle against cancer. Ms Y, who suffered from cancer of the ovary, illustrated the typical pervasive adverse effects of cancer.

> [I] feel that my condition must be getting worse. It seems natural. It has to be like that, the cells have spread. That means it (cancer) has won. This is the normal process of cancer: to conquer the whole body. It wins and causes death.

> Yes, I wish to win the battle.

The patients also emphasised that each previous experience was unique. Although they had one thing in common: they all had cancer, their responses could be very different. A seventy-year-old patient described his experience clearly. He emphasised that everyone may have different responses to illness, as he referred to cancer. The disease process and medical procedure could affect the response.

> Everyone is different. There may be a hundred (of us); our experiences can be different... Oh yes, we have similarities, we have something quite alike but we would never be the same. The illness is the same but our feelings can be different. For example, my feelings are different from his (he refers to his fellow patient who was discharged home today, but has just been re-admitted). Today's feeling is different from yesterday's. I was told that I would have an operation today. It is a minor operation but I am more anxious today.

Awareness and acceptance

The patients who knew the causes of their cancer seemed to have a better acceptance of their condition. Twelve patients explained that they were aware of their impending death because they had an understanding of the causes of their illness. For example, smoking was the main cause of carcinoma of the lung. Some patients identified other causes of illness, such as emotion and lack of intimate social relationships. For example, an elderly woman explained that her illness was related to her unresolved anger with her friend who had deceived her and taken her money. She said she had lost about HK$

200,000 on this occasion. She was very angry, so she acquired cancer. She could not accept the truth of having cancer. Fortunately, she had a supportive family, which facilitated her gradual acceptance of reality.

> My illness was due to my anger (she paused and sighed deeply). I used to give money to a woman for saving (this is a similar idea to keeping money in the bank but on a private basis). She has deceived me. She has taken my money and run away. I have not told anyone about this incident and my family doesn't know about it. There was nobody I could tell because I have been separated from my husband for over ten years. It would not matter if it was 10,000 dollars but it was as much as 200,000 dollars.
>
> Nobody shares with me and I sit facing the two walls in my house. My son came back (from work) and comforted me. He said, 'Don't cry, Mum, don't feel bad... please don't. Mum, can you eat a little bit? Mum.' I replied to him that I could not take anything.

On the other hand, three patients did not understand why they had acquired their illness, while some expressed that they understood their own conditions and accepted their limitations. Based on the findings of this research, the degree of acceptance and awareness varied from individual to individual and it also changed from time to time during the illness. Acceptance of having cancer and death seemed to relate closely to patients' physical condition and consequently contributed to their sense of hope. Acceptance could take several months and years to achieve. Mrs. L, a housewife, was a typical example. She was in her fifties with cancer of the lung. She appeared cheerful and she accepted her condition during the initial interview because she had a supportive family. The next interview took place eight months later, one month before she died. She was re-admitted for treatment of her symptoms. She told me sadly and unwillingly that she had thought of doing 'silly things' (committing suicide), because her symptoms (mainly dyspnoea) could not be relieved and she felt that she could no longer endure the suffering. She was very sad and reluctant to talk. She replied 'no, [I] don't know' twenty-five times. In addition, most of her answers were short and she had avoided eye contact with me during the interview.

It is also essential to bear in mind that emotional responses towards cancer can be lasting after the episode of receiving the 'bad news'. The word 'cancer' definitely carries a psychological impact on people though they may know very little about cancer. [21] For example, during the early phase of data collection, a thirty-four-year-old woman agreed to an interview. She was an accountant and suffered from cancer of the lung. When I informed her that I was visiting cancer patients, her expressionless face suddenly turned ashen. Although the conversation went on for a couple of minutes, it had to be terminated as she said she felt a bit 'dyspnoeic'. From that time onwards, I learnt that I had to be very cautious when I mentioned the word 'cancer' during my interviews.

Being aware of dying

Awareness of dying

Glaser and Strauss [4, 22-24] have contributed extensively to the study of death and dying. Their field study on 'awareness concepts' has deepened our understanding of the social contexts of dying. 'This is an awareness that most, if not all new, hospice patients must face. Hard-core denial of facts related to illness and its progress is incompatible with requirements of good coping' (p.68). [25] If health care professionals and the patient share the 'bad news' with openness and respect, this will lead to 'creativity and the healing of relationships'. [26] Openness means that the information possessed by medical practitioners should not be concealed from patients (unless they want it to be). [6]

Many hospice patients identified the need to know the truth about their diagnoses so that they might develop an awareness of dying. Awareness of dying is a complex experience. One may find it difficult to be completely sure of the level of awareness. Fifty-eight percent of the patients used the word 'death' directly in the conversation. These patients indicated that they were aware of death. The inclusion of the word 'death' in the discussion may be considered quite specific evidence of death awareness for hospice patients in this research, since they normally considered death a taboo subject. Meanwhile, some patients were not comfortable using the word 'death'. Therefore, they used other terms to explain the situation. The terms or phrases described either deterioration of their physical conditions or the act of 'passing away'. Examples of these terms are: critically ill, not getting well, would not be going home, disappearing, sleeping, and passing away (Table 4.2). This phenomenon is not confined to dying people but is also a common practice among Chinese. These patients could be in any context of death awareness. Therefore, accurate and sensitive assessment was required to identify their context of awareness.

Table 4.2
Examples of terms used by the patients to explain 'death' in this research

I have quite severe dyspnoea, I am afraid I cannot answer your questions because I am *not feeling well at all*. I am sorry about that (1).

I was *critically ill* recently (11).

Yes, you see that I am still dyspnoeic. They wanted me to go. What can I do...? I don't think that *I would not be going home at all* (2).

The old man *emigrated* (to heaven) after breakfast (2).

I would not mind *leaving* any time (22).

My life may *end*. It was possible that my life will end. Yes, I thought, my life will end and I have to *leave* soon ... (13).

I practise ancestor worship. I will *sleep and pass away...* Death of man resembles *the fading away of a light* (29).

Among the patients who talked about death openly, a majority had made adjustments to maintain their hope and preparations for death. On the other hand, thirteen patients who did not mention the word 'death' also talked about various issues relating to their illness and future. Their concerns about themselves and their relatives were similar to those of patients who talked openly about death. For example, four of these patients maintained their hope for a cure by searching for alternative treatments or made adjustments). Six discussed their preparations for death. Six also hoped to be able to choose who was with them when they died or where they died. Four of them wanted to have control over their pain and suffering and eight wanted to have connectedness with their families. In other words, these patients, who did not discuss death openly, indicated that they knew they would die soon. Therefore, it can be concluded that patients in both groups presented evidence of awareness of dying, which is an important initial basis for discussion of Good Death.[2]

As discussed previously, the medical practitioners and the family had more control over the information on the patient's condition and thus his or her death awareness. Family members often made decisions for Chinese patients. [8, 16] They decided what the patient should know, including the diagnosis and prognosis. Some family members believed that if the patients did not know their diagnoses, they could always retain the hope that they might not have cancer. [17, 27] 'For them, to suffer the uncertainty was preferable to the risk of losing their hope'. [28] However, the viewpoint of the patients could be different. An example was a patient who did not know his diagnosis at the time of the interview. His family preferred not to let him know the truth. Some patients also felt frustrated because they were not informed clearly about their diagnoses. The followings are some examples of patients' responses.

> The medical practitioner did not explain. If the medical practitioner had told me the diagnosis, I would not be so confused.

> I am worried. The medical practitioner has not mentioned what happened to me. I cannot share it with my family because I do not want them to worry.

The contexts of death awareness

It is essential to understand the awareness contexts because of its effect on the interaction among patient, family, and hospice staff. Awareness contexts are defined as 'what each interacting person knows of the patient's defined status, along with his recognition of the others' awareness of his own definition' (p.10). [4] There are four types of awareness context: closed awareness, suspected awareness, mutual pretence, and open awareness.

In closed awareness, the patient does not recognise that he or she is dying, but everyone else does. [4] In this research, an old man with cancer of the lung was the only patient who was kept in closed awareness. His family preferred not to let him know the truth so they did not inform him that he had cancer. When his family disclosed the truth some time later, he appeared unhappy and withdrawn. He did not express his disappointment openly to anybody but he showed his resentment by withdrawing from his family and keeping quiet. He died several days later. His death was an unexpectedly quick one. The old man may have lost his trust in both his family and the hospice staff. Meanwhile, no patient pretended they did not know that they were dying (pretence awareness), and none of them suspected what others knew and attempted to verify the suspicion that they were dying by tricking their family and staff (suspected awareness). A few patients were suspicious about their diagnoses but they clarified their suspicions with their medical practitioners. In this way, they developed an awareness of dying. In other words, all the hospice patients in this research, except one, understood that they had a life-threatening illness. Their responses were negative, as they perceived that they would die soon. Even when they had an open awareness, the degree of acceptance of cancer (and death) varied. Consequently, some patients were ready to talk about death with openness, while some were not.

The open awareness context is complicated and Timmermans [29] suggests splitting it into three different contexts: active, suspended, and uncertain. In the active open awareness context, the patient (or relative) accepts the impending death and prepares for it. In this research, nineteen patients belonged to this context. They used the word 'death' directly in conversation although four of them also used other terms to illustrate their ideas about death simultaneously. They admitted that they were aware of death and discussed issues of their impending death openly. This is an unexpected finding, as death remains a taboo subject in Asian cultures such as Hong Kong. Among them, twelve also mentioned the word 'cancer'. In other words, more than one-third of the patients mentioned both 'cancer' and 'death' during the interviews. These patients openly acknowledged their awareness of both their diagnoses and prognoses. Further, a majority of them made adjustments to maintain their hope and made preparations for death. While the patient may not hope for a recovery, this does not imply that the patient has to abandon hope and simply wait to die. [29] For example, a few patients found peace of mind in thoughts of an afterlife.

> I have lots of things to think. I will go to a place where is dark. A bright world will follow and this makes me happy.

Consistent with Seale's [30] study, hospice patients in this research were more likely to know that they were dying than patients receiving conventional care. The current development of hospice care makes it easier for patients and family members to prepare actively for death.

In the suspended open awareness context, the patient and family ignore or disbelieve the message, which is communicated by the medical practitioner. The medical practitioner who makes blunt direct statements increases the chance that the information may become blocked. The 'bad news' has been given, but its consequences have not been fully assimilated. If the context of suspended open awareness is the preferred level, disbelief will become permanent. [29] In this research, some patients did not want to know more about their condition. They thought they had enough to cope with and could not take in any more information. Their minds were so full of their own conceptions and beliefs that there was no room for anything else. [31] For instance, Mrs. M was divorced and had raised her five children all by herself. She claimed that she had a tough life and she responded angrily to the news that she had cancer. When I asked her how much she knew about her situation, she denied it bitterly and did not want to know anything further. Similarly, a few patients refused to find out further details about their illness. They simply could not accept the truth of having cancer.

> I do not like to ask. It is purposeless. Not knowing is better than knowing (the truth). I do not want to know too much. My son knows everything and he will make decisions for me.

> I know nothing about my diagnosis. There is a lump in my lung. He (the medial practitioner) asked me to have an operation. I refused. I did not have any oral medication or injections.

In the uncertain open awareness context, the patient (or family member) dismisses the bad parts of the message and hopes for the best outcome. Uncertain open awareness occurs when the medical practitioners withhold information, and soften the plain and full clinical truth. They may admit uncertainty about the diagnosis and prognosis. In this research, some patients complained that the medical practitioners withheld information and used other terms to replace the word 'cancer' when they disclosed the 'bad news'. However, these patients did not remain in the uncertain open awareness context. Three asserted their control of information and clarified their suspicions of the diagnosis or poor prognosis with the medical practitioner. The following are some examples.

> At the beginning, he (the medical practitioner) said I had a terminal illness, my God, it was incurable ... he (the medical practitioner) was

crazy! He said I had a terminal illness. I asked if it was cancer. I did not eat for three months. I cried.

This is the normal process of cancer: to conquer the whole body. It wins and causes deaths, it (cancer) is basically more violent than me. I cannot win the battle. I cannot accept it. The medical practitioner felt that he could do nothing for me. I felt that they were not all right. They did nothing to help me and they gave up. The medical practitioner said, 'What can we do (about the relapse)?' I then replied, 'The worst thing is to die'. The medical practitioner then replied, 'You say it yourself now'. His statement was very unkind.

Glaser and Strauss's [4] theory of awareness of dying suggests that dying patients should know the truth about their illness, including the diagnosis and prognosis. In other words, people with terminal cancer need to have knowledge of the diagnosis of cancer and the prognosis of imminent death. [32] Based on the finding of this research, however, the hospice patients viewed 'the truth' of their condition in a different way. They indicated clearly that they needed to know the truth about having cancer but they did not specify the need to know the prognosis of imminent death as a consequence of having cancer. In fact, many of them developed an awareness of dying when they learnt that they had cancer (or a life-threatening illness) because they often associated cancer with death. It is important for health care professionals to recognise that the meaning of 'truth' may vary from culture to culture and from individual to individual.

Openness and awareness

Although the literature indicates that most people prefer to have an open awareness than to be placed in the other three awareness contexts, [4, 33] this can present the staff and relatives with many problems and questions. These problems are, first, the patients, their families, or health care professionals may not support an open awareness context. Second, some people, including the patients and their families, have different capacities for coping. Some have not learnt to value the period of dying as it is now experienced by many people. [34] Although some patients were willing to talk about their concerns regarding their death, they could not find a listener.

Some patients expressed to me that they did not know to whom they could talk (and that the nurses were always busy). The situation was especially difficult if the patient had not maintained an intimate relationship with his or her family.

Even though the patients had an awareness of dying, some might prefer not to discuss death openly. For some patients, death was essentially a private process. They perceived death as a personal and private matter, and would only discuss it with their families. Some people do not wish to talk about all things with all people openly. They select the 'right' person for particular kinds of confidences and discussions. [35] Some patients had not indicated their death awareness because they could not cope with the confrontation with death. They had to leave their loved ones behind, which might create separation anxiety.

The 'timing' of the interview may have been another reason why patients did not talk about death.

> Some days are better than others for raising some topics, and some days "talk of death is depressing" (p.29). [35]

At other times, a patient may have an immediate need to talk about dying and death. Four patients were interviewed three days before death, seven within one month, and two within three months before death. These patients may have experienced mixed feelings about their imminent death, and so were not happy to talk about it with openness. Further, their preference to not talk about death should be respected so that they may experience a sense of control. On the contrary, two patients appeared exceptionally 'peaceful' and contented, although most patients appeared rather ill and upset for the reasons discussed. The situations of these two patients will be discussed in Chapter Ten.

The other reasons for this phenomenon was that death remained a topic of taboo for patients and their families if they did not have an open awareness of dying. [36] In ancient China, illness and bad death (death which was not a natural death) were perceived as suffering and punishments from heaven. [37] Today, some Chinese continue to view death and illness as a 'curse' or 'bad fate'. Therefore, the medical practitioner, the family, or the patient may have tried to 'soften' the clinical truth. Clearly, discussion of death-related issue has not been easy for the dying, their families, and health care professionals in contemporary Chinese society. [38]

Therefore, not everyone is 'empowered' by openness and frank discussion of death and dying issues. 'Some people prefer a more subtle exploration of these issues that complements and respects their individual cultural prohibitions and prescriptions' (p.101). [35] Those carers who experience tremendous discomfort with death may also find it difficult or impossible to talk with a dying person. Therefore, it was not surprising that only twelve patients felt comfortable talking about various issues of cancer and death openly. Despite the fact that some patients did not mention the word 'death' openly or that their awareness of dying was less certain, their dying experience might not necessarily be a negative one.

The taboo of death in contemporary Chinese society

As discussed in the previous section, hospice patients may be under additional emotional strain because death has for so long been a subject of social taboo. Death is often considered a forbidden word in Chinese culture. Many Chinese avoid talking about death openly. There are ample examples in the daily lives of Chinese. For example, for centuries the Chinese have used numbers and numerology to predict the future, to interpret dreams, and to justify superstitious beliefs and practices. Even the sound of the numbers can suggest good or bad luck. Therefore, Chinese dislike the number 4 simply because it has a similar pronunciation to the word for 'death', *si* in Cantonese (*Ethnic Chinese in Hong Kong*). [39] Some builders in Hong Kong deliberately skip the floor numbers that contain '4', for example 4, 14, 24, and 34. That means the fifth floor follows the third floor instead of the fourth floor. It is because Chinese do not often like to live on a floor with the number 4 or to have a vehicle with the number 4 in the registration number. [8] The Chinese also avoid mentioning the word 'death' on many important occasions such as Chinese New Year.

On the other hand, most Chinese value longevity. According to the *Book of History*, longevity is the first of the Five Blessings from heaven. [37] Traditionally, Taoism believes in longevity and immortality. In Chinese history, the emperor was addressed as '10,000 years old' to signify his long reign and longevity. The first emperor, Qin Shi Emperor was the first to be addressed in this way. Several emperors, such as Hang Muk, had strong faith in immortality. Therefore, they sent out people to find the drugs (or herbs) that would render them immortal. Some of these people went to places outside China such as Japan and Southeast Asia. When they could not find the herbs or drugs, they were afraid to return to the country and be punished. So, they settled down and lived in those lands. Hence, Taoism reinforces Chinese people's belief in immortality.

There are also fairy tales about longevity such as the story of the Mid-Autumn Festival. Today, the custom is still practised and people in Hong Kong are offered a public holiday to celebrate this festival. The fairly tale relates that Chang E took a tablet to make her immortal. Then she flew to the moon and has stayed there since then. Other evidence is the belief in the God of Longevity, who can offer people long lives. The God always holds a peach, which is a symbol of immortality, long life, and prosperity. [40] The endurance of such legends also explains the continuous development of Taoism in Chinese communities.

As long as the Chinese hold the value of longevity and immortality, they will probably continue to keep death as a social taboo, and will maintain their health in a unique way. For example, some Chinese practice Tai Chi and Qigong, which help to maintain their body-and-mind balance. Some patients in this research, sought Chinese medical treatment and food therapies when told by the medical practitioner that their illness was incurable. The Taoists are eager to find ways to achieve eternal life. Therefore, as an example of funeral rituals, some Chinese use birds to resemble life after death. They believe that a dying person does not die but he or she will be carried by the birds to heaven to live an afterlife.

In summary, medical professionals often controlled information about patients' conditions and thus their death awareness. Although medical practitioners may have different ways of disclosing the 'bad news', most of the patients developed awareness of dying after receiving 'bad news'. Some could accept it and discussed death with openness, while some preferred not to talk about it. Both groups of patients presented similar evidence of death awareness, which was important for achieving a Good Death. Chinese cultural values such as longevity and immortality may continue to sustain the taboo of death in the Chinese communities. Some Chinese also believe that illness and bad death are suffering and curses from heaven. Therefore, some families were reluctant to discuss the potentially fatal condition with the patients because they were also experiencing anticipatory grief. It was evident that mutual trust and connectedness between health care professionals, the dying persons, and their families would allow them to accept their impending death at their own pace. The value of truth-telling to establish such connectedness is therefore the starting point for promoting a Good Death. Accordingly, the following clinical implications are suggested.

Clinical implications

Goal:
To promote truth-telling between hospice patients and health care professionals.

Provide community health education on life, death, health, and illness experiences such as cancer

Death is clearly a social taboo subject in contemporary Chinese societies. However, many teachings of traditional Chinese philosophies and religions, such as Confucianism, Taoism, and Buddhism, have a more optimistic and holistic view on death and dying. They encourage people not to fear death and suggest various ways to live a good life and to die a Good Death. Therefore, the indigenous teachings and inspirations of these ancient philosophies can provide a fundamental and substantial background for discussion of life, death, and Good Death in Asian communities. The general public also requires health education so that they will have a better understanding about health and adjustments to illness such as cancer, as examples of human experience rather than patho-physiological information. People with cancer need to have more specific knowledge about their condition. In this way, patients are empowered with the necessary knowledge, strength, and will to participate in making decisions regarding their care plans. Also, they are able to strengthen their sense of hope and control over their lives.

Formulate a standard protocol for 'breaking bad news'

The problem of 'awareness' can be a moral one, involving professional ethics, social issues, and personal values. [4] Therefore, the decision 'to tell or not to tell the truth' to cancer patients has been an ethical dilemma for health care professionals in Asian cultures. Unless something is done to improve the information-giving process, the promotion of truth-telling of information may not be successful. Therefore, it is essential to formulate a protocol to guide the procedures for 'breaking bad news' and enhance diagnostic clarity. [41] In principle, medical practitioners have to recognise the value of truth-telling so that they will not conceal information from the patients. 'The information is not only that someone has cancer but about its likely course of development and the treatments worth considering' (p.46). [6] More importantly, they also need to recognise the culture-specific needs of patients. Medical practitioners control the amount of information they disclose and thus, the outcome of the procedure. Therefore, it is just as important that patients have a sense of control over the information that they receive. Patients should be encouraged to ask questions. They must have this information before they can make essential decisions during the course of their illness.

Provide psychosocial and spiritual support to patients and families as soon as they receive the diagnosis

It is important to include the patients' primary caregivers or next-of-kin when the 'bad news' is announced unless the patients prefer otherwise. Further, immediate emotional and spiritual support services have to be available when the patients and their family members receive the 'bad news'. Therefore, a member of the health care team should remain with the patients and the family until their emotions become settled. The patients are reassured that they will receive continuous help, such as referral to a counsellor or self-help group, at the most critical stage of their illness.

Assess and record patients' levels of information needs and schedule their care plan accordingly [43]

A person needs to have an awareness of dying before he or she can achieve a Good Death. Since one's death awareness relates closely to one's understanding of a diagnosis, it is essential to assess and record the information needs accurately and sensitively. Health care professionals can identify the evidence of awareness of dying in several ways: the word(s) that the dying persons use to describe their condition; their future (such as how long they will live); their social activities after learning of their condition, such as their adjustments and/or preparations. In this way, the individual's information needs and care plan can be scheduled.

Table 4.3
Categories and significant statements of being aware of dying (Death awareness)

Categories	Significant statements
Being informed: receiving 'bad news'	I was shocked. Cancer is horrible. It is a terminal disease. I think I am young and my burden of living has just been relieved. I had just relaxed a bit (pause and sigh) then I got this illness (12, p.5).
Being aware of the diagnosis of cancer	It was not the medical practitioner who informed me of the diagnosis. I said to the medical practitioner that I had cancer. I guessed I had cancer because the symptoms could not be relieved for some time. I knew that it was cancer because no medical practitioner could treat me well (6, p.3).
Being aware of dying	My pain was unrelieved. The medical practitioner dared not say anything... He kept silent... (6, p.2). I did not have much feeling. The only way is death (6, p.3). I have lived long enough; I do not want to live any longer... I am suffering. I do not know how to say, it (my death) should be quick... I feel very painful. I am more or less like a lump of rice (stupid fool) (22).

Table 4.4
Summary of Being aware of dying

Related issues	Clinical implications
1. Being informed: receiving 'bad news' • Perceptions of the 'bad news' • Communicating the 'bad news' • Accepting the 'bad news' 2. Being aware of the diagnosis of cancer • Knowing the diagnosis • Understanding cancer • Response to cancer • Awareness and acceptance 3. Being aware of dying • Awareness of dying • The contexts of death awareness • Openness and awareness • The taboo of death in contemporary Chinese society	Goal: Promote truth-telling between patients and health care professionals 1. Provide community health education about life, death, health, and illness experiences such as cancer. 2. Formulate a standard protocol for 'breaking bad news'. 3. Provide psychosocial and spiritual support to patients and families as soon as they knew the diagnosis. 4. Access and record patients' levels of information needs and schedule their care plan accordingly.

Summary

Most patients considered receiving a diagnosis of cancer as one of the significant points of psychological distress in the course of their illness. For a few patients, the emotions towards having cancer lasted until they died. While a majority of patients in this research preferred to know their condition, their carers, including health care professionals and their relatives, were clear that knowledge about having cancer often created an emotional impact on the patients. Consequently, the decision 'to tell or not to tell' the diagnosis to the cancer patients remains an ethical dilemma for most health care professionals. The episode of receiving 'bad news' becomes a crucial moment when people with terminal cancer, develop their awareness of dying. Health care professionals have to realise that there must be an awareness of dying if a person desires to achieve a Good Death. Only if dying persons possess the knowledge of their imminent death, will they be able to incorporate this knowledge to make appropriate adjustments and/or preparations for a Good Death.

On one hand, some patients preferred to have an awareness of their social role as a 'dying person'. Most if not all patients were informed about their conditions. Half of the patients openly talked about their cancers and more than half of them discussed various issues related to death. Thus about one-third of the patients talked about death and cancer with openness. These preliminary findings may reflect the progress of hospice work in Asian countries. Indeed, the hospice movement has helped to open the discussion of death in health care institutions since the 1980s.

On the other hand, death is clearly a social taboo and many Chinese avoid and refuse to talk about death. In this research, thirteen patients did not mention the word 'death' and sixteen of them did not mention that they had cancer. Nevertheless, they talked about their illness and future using the expressions that they preferred. The role of health care professionals is not to change the patient's viewpoint but to acknowledge and support the patient through the various stages of adjustment to illness. [42] It is important that they will also respect people who show awareness of dying as much as those who do not present clear evidence of this awareness. Both groups of people can have a positive experience when they die.

In order to facilitate patients' achievement of a desirable Good Death, it is important to promote truth-telling between patients and health care professionals. I suggest that this has the following implications:

1. Community health education about life, death, health, and illness experiences is essential. The philosophy of truth-telling needs to be emphasised. From the perspective of the hospice patients in this research, 'truth' refers to having cancer.
2. A standard protocol for delivering the 'bad news', in which the medical practitioners will communicate the fact with a hopeful and compassionate attitude, is suggested.
3. Psychosocial and spiritual support should commence as soon as a person knows the diagnosis. In this way, they will accept their condition at their own pace and will be willing to control the quality of their own life in achieving a Good Death.
4. Finally, it is important to keep an accurate record of patients' levels of information needs so as to schedule their care plans accordingly.

5
Maintaining hope
(Hope)

Introduction

'*WHERE THERE IS* hope there is life, and the role of health care professional is to nurture both'. [1-2] The presence of hope is extremely important for terminally ill patients, regardless of physical limitation or proximity to death. [3-4] This view was agreed by both caregivers such as nurses. [5-7] and dying persons. [3, 8] Consistent with some previous studies, patients in this research identified maintaining hope as an essential element if they desired to die a Good Death. They needed to express and develop a hope in respect of the future, whether that is for themselves or for their families. Thus, they were motivated to seek various treatments and carry out strategies to achieve a new goal to live. In this chapter, discussion will focus on four topics of maintaining hope: 1) concepts of hope, 2) having treatment 3) adjustment, and 4) hope and the course of illness.

Concepts of hope

Despite previous research efforts, 'the domains of hope and how persons maintain hope while confronting adversity are not well known'. [9] At present, the concept of hope remains poorly understood. Fromm [10] has presented a philosophical view of hope. He states that 'hope is a shared human experience essential for life. Understanding it is difficult as it is so integral to human life. It is like a fish trying to understand the meaning of water. Water might be the last thing a fish is concerned about until it is taken out of it. Hope is so vital to life, that its loss is equated to the loss of life itself (cited by Flemming, [11] p.14). In reality, people with terminal cancer, consider the social function of an individual as manifestation of hope. Thus, 'the meaning of hope was identified as involving and maintaining existing functions, without further deterioration'.[11] For Hunt, [12] hope is a belief that the present situation can be modified and there is a way out of difficulties. From these descriptions, a person's hope relates to his or her current unfavourable situation. The presence of hope will motivate him or her to overcome the existing difficulties or to prevent the existing situation to become worse. Better still, he, or she often perceives a near future and not a dead end. Consistent with Flemming's [11] study, many patients hoped that perhaps there might be some new treatment, which would cure or prolong life. This is the hope for physical restoration. In this research, twenty-three patients underwent some forms of treatment. Some also made adjustments to maintain their hope to prolong their lives. They hoped that their cancer could be in control and their condition would not deteriorate. In other words, they hoped to live longer.

Next, there is the hope for the ability to love and be loved. [13] Consistent with Flemming's [11] study in Britain, many hospice patients in this research required social and emotional support to sustain their hopes. Half of the patients reported that they obtained support from the hospice staff, including medical and nursing staff. Social support of the hospice staff was important because 'the positive presence and interest of both nursing and medical staff; and the perceived existence of a positive future for the patient and his or her family'.[11] In addition, many patients felt that they were important in the family and they had harmonious family relationship. It is the presence of such support that renders dying people hopeful.[14] Furthermore, maintenance of 'the people's perception of control over loss helps to preserve hope.

The greatest threat to loss of hope is the loss of control over present circumstances, which threatens the existence of a future. For example, about half of patients in this research maintained a sense of control by asserting that they preferred to stay in the hospice unit until they died. Ten patients hoped that their relatives would stay with them at the moment of death.

Finally, hope can include spiritual contentment, not just in a formally religious sense, because hope involves faith, trust and peace of mind. [15] Overmyer [16] stresses that the deepest hopes are expressed in religious beliefs and activities. This is the hope that one might find meaning in life and meaning in the mystery of death. For example, The Bible states, 'And we rejoice in the hope of the glory of God. Not only so, but we also rejoice in our suffering, because we know that suffering produces perseverance; perseverance character; and character, hope. And hope does not disappoint us, because God has poured out His love into our hearts by the Holy Spirit, whom He has given us'.[17] Thus, Christians hope to have steadfastness - the ability to remain under difficulties without giving in. Such perception of hope often leads to exploration of views and beliefs regarding life after death. [13, 18] For those people with religious faith, their concepts of Good Death appear to follow the more religiously oriented belief of hope in entry into the heaven. [19] In this research, twenty-seven patients had religious faith or Chinese popular beliefs. Six patients were Christians and five were Buddhists. Not every patient of the 'religious group' related his or her hope with faith and only two Christians and one Buddhist had made such association. Eight patients hoped that they would go to heaven after they died. Just a few patients discussed the idea of an afterlife as another source of hope. Some had shown better acceptance to the timing of their death because they accepted death as a natural part of their lives.

If the hospice patients have a hope in respect of their future, they would be happy and contented because 'hope is itself a species of happiness, and perhaps, the chief happiness which this world affords'. [20] From the review of literature; the concepts of hope includes physical restoration or a cure, social and emotional support, a sense of control and spiritual contentment.[13] Therefore, maintaining social relations, experiencing personal control and accepting the timing of one's death are important elements to die a Good Death from the perspective of the hospice patients.

Having treatment

Conventional treatment

The hope for a cure and physical restoration is a natural one. Most patients received conventional medicine during their courses of illness. Conventional medicine refers to mainstream medicine as practiced according to the medical practitioner-scientist mode. Conventional medicine is governed by standards of practice that become acceptable by medical practitioners because the methodology of scientific inquiry has screened out unacceptable practices. [21] Most of the patients had chemotherapy, surgery and or radiotherapy. Only a few patients did not receive any active treatment as their cancers were advanced. Then, they had palliative treatment to relieve their symptoms. For example, one patient had physiotherapy to relieve his leg oedema. The hospice patients often conformed to medical treatment. They hoped the medical practitioners would cure their illness. Therefore, they perceived medical treatment the main source of hope. The following example is an illustration. The patient developed new hope because she felt that she could restore her health.

> During the course of chemotherapy, I gave myself a hope because the tumour was surgically removed. I followed the instructions of the medical practitioner. I have been conforming completely to the medical treatment for the whole year. I would like to have new life and new hope. Then I followed up at Sai Ying Poon Clinic. I have been very happy because I was all right.

Although the hospice patients in this research perceived that they might have a premature death, they also needed a choice to live. They needed to maintain hope to live and not to die soon. This need could be strengthened by their traditional Chinese belief of longevity and life after death. Therefore, many patients continued to explore different forms of treatment, such as Qigong and acupuncture to cure their cancer or restore their health. [22] Chinese medical treatment was a popular choice. In U.K. for example, Smaje and Field [23] observe that the Chinese do not use General Practitioner services as most minority ethnic groups. In other countries, such as UK, Canada and Australia, alternative therapy has received more attention. Massage and aromatherapy are common examples.

Table 5.1
Strategies of maintaining hope

Type of strategy	Frequency	Patient's file number
Having treatment	9	2, 3, 16, 17, 24, 25, 27, 28, 32
Adjustment	16	3, 4, 5, 6, 8, 10, 11, 12, 13, 14, 17, 18, 20, 21, 22, 30
Total	23	2, 3, 4, 5, 6, 8, 10, 11, 12, 13, 14, 16, 17, 18, 20, 21, 22, 24, 25, 27, 28, 30, 32

Traditional Chinese medical treatment

Traditional medical treatment more accurately describes the indigenous health care practices that can be found in a specific culture. [21] Evidently, most Chinese have faith and trust in traditional Chinese medical treatments as alternative medical therapies[24] despite the fact that Chinese medical treatments have less scientific evidence. 'Alternative medical therapies', which refer to those therapies that are not recognised as mainstream care.[25] Examples of Traditional Chinese medical treatment are Tai Chi, vegetarian diets, acupressure, acupuncture and meditation.

Several factors encourage the trend to using Traditional Chinese medical treatment. First, Traditional Chinese medical treatment encourages culture-specific traditions in maintaining health and treating illness which are carried from the old world into the new. [21] Traditional Chinese medical treatment has a long history of over 3,000 years. The practice of Traditional Chinese medicine is based on the Taoism's philosophy of life. This philosophy has evolved over thousands of years and is detailed in ancient Chinese texts. Second, Chinese medicine is good for a wide range of health problems, in particular, bone fractures, nervous system disease and chronic illness, such as cancer.[26] Third, it has more therapeutic effects than side effects to the body as it works by maintaining a balance of 'hot' and 'old' energy within the body. This is Taoist philosophy of health. Fourth, reasons for seeking Traditional Chinese medicine also included dissatisfaction with the treatments offered by conventional medicine and the growing trend that consumers are better educated and demand more involvement in the treatment decision- making process. [27]

Complementary and alternative medical therapies are emerging as a significant force that is shaping the delivery of health care. In the United States, for example, 34% -40% of adults have used some form of alternative or non-traditional health therapy in a previous year.[28] In Chinese communities, taking Chinese herbs has been one form of Taoist practise that enables people to maintain health and achieve longevity. Today, many Chinese go for Chinese medical treatment before or after the western medical therapy. For example, they take Chinese herbs and or food remedies. [24, 29] More importantly, it offers a new hope and a choice to the patients with incurable cancer. Therefore, many cancer patients consult Chinese medical treatment. [29-31] This finding is further substantiated by a recent survey to study the current situation of health-seeking behaviours of Chinese. The results reviewed that more than half of the participants considered solely the Chinese medicine and about one-third of them used both Chinese and western medicine simultaneously. [24]

Consistent with some previous studies, [29, 31] many patients took Chinese medicine to restore their physical health. Nine patients had Chinese medical treatment (Table 5.1). Six of them even sought treatments in China. Five patients were contented because they were 'cured' after trying Chinese medical treatment. A few claimed that the treatment was most helpful in the course of their illness.

As compared with Wong's [24]study, fewer patients reported that they had received Chinese medical treatment. This may be due to several reasons. First, some patients did not feel comfortable to report the truth of having Chinese medical treatment. They worried that their medical practitioners might perceive their consultation with Chinese medical practitioners as a mistrust of the Western medical treatment. Medical practitioners often object patients to 'shopping around' for impossible cures. [32] Second, there may be problems of compatibility between Western and Chinese medical treatments. Some Chinese patients were advised not to take both types of treatment. Therefore, they consulted Chinese medical treatment privately. Third, they did not want to disclose the information about their financial situation because consulting Chinese medical treatment required a lot of money. The consultation fee for Chinese private medical practitioner is almost three times that of the government health services. Some Chinese drugs are expensive too. The following description is an example.

These Chinese drugs are very expensive. The formula consists of Ning

Chi and horns of the deer. It costs about HK$ 5,200 per 150 tablets. The other type of natural Ning Chi is HK$ 6,000 per 100 tablets. (Then he listed other seven types of Chinese drugs). It is sold in a shop near a market in Sheung Wan. I take it regularly.

Therefore, having cancer can have a financial implication for the patients and their families. Most patients relied on their children for financial support. In other words, those patients who could afford to consume Chinese medical treatment, were likely to have a good family support. Consistent with other local studies on Chinese hospice patients, [31] several patients spent a lot of money for their treatment in China. When they used up their money, they returned Hong Kong and continued their western treatment in the government hospitals. In other words, the financial status of the dying person can influence the reality of his or her hope.

Adjustments

According to Erikson,[33] adjustments to loss is one of the developmental tasks of older adulthood. People with terminal cancer often hope for physical restoration and that their lives may be prolonged. With these goals in mind, sixteen patients made some adjustments. There were three main types of adjustment. First, they adjusted to the hospice environment so that they would receive appropriate health care service. Second, they changed their lifestyles to maintain their health and prevent it from deteriorating. Third, they made some psychological adjustments (Table 5.2). Among these sixteen patients, two of them also received Chinese medical treatment.

Adjusting to the hospice environment

According to Glaser and Strauss, [32] health care professionals often judge the conduct of dying patients by certain implicit standard. For example, the patient should maintain relative cheerfulness and

Table 5.2
Strategies of adjustment

Type of strategy	Frequency	Patient's file number
Adjusting to hospice environment	7	4,5, 8, 11, 14, 17, 22
Changing life styles	8	3, 5, 8, 12, 17, 18, 20, 22
Psychological adjustments	9	6,10,11,12,13,16,17,21,30
accepting changes of their body image		6,11,21,30
thinking positively		10,11,12,13,16
living day by day		10,11,12,17
selective forgetting		6,11,13

calmness. He or she should continue to be a good family member and should face death with dignity. He or she should co-operate with the staff members who care for him or her, and if possible, he or she should avoid distressing or embarrassing them. A patient who does most of these things will be respected. For the hospice staff, this is 'an acceptable style of living while dying' (p.86).[32] Glaser and Strauss's descriptions accurately reflect the current situation of most clinical settings in Asian countries. Accordingly, the hospice patients made several adjustments to follow the hospice routine or standards so that they would receive appropriate health care. They wanted to maintain hope for a cure or prolonged life. Seven patients were willing to share with me the strategies they had used so that they could receive the health care they needed and be able to restore their physical health as soon as possible.

The hospice environment

The patients had identified several problems of the hospice environment. First, they highlighted that nurses were too busy, so they had little time to communicate and listened to their needs. Second, some older patients could not differentiate nurses from health care assistants because they both wore uniforms. Therefore, these patients had problems of requesting the right person for assistance. The third problem related to the work schedule of the hospice unit. Health care professionals and visitors could attend the patients any time during the day. Their visits may disturb the patients' plan for rest. The following is an illustration.

At one field visit, an elderly patient stayed in his bed because he was weak and tired. Some volunteers visited him and stayed for a short while. Then a student social worker came to his bedside and talked to him. This was her field practice. When the student left him, a health care assistant entered the unit for some routine work. The patient then told her that he had severe pain. She agreed to report his situation to the nurses. Afterwards, one nurse came to him and assessed his pain and then gave him some oral drugs to relieve his pain. The patient also requested the nurse to change his position. He felt much more comfortable when he could stay in a position which was best for him.

Strategies used to adjust to the hospice environment

The hospice patients were expected to appear settled in well in the unit even they could not be 'cheerful'. [32] Most patients had to carry out some strategies to adjust to these hospice expectations. For example, a 77- year old patient, with cancer of the lung, was weak and dependent. After an assisted bath in the morning, he was kept sitting in an armchair until lunchtime. He would then be helped to rest on the bed after his lunch. This was a routine for bedridden patients. He avoided 'bothering' the hospice staff to assist him to the toilet by reducing his food and fluid intake. He described his adjustment as follows.

> I dare not drink more than what is enough because I do not want to void urine. I am afraid to wet the bed, as I cannot control my bladder. I will be told off by the staff if I wet the bed.

Incontinence is a common problem for hospice patients. Three hospice patients felt embarrassed because they developed incontinence when they became very weak. A few of them had to put on disposable nappy and they felt that this was a humiliating experience. Evidently, the patients' self-esteem and identity were greatly affected. One patient described her feeling precisely. 'I am just like a big baby because I cannot go to the washroom myself. When I have my bowel movement, I feel shameful to contaminate my clothing'.

The patients were expected to co-operate with the staff members who care for them. They should also avoid distressing or embarrassing the staff. However, some patients may have grievances and complaints about the hospice environment or routine work. Some patients learnt to play the passive, dependent and obedient 'sick role' but some refused to do so. Two patients complained to me that they were embarrassed when they had assisted- bath. The first patient was a 70-year old woman. She described her frustration after the bath. 'I did not have any assisted- bath for my whole life. I (my whole body) was exposed'. She was very unhappy but she did not express her grievances to the hospice staff. She learnt to adjust to the hospice routine because she needed to stay in the hospice unit. The second patient was a middle-age man. He was more concerned about the situation as a female health care assistant, who was of similar age as his, assisted him to have a bath. After the bath, the health care assistant complained that he was not co-operative. In addition to the embarrassment, he was unhappy because the health care assistant teased him for not able to self-care. He aired his grievances to the hospice staff. However, hospital staff generally likes patients and families who never complain. [32] Therefore, patient was considered a 'difficult patients' in the unit.

The success of hospice patients' adjustment to the hospice environment depended largely on their social relations with the medical and nursing staff. This finding is consistent with Flemming's [11] study. In addition, the social relation with the supporting staff such as the health care assistants was particularly important. It is because they had more direct interaction in the hospice unit. The hospice patients have to adjust to the hospice environment to maintain their hope to restore their physical health.

Changing life styles

Eight patients adjusted to the changes of their bodies by changing their life styles which included changing their diet, rest, sleep pattern and physical exercises. Some patients changed their diets and took natural food such as cereal, green vegetables and some preserved vegetables. In addition, some hospice patients took different recipes of soup, for example, swallows' nests or shark's cartilages. These foods are nutritious and rich in protein. This is commonly known as 'food therapy'. Apart from changing their diets, some patients spent more time sleeping and resting. Several patients were keen to have more physical exercises including deep-breathing exercises. These exercises would help relieving the physical symptoms. They hoped that by changing their lifestyles, their health could be restored to fight against cancer.

Psychological adjustments

Having cancer can bring people many losses. The problem list of unexpected losses can be long too. These losses include control, independence, productivity, security, various types of psychological, physical and cognitive abilities, predictability and consistency, experiences, future existence, pleasure, ability to complete plans and projects, dreams and hopes for the future, significant others, familiar environment and possessions, aspects of self and identity and meaning. Death itself is the supreme loss. [34] Therefore, nine patients made some psychological adjustments to maintain their hope to live and to have peace in mind. They used several strategies, which included accepting changes of their body image, thinking positively, living day by day and selective forgetting.

Accepting changes of their body image

The change of body image commonly occurred as a result of operation and or loss of body weight. The change of physical appearance has a negative impact on the cancer patients' confidence and will to live. In a recent study on Chinese patients with nasopharyngeal carcinoma, three-quarters of the sample reported that they were stressful. The stress came from the loss of physical beauty because they lost their hair and their skin was darkened but the gender of these patients was not specified. The finding of this research is consistent with Cheng's [29] study. Four female hospice patients suffered from permanent facial disfigurement and they had to learn to accept changes of their body image. Furthermore, a majority of patient lost about one-third of their body weight because of their illness and anorexia. Therefore, these patients had to adjust to the changes of their body weight, body image and consequently their physical functions. The followings are some examples.

Mrs L was 70-year old with cancer of the lung. She used an old photograph to show me the contrast of her appearance before and after the diagnosis of cancer. She was good looking before she had cancer. This patient learnt to accept the changes of her body image by sharing her past with others. Sharing has given her psychosocial and spiritual comfort to face the changes.

> Now I am so ill ... I was 140 pounds (sighed for a few seconds). I was a 'nei nei' (rich and fat woman) ... Now (I) look like a vampire (sighed again). No, I have not checked my weight and I can't be bothered. My skin has wrinkles and [I look] like an old woman. (Then she took out one photograph from her bedside drawer). Yes, this was taken in the past (she made a deep sigh again, with anger). This is my sister-in-law. She was also good looking. I am so thin now ... It is so sad ... (sigh for the third time). I like to follow the fashion and my sister-in-law has a good taste too.

Another patient felt angry about the alteration of her body image. She realised that she had to come to term with the reality and accepted the changes.

> I have been a healthy person with a good round face. I have been healthy, independent and optimistic. I was a volunteer in a women's society too because I have been social and active. For example, I taught the old people to make the dumplings. Now I feel clumsy (dependent) since I was not able to walk. I am very angry ... but I have to learn to accept these changes.

People who had cancer of the limbs or the head, they had higher risks of developing disfigurement after the operation. They had to use an extra effort to adjust to the immense changes of their bodies and body functions, as a result of having cancer and its treatment. An elderly woman was another typical example. She was 66-year old with cancer of the palate. She was a business woman who operated a restaurant before her illness. She developed a serious facial disfigurement after an extended surgery. Her eyes were protruding. Her mouth also looked awkward because her mouth could not close 'properly'. On top of this rather 'horrified' physical appearance, she could neither see nor hear clearly. She also had an open-wound in her mouth, which produced profuse foul-smelling discharge. Therefore, she could not swallow and speak properly. She could only murmur a few words to the people around her. Evidently, she suffered enormously spiritually, emotionally and physically. Understandably, it was difficult for her to accept these enormous changes. She had thought of suicide soon after her surgery. Fortunately, she had established a close connectedness with her family that supported her adjustment to these changes. Of equal importance, the hospice staff had shown acceptance to her and looked after her without prejudice. In this way, the staff had helped the patient to maintain hope for the ability to love and be loved.

Altered body image is a common problem for cancer patients. Thus, several patients of this research had this problem. Therefore, they made psychological adjustment to learn to accept the changes of their body image by sharing their emotions with others. Just important, they felt being loved and accepted because they maintained a harmonious social relation with the caregivers. The social connectedness and respect had facilitated them to develop hope to live.

Thinking positively

Some people used other people, rather than objective criteria, as a basis for comparison. [35] In this research, five patients compared their current situation with people who were in 'less favourable' situation in order to maintain some positive feelings. This strategy of psychological adjustment helped them to maintain a hope in respect of the future, as they perceived others' situation could be worse. The followings are some examples.

An elderly patient with cancer of the colon, had a hope to cure after taking some Chinese herbs. He related his condition to his son and his sister. He felt better because he was still alive at the age of over 80. His son died at young age. Realistically, he was ready to die because of his old age. However, he still believed that he would be cured because his sister was cured after taking Chinese medicine.

> My third son died of leukaemia when he was over 40-year old. I have cancer of the colon but I am cured! My sister, who stays in Taiwan, has cancer of the liver. She has taken these drugs and she was cured. I have another relative who took it as well and he was cured too. My sister gave me a phone call and told me that I should not have any surgery... I am not afraid, I am over 80 now and it's time to die.

One patient compared himself with those who died in an accident. He also pointed out the inevitability of death.

I talked to my friends and they said I was unlucky, because some people might die in an accident. Then I felt better. Good persons and healthy persons will die without a warning. Everybody will die. Nobody knows about tomorrow, isn't it right? Don't you think so? A healthy person may die without notifying others. I have discussed about this with my friends. They were sad about the bad news but they advised me not to think about it too much. People might drop death while they are walking in the street. A healthy person can die any time. Therefore, one should think positively.

Another patient compared himself with those persons who died at young age. 'Some people died at the age of 10 or so and they were worse than me'.

According to people with terminal cancer, the greatest threat to loss of hope is the loss of control over present circumstances.[11] Therefore, two patients felt that they should choose to live happily if they were given a choice. It was important that they perceived a sense of control and hope to live.

No matter what happens to my illness, I will live happily. One can make a day happy or sad. This encourages me to be happy.
I have thought of many things when I was diagnosed to have the illness. Now I can accept it more. Why should I think of too many things? If (I) can either live happily or unhappily every day, why shouldn't (I) live more happily?

Some patients tried to think of their future with optimism. This strategy of psychological adjustment may relate to one's optimistic personality.

Yes, I lost myself (personal identity). I have lost myself. I do not feel sad about it because I have accepted it. I have mixed personality. You can say I am optimistic but I am also an introvert. I am both (introvert and extrovert). I can be very optimistic. I like to think. I do not blame on other people or other thing. I think I acquire it (cancer) myself. Everything is acquired. If I do not have this illness, I may have another [illness] in the next year or so.

Several patients adapted the strategy of thinking positively in order to maintain their hope to live. They maintained hope by subjective comparison, feeling in control and being optimistic.

Living day by day

The idea of this strategy is quite similar to the concepts of bargaining, [36] mitigation and accommodation. [37] Consistent with Young and Cullen's study, [34] four patients considered the strategy of living day by day as way to maintain their sense of control and hope. They learnt to live 'one day at a time'. They also accepted that they required some assistance from people around them to strengthen their capabilities to control and to be less dependent until they died. The followings are some examples.

> I do not think about 'those things', those unhappy things. I will think about eating, I will think about what I want to eat ... I will think about where I will go when I am getting better... I just live day by day.

> The day passed one after the other. This is reality. I feel tired day by day and I cannot control it. I have nothing to do now. I live one day at a time.

When death became imminent, some patients realised that they might not live long. They chose to live one day at a time which allowed them to gradually detach from the secular world.

Selective forgetting

While some patients could remember clearly the details of what happened during the breaking of the 'bad news', three patients chose to forget the details. In this way, they were able to maintain their hope for a future. For example, an elderly patient asserted that she forgot the date of when she was diagnosed, which medical practitioner she attended and when she was admitted. She explained that she was forgetful. Another patient preferred not to think about her condition. This patient was asked if her insomnia and sadness were due to her worries, she replied five times that she did not like to think about it. She explained that she did not know how to communicate and she was not good in thinking. It seemed that she did not want to face her illness and death. One way of psychological adjustment was to put the problems aside until one was ready to face them again.

> I forget when I was diagnosed and the name of the private medical

practitioner. I am rather forgetful. The medical practitioner did not tell me the diagnosis.

I make an effort not to remember things. I do not remember it.

Table 5.3
Categories and significant statements of Maintaining hope alive (Hope)

Categories	Significant statements
Having treatment	Physiotherapy helps to improve my condition. I like it because it reduces my leg oedema (3, p.1).
	I have cancer of the colon. I have cured. I take Chinese herbal medicine: Ning Chi, Wan Chi (24)
Adjustments *Adjusting to the hospice environment*	I did not feel happy (if I have to bother people to look after me), so I would not make too many requests. I dared not make too many demands (22)
Changing life styles	I lived in the hospital for over twenty days. I walked up and down the stairs. Later, I carried out physical exercises near St. Joseph College that was near this hospital. How could I lose what I have done over the years? I seemed to lose everything momentarily. No, it could not be like that! I needed to be strong. I lose everything in these several days. I must do some exercises. Initially, I exercised in the morning and in the evening too. Later, I even joined the aerobics. Every body said that I was 'fit'. My condition was good and then I went to swim because I like to have a healthy body (12, p.6).
Psychological adjustments	After the second operation, I did not want to go outdoors. Later, I thought it over. I asked myself, 'Am I not going out for the rest of my life?' I was not used to it (my appearance). I felt very sad. Everything affects me: my outlook has changed and my illness has changed too. I begin to accept myself and will not care too much about how people think about me (30, p.9).

Hope and the course of illness

People may overlook the fact that hospice patient's goal is constantly being revised. Quite often, the nature of hope of a dying person changes due to deterioration of his or her condition. Clearly, the strength to maintain hope was largely affected by his or her physical condition. Therefore, most patients felt anxious and depressed when their cancer relapsed. This was another important reference point of the course of their illness. This finding is consistent with Cheng's [29] study. She reported that 80% of her participants had fear of relapse. It was because recurrence of cancer would mean that their battles with cancer were defeated and they had to be confronted with their imminent death. The followings are examples of two patients who experienced relapse of cancer.

The first patient was a 53- year old woman with ovarian cancer and lung metastasis. She felt contented because she had overcome a lot of life crisis in the past. She liked her new job and she was ready to retire and enjoy the rest of her life. Therefore, she responded to having cancer with a lot of anger and frustration. She did everything to fight against her cancer to restore health. She was happy for her initial 'successful' adjustments because she hoped to live and not to die. When she developed metastasis of the lung, she had difficulty to redefine her goal and she committed suicide.

> There was eight months in between (the time between she was diagnosed and the relapse). I felt so shocked when I knew the diagnosis. The experience was liked the thunderstorm. I have given myself courage, I used to have a strong will, and I have been brave. I also thanked God for giving me new treatment and new hope. The metastasis was unexpected. I was totally shocked. In 1994, I have fought against the battle with cancer with all my strength... I cannot win the battle. I cannot accept it. The medical practitioner felt that he could do nothing for me. I felt that they were not all right. They did nothing to help me and they gave up. The medical practitioner said, 'what can we do (for the relapse)?' I then replied, 'the worst thing is to die'. The medical practitioner said 'you say it yourself now'. His statement was very unkind.

The second example is a 48 - year old man with cancer of the lung. He was a clerk and had worked hard for most of his life. He had a misconception that radiotherapy may give rise to many complications.

Therefore, he refused to have radiotherapy, instead, he undertook a course of 'ultraviolet light therapy' in a private clinic. Unfortunately, his cancer progressed very quickly and metastasised to his spinal cord five months after the diagnosis. When he realised the rapid deterioration of his body, he went back to see the medical practitioner. He was very upset with relapse of cancer. Worse still, he could not walk after the relapse. Therefore, he had thought of suicide at that particular depressed moment. Fortunately, he had searched the meaning of life (and death) and changed his philosophy of life with the influence of his family and volunteers. He felt spiritually contented and he was able to hope for a Good Death.

> I was diagnosed in February. In July, I felt that something wrong with my spine. On 13th July, when I went to the washroom in the evening, I fell down and my knees were hurt. Then, I was sent to the hospital for x-ray. It was confirmed that the cancer cells have gone to the spinal cord - the 3rd to 4th lumber spine so that my lower limbs were affected. At that time, I was very upset. It was all right to have cancer. When I knew that I could not walk, I almost wanted to die. The feeling was worse than dying: I felt helplessness and very depressed. I did not want to talk to anybody. I could not sleep for 2-3 days. Later, I was referred to the hospice unit. The staff often came and comforted me. They helped me to accept the reality. Now I will not mind to die or to live. To think it positively, I have gained some days. Yes, I have changed my philosophy of life.

Having cancer can bring people many losses including loss of hope for a future. It is important that health care professionals would show genuineness and compassion to the patients. These patients had to learn to accept the losses, which included their loved ones and eventually their lives.

Clinical implications

Goal:
Instil and nurture realistic hope for the patients

Redefine hope

Hope is a response to a threat that results in the setting of a desired goal. [38, 42] Health care professionals can help hospice patients to remain hopeful by redefine hope with them. Then the patients may hold a future in which their pain and other symptoms can be controlled. Health care professionals can discuss different kinds of hope with them - hope for cure, hope for freedom from pain, hope for accomplishing something before dying, hope for being loved, accepted and valued and hope for dying a Good Death. Hope is a personal thing unique to each patient. It is usually difficult to articulate, but is always worth speaking about. [39]

It is also important to recognise those hospice patients' hope changes day by day. Health care professionals can facilitate them to plan for new but attainable goals [34, 39] and readjust their goals as their condition change. In this way, they will be given a sense of hope and control.

Assess the sources of hope

Hope initiates a systematic goal-directed and action-oriented process. This process involves assessment, planning, selection, and use of all internal and external resources and supports that will help in achieving the goal. Hope also requires revaluation and revision of the plan while enduring, working and striving to reach the desired goal. [38]

Health care professionals can assist the patients to access the source of hope and their meaning in living (and dying) in everyday experiences. It is important to identify the sources of hope of the patients from different perspectives: personnel, financial resources, religious beliefs and coping mechanisms. Therefore, patient's assessment has to include an alternative form of treatment, status of symptom control, social relations and spiritual adherence. In this way, health care professionals can guide the patients and the family in finding the sources of support for their uses. Since faith in god(s) may give the patients a sense of hope and a source of unconditioned acceptance, health care professionals can arrange for a visit by a religious representative and prayer. It is also helpful for them to be familiarised and sensitive to the reactions of hospice patients when they go through their dying process. The patients will attempt to view their future with hope even they have experienced disease progression. Hope comes from within the person, but encouragement from others is important in fostering patients' confidence in the future.

Help patients to identify alternative therapies

The hope for a cure is a natural one and the hospice patients require a careful discussion of the treatment options open to them and a clear explanation of the nature of palliative care so that hope is not unrealistic.[13] Health care professionals can help patients and their families to identify various possible alternative therapies that are currently available. It is encouraging to see that formal programs on Traditional Chinese medicine are established since 1998. Complementary treatments such as Qigong, massage and acupuncture, have become popular in caring for the dying people. It is good to see that Traditional Chinese medicine is introduced in some major hospitals in some Asian countries such as Hong Kong. Evidently, cancer treatment has an economic impact on the hospice patients and their families that demands more attention and support from the Social Welfare Department and Department of Health in their countries.

Facilitate patients to have a hopeful attitude

Hope can be inspired through effective communication. Cousins [40] emphasises that words used by medical practitioners and nurses have a profound effect on the well being of the patients. The words of the medical practitioners and other health care professionals can give hope to the cancer patients, but they can also take away the hope from them when they disclose the 'bad news' with little empathy [41] Therefore, it is essential for health care professionals to have hope, love, and confidence within themselves.

It is equally important to have an understanding of the critical requirement that characterised 'hope-full' interactions: being known as human, connecting, descriptive, welcoming, and informing. [41] 'Connecting' refers to the rapport between the patients and the health care professionals in which the patients perceive the true caring of these professionals who are listening, understanding, and supporting and encouraging them as human being. 'Welcoming' refers to similar rapport in which the patients feel that the health care professionals is easily accessible. These strategies will remind hospice staff the importance of maintaining patient's connectedness and the need of being informed.

Summary

People need to be hopeful. When people are confronted with incurable cancer, they lose hope for a future and this is an ultimate lose of human being. However, the sense of hope is extremely important for them. Kubler-Ross [36] observes that dying person needs to have hope throughout the trajectory. Health care professional need to have a sound knowledge on hope so that they may assist the hospice patients to instil realistic hope and attainable goals at the end of their life journey.

The findings of this research have presented the diversity of hope and the meaning of hope from the hospice patients' perspective. First, there is a hope for cure and life can be prolonged. A majority of patients conceptualised hope in this context. Second, dying individuals need to have social and emotional support to sustain hope. The patient needed to love and being loved. Their relationship with the hospice staff and the family was also important. Third, the presence of personal control reinforces the sense of hope. Lastly, hope can include a spiritual element. Some patients were stimulated to search for meaning of life and death, particularly when they felt that death was near. This stimulation may lead them to explore the notion of life after death. With this sense of hope, a dying person will feel happy,

Table 5.4
Summary of Maintaining hope alive (Hope)

Related issues	Clinical implications
1. Concepts of hope • Physical restoration • Social connectedness • Personal control • Spiritual contentment	Goal: Instil and nurture realistic hope for the patients 1. Redefine hope 2. Assess the sources of hope
2. Having treatments • Conventional treatment • Chinese medical treatment	3. Help the patients to identify the possible alternative therapies
3. Adjustments • adjusting to hospice environment • changing life styles • psychological adjustment	4. Facilitate the patients to maintain a hopeful attitude.
4. Hope and the course of illness	

contented and he or she will have peace in mind.

In this research, twenty-three patients reported that they had done something to maintain hope. Nine patients had alternative medical therapy. Most of them had received conventional treatment to control their cancer. They also hoped that they could continue palliative treatment even medical practitioner told them that was no more treatment available. Therefore, most of them sought alternative therapy. Chinese medical treatment was a popular choice of alternative therapy as most Chinese have faith and trust in this treatment modality.

Some patients also carried out strategies to adjust to the changes of their bodies and body image. They hoped to restore health and re-establish strength to fight against cancer. These strategies included adjusting to hospice environment, changing life styles and making psychological adjustments. Their strengths to keep their hope also alive depended on the social support from the caregivers and their perception of control over loss. For a few patients, their hope built on their faith and spirituality such as confirming the meaning of life and death.

For clinical implications, it is important that health care

professionals, especially medical practitioners, will not take away the hospice patients' hope when they disclose the 'truth' of the patients' condition. Health care professionals can continue assisting the patients to foster realistic hope for a future. First, they can facilitate patients to redefine hope. They have to know their patients' hope. Second, they have to assess different sources of hope for the patients and the families. Third, they can facilitate patients to identify various alternative therapies. Finally, they can help them to sustain a hopeful attitude. It is equally important that health care professionals to have love, hope and confidence within themselves.

6
Being free from pain and suffering (Comfort)

Introduction

IN THIS RESEARCH, most hospice patients associated cancer with death. More than one-third of them avoided using the word 'death', and some of them had difficulties facing death. To face a cancer death is not easy because people generally predict it will be painful. Therefore, when the patients were asked what their main concerns were, they gave freedom from pain and suffering as the most common answer. They identified control of pain and suffering as an essential element of dying a Good Death. Control of pain and symptoms is the most crucial element of the hospice philosophy.[1] In this chapter I present my findings on being free from pain and suffering. The chapter will explore the concepts of cancer pain and the effectiveness of pain management; the concepts of multi-dimensional suffering; and the final topic of unresolved pain and suffering, including observations about suicide and euthanasia.

Being free from pain

Cancer pain

Pain has been defined in various ways. For example, one definition is 'an unpleasant sensory and emotional experience associated with actual or potential tissue damage or described in terms of such damage'. [2] Pain comes from the Greek word 'poine', meaning penalty. Therefore, it is predominantly an emotional and subjective experience which has a physical consequence of actual or potential tissue damage.[3] The way one defines pain influences not only one's attitude towards pain but also one's approach when one cares for others in pain. [4]

From the patients' subjective descriptions, a majority reported that they were in pain, with more than half of them experiencing moderate to severe pain. In more detail, most of them experienced pain, nine patients experienced a mild degree of pain; nine experienced a moderate degree of pain, and nine experienced uncontrollable, intolerable, and severe pain, which was not relieved by medication. Therefore, more than half of the patients addressed the importance of pain control. Being free from pain (comfort) became their most immediate concern when they were dying. Nevertheless, not every terminal cancer patient experiences pain, and six patients in the present research experienced little or no pain. Those who were in pain simply hoped for a painless death.

This result is consistent with the findings of some previous studies in the Western countries, which indicate that fifty to seventy-five per cent of terminal cancer patients experience pain. [5-8] It also substantiates the findings of some local studies that focus on hospice patients. [9-11] For example, Yeung [10] reports that three-quarters of her patients experienced pain and eighty-seven per cent had discomfort and symptoms during their stay in the hospice units.

According to Ahles and Martin, [6] forty per cent of all patients with metastatic cancer experience moderate to severe pain. In this research, two-thirds of the patients had developed metastases and most of them experienced moderate to severe pain. Therefore, the problem of pain control appeared to be more serious. Further, some patients, who experienced severe pain, had the same diagnosis of cancer of the lung with pleural metastasis. This finding also parallels the local study by Sze and his colleagues [12] on hospice patients, which finds that people with primary tumours of the lung often experience pain.

'Total pain'

Cancer pain can be perceived as a physio-pathological process, and a psychological dimension often follows. Unrelieved physical pain and non-acceptance of death are often attributed as the causes of psychological pain.[13]

Most patients were anxious about the uncontrollability of pain. They worried about their pain every time the effects of their analgesic medication began to wear off. They also feared pain, as it was chronic and tedious. It was the chronicity that made pain so intolerable and depressing. When the hospice care professionals did not address causes of anxiety, it would further create anger, hostility, loneliness, and consequently depression.[14] Increased anxiety and depression will serve to further intensify pain[15] and absorb one's whole attention. [16-17] This represents the progression of pain to suffering and 'pain of the soul'. [18] This is the concept of 'total pain' that was first described by Saunders. [19] Total pain addresses pain from four dimensions: physical, emotional (psychological), social, and spiritual. To relieve pain, one has to consider each of these dimensions. 'All this calls for great competence in the analysis and the relief of various forms of suffering that make up the "total pain" of a terminal illness'. [20]

Ineffective pain management

The patients in this research referred their pain experience to physical pain more than other aspects of pain. When they had emotional disturbances, many of them used the word 'suffering' to describe their feelings. A majority of patients suffered from pain. If one of the goals of hospice care is to help patients to control pain, one may query what happens to such patients. The following discussion attempts to explore the causes of ineffective pain management from the perspective of literature and the patients. Future studies are necessary to obtain the appropriate information. It was noted that some patients endured pain and some health care professionals may have performed inconsistent assessments. Other contributing factors were inadequate medical intervention and ineffective communication between patients and health care professionals.

Enduring pain

When a Chinese patient requests pain relief, it may mean that he or she has reached his or her threshold of pain tolerance. It is at this point, if not before, that pain has resulted in suffering. Consequently, many patients in this research endured pain, and did not call for nurses' attention to relieve their distress. Some of them reported their pain to health care assistants. They did not want to add to the nurses' existing workload. Even when they were in a state of severe pain, they might not report it until they could tolerate it no longer.

There may be many reasons to explain why the patients did not report their pain to health care professionals. First, they wanted to be 'good patients' and therefore did not want to bother the hospice staff.[21-22] Chinese patients generally feel the needs of the group to be more important than those of the individual. Therefore, they believe it is best not to call attention to oneself. [23] Second, some of the patients did not like to take Western medicine, so they delay reporting their pain. According to the Taoist health model, health is a balance between 'Yin' and 'Yang' energy. Some patients believed that Western drugs were 'Yin' and would cause 'cold' or harmful effects on the body. Third, some patients perceived pain as a sign of physical deterioration.[14, 24] They did not report their pain because they may have hoped that their conditions were not deteriorating. Lastly, some endured pain because they perceived it as an inevitable part for having cancer and/or it was their fate to have pain.

Inconsistent assessment

Cancer patients often expect the medical practitioners and nurses to help them relieve their pain and symptoms, but they seem to provide little help with their physical suffering.[7] Several authors make the criticism that health care professionals, in particular nurses, tend to conceive suffering as a patient's condition and an essential human experience. [25] Therefore, they may not pay adequate attention to solving the problem of pain. Consistent with Chao's[7] research in Taiwan, the present research indicated that nursing care for people with terminal cancer was relatively inadequate. For example, several patients in the research showed gratitude to medical practitioners who prescribed drugs to control their pain, but very few of them gave credit to nurses. Lack of knowledge about pain assessment is also a common barrier associated with inadequate pain treatment.[26] Similarly, lacks a central policy to ensure the level of competency of pain assessment for nurses is another factor. A seventy-year-old patient illustrated the situation.

> Medical practitioners help me to relieve pain. Nurses cannot make any decision to help my pain. They often ask me to report my pain to the medical practitioner. The nurses are very busy and they have no time to talk to me. If they could spend fifteen minutes with me everyday, I would be satisfied.

Inadequate medical interventions

One possible explanation for the failure of pain relief is ineffective medical intervention. First, pain was not improved because knowledge of drugs is not adequately applied. [27] Some medical practitioners may fear contributing to addiction, despite strong evidence that addiction was not usually an issue for patients with cancer pain. [28] Second, medical practitioners may have underestimated the problem and failed to treat pain in a sufficiently aggressive manner.[29] Third, the patients failed to comply with the recommended regimen. [27, 30] Since pain is a unique human experience that affects the whole person, effective use of morphine is not sufficient to improve the overall care of terminally ill cancer patients. The caring art of medicine has to be restored along with the sensitive application of scientific methods. In this research, very few patients reported that they had received non-pharmacological interventions. Nevertheless, reports of some local self-help groups indicate that complementary treatments such as Qigong, massage, meditation, music therapy, and aromatherapy have become popular in caring for dying people.

Ineffective communication between health care professionals and patients

Another reason for ineffective pain management is insufficient communication and understanding of the nature of pain. [31] Poor communications between patients and health care professionals, either under-reporting by the patients or under-assessing by nurses or medical practitioners may be reasons for ineffective pain management. [31] Therefore, the patients may have endured pain, while health care professionals did not manage the pain or communicate effectively. Moreover, Dunlop [32] observes that the effectiveness of communication may be due to differences in socio-economic background. Health care professionals, especially medical practitioners, tend to come from a higher socio-economic group. They probably have limited personal experiences of suffering. Younger staffs are unlikely to have experienced a major illness, and their families may still be alive. A few patients commented that some nurses were too young. A first-person experience of illness is not always a prerequisite for working in the field; however, if handled correctly, personal experience can improve empathy when balanced with self-awareness. Patients and their families will know they are heard and valued when they feel an empathetic response. [33] Furthermore, they hope that nurses (and medical practitioners) will spend more time with them, because they need to communicate their needs. 'Caring may mean being connected and having persons, events, projects and things matter'. [34]

Being free from suffering

Concepts of suffering

The Chinese word for suffering is composed of two words: 'pain' and 'bitterness'. The hospice patients in this research mentioned the word 'suffering' more often than the word 'pain' when they hypothesised their Good Death. Some patients used these two terms interchangeably. The patients often used the term 'suffering' to describe the intensity and dimensions of their emotional experiences.

Several definitions of suffering consist of the word 'pain'. For example, 'pain is capable of producing physical and/or mental suffering qualities'; [4] suffering is serious pain that a person feels in their body or their mind. Suffering is 'a state of severe distress associated with events that threaten the intactness of the person'. [35] In addition, a person's personal identity can be threatened. Noticeably, these authors agree that suffering has the quality of pain. It is a serious, severe and stressful human experience that affects a person's body and mind. Consequently, it affects his or her personal identity and integrity.

The multi-dimensional suffering

Although suffering is assumed to be a universal human experience, ways of responding to suffering in oneself and in others may vary considerably across cultures. Fourteen patients stated that they wanted minimal suffering. Consistent with the findings of Brallier [36] and Beneliol, [37] the suffering of the patients in the present research can be viewed from four dimensions: physical, psychological, social, and spiritual.

Physical dimension of suffering

'Physical suffering' usually refers to symptoms.[36] These are bodily changes that interfere with one's physical and mental access to the world.[37] Some common symptoms include fatigue, dyspnoea, anorexia and insomnia, decreased mobility and constipation. In this research, twelve patients had anorexia, fatigue and dyspnoea. Eleven patients suffered from loss of body weight. In addition, oedema, insomnia and decreased mobility were common (Table 6.1). Other less common symptoms were confusion, incontinence, dermatitis, sputum, tremor of hands or legs, abdominal discomfort, sore mouth, diarrhoea, dizziness, fever, loss of teeth, nausea and vomiting, convulsion, poor vision, and wound bleeding.

Three patients wanted to be less dyspnoeic, to have less cough and sputum, and a better appetite. In other words, they hoped to be as comfortable as possible. For example, four wanted to die while they were asleep. They found it easier to express their physical symptoms than emotional upset or suffering.

Consistent with some previous studies,[7, 38] nearly half of them had three or more symptoms. More than two-thirds of the patients had more than one symptom: four patients had five symptoms, six patients had four symptoms, five patients had three symptoms, and nine patients had two and one symptom consecutively (Table 6.2). Very often, symptoms were interrelated. For example, a patient who

Table 6.1
Summary of common physical symptoms (*n*=33)

Type of symptom	Frequency	Patient's file number
Fatigue	13	3, 4, 5, 11, 15, 16, 17, 18, 20, 22, 24, 26, 30
Anorexia	12	2, 5, 8, 10, 11, 15, 17, 19, 21, 25, 28, 33
Dyspnoea	12	1, 3, 8, 9, 10,17, 18, 20, 22, 28, 29, 32
Loss of body weight	11	2, 7, 10, 14, 16, 18, 20, 21, 22, 24, 31
Decreased mobility	10	4, 5, 6, 14, 17, 21, 22, 23, 24, 31
Oedema	9	1, 3, 11, 12, 13, 14, 16, 22, 27
Insomnia	8	3, 5, 7, 8, 13, 15, 18, 20
Constipation	6	1, 6, 18, 20, 28, 32
Incontinence	5	8, 9, 11, 16, 17
Confusion	3	6, 11, 15

Table 6.2
Frequency of symptoms (n=33)

No. of symptoms	Frequency
5	4
4	6
3	5
2	9
1	9

suffered from carcinoma of the lung had a productive cough and dyspnoea that affected his body weight. Although his appetite was good, he could not take in too much food because of his nausea and vomiting. These findings echoed the findings of many previous studies. [39-41] The patients worried most about the controllability of their symptoms. It should be emphasised that these data were obtained from interviews and no specific instruments were used to measure the severity of pain and symptoms. It was not the purpose of the research to include detailed descriptions of the patients' symptoms.

Psychological dimension of suffering

Suffering was certainly an experience that involved more than just physical symptoms. The psychological dimension of suffering refers to feeling a loss of control. Suffering is due to a disconnection between identified purpose in living and a sense of belonging to an ordered world.[37] A person will experience a sense of alienation when he or she is redefined as being a 'cancer patient'.

The following patient suffered because of losing control and independence. She was eighty years old and had cancer of the lung. She was an able and independent person and she had done everything by herself before she had cancer. Because she was ill, she had to rely entirely on others to make her comfortable. She pointed out clearly that suffering to her meant the loss of control.

> (I) suffer a lot. I cannot get what I want! (When) I want to drink water, I have no water. I want to change my position, but I cannot do it myself. I feel sad. Every day is like that. The staff are helpful, but I do not feel comfortable calling them (to help me) all the time. I call them two or three times a day. If I call them more often they will not be happy. They will not be interested and they will answer me unwillingly. If you ask me, what do I want? Yes, I want water, please give me water. I want to change my position, please change my position, and cover me with enough clothing. Now, I cannot get what I want because I cannot move! This is what I mean by suffering.

When the patients experienced uncertainty about future, they did not have a sense of control. Uncertainty could come from waiting for the results of laboratory tests, undergoing investigation, and waiting to die. Therefore, some patients considered that having cancer was itself a suffering. The progress of cancer and the side-effects of cancer treatment lengthen the list of aspects of suffering.

Social dimension of suffering

The social dimension of suffering refers to interference with interpersonal relationships and connections to other people.[37] This results in the presence of loneliness due to some degree of social isolation and disconnection. Maes [42] stresses that suffering is always interpersonal for human beings. At the core of suffering is the sense of being cut off from normal human relationships. For example, poor communication and relations among the patients, family, and staff were often the key to problems. [36][37] All these social problems can cause anxiety and insomnia, thereby exacerbating the feeling of pain and suffering. This is important for the Chinese, as they generally believe in the Confucian value of harmonious family relationship. Therefore, maintaining social relations (connectedness) is essential for a Good Death. Furthermore, the social experience can be a manifestation of spiritual integrity in Chinese culture.

The following is an example. An elderly patient mentioned three times in an interview that he hoped to have minimal suffering when he died. During the interview, he described little about his emotions on hearing the diagnosis as it had happened just a few days previously. Rather, he reflected on his discontentment over other things such as his financial situation and his family relationships. These were probably his two major concerns before he died. He stated that he had worked as a tailor for his whole life and had been responsible for his family. In his terms, he had maintained the Confucian values of commitment to his family. He had a good relationship with his children, but not with his wife, and the inharmonious marital relationship had created his feeling of suffering.

Several single mothers in this research experienced the social dimension of suffering. They suffered from social pressure when they were young. The following is an example. She stated that she had a tough life and had suffered a lot. She was fifty-two years old with cancer of the cervix. She was divorced and did not mention her ex- husband. She had previously worked in a garment factory, and had started smoking to relieve her anxiety and tension. She reported that she experienced some degree of social pressure, since women tended to stay at home and look after their children in Hong Kong in the 1960s. To be a 'single mother' was not a common social phenomenon and she was not well accepted by the Chinese community at that time. She felt that she was isolated and experienced low self-esteem. Thus she valued filial affection from her children most highly. For the patients in this research, filial piety was regarded as the starting point of compassion, connectedness, and spiritual comfort, which began at home.

The following conversation illustrates the complicated nature of suffering. An elderly woman mentioned the term 'suffering' ten times during an interview. She had covered many aspects of suffering, which included experiencing physical symptoms, maintaining a living, and raising her child on her own. Her meaning of life appeared to be related to her only son. Her experience provides a better understanding of 'suffering' from the perspective of Chinese hospice patients. The following is a transcript of her conversation.

R: My husband passed away long time ago, around the time of the Japanese War.

r: Did you raise your child all by yourself?

R: Yes, (I) have had a lot of *suffering*.

r: Suffering. You must be very capable. You had to work and raise your child.

R: Yes, it was better after the war. I worked as a hawker. I had to do everything to earn a living.

r: So you earned your living ...

R: Yes.

r: You have one son.

R: One son.

R: Yes. At that time, (I had) a lot of *suffering*. I might earn something in the morning, but it would not be enough for the evening.

r: Do you consider your son a filial son?

R: He is all right. He likes to study. He graduated from a university in Taiwan. He is now running a private school.

r: How big is the school?

R: The school is about 1,000 square feet. He teaches every subject and he has to go in and out frequently, and he *suffers* a lot ...

R: I was admitted in May/June last year. I *suffered* a lot; I had dyspnoea and pain. Early last year, I did not feel such pain. They asked me to go for a follow-up on 5th January ... I waited until the date came, and I was in a lot of pain and *suffering*, so I was admitted for treatment ... Another time, I developed dyspnoea in the nursing home, I was *suffering* a lot so they sent me to the hospital.

r= Researcher R= Patient

Spiritual dimension of suffering

When patients had come to term with their serious illness and imminent death, many of them began to think more deeply about the meaning of life. This is the spiritual dimension of suffering: the process of dying which involves defining or clarifying the meaning of one's own death.[36] Benoliel [37] explains that there are discrepancies between a person's ideals and principles and his or her actions, which cause a loss of personal integrity, which in turn will create suffering. In this research, a few patients had a profound sense of guilt and failure about the past. Some regretted that they had left something undone or had failed to be reconciled with their family members. Sixteen patients felt extremely disappointed and hopeless when their symptoms could not be controlled. They had felt deeply that their lives were meaningless. The following are some examples.

One female patient, who usually appears cheerful and relaxed, wished to die when she became very dyspnoeic. She was very depressed because she suffered a lot from her uncontrollable symptoms, and her hope to recover began to diminish. She could not find any meaning for living. She expressed to me that she had thought of 'doing silly things' (committing suicide) when she was experiencing unrelieved dyspnoea. During her final days, she felt that her death was lingering, and she felt helpless. More important, she did not have a sense of control over what lay ahead. I anticipated her suffering, because she had previously been an optimistic person. Another patient felt that she had been defeated in the battle against cancer. She had also lost faith in God and suffered spiritually. She described her experience in the following words.

> One energetic and lively person has to be admitted to hospital and receive so many 'lousy' investigations. I feel I am suffering. I am a nurse. There will be many tests. I just feel anxious... There's been mental suffering and physical suffering. I have done a lot but I still have metastasis. I still have metastasis. I have done my best. I said I could not be defeated after these several days of hospitalisation. (I cannot be) Just defeated like that! Defeated! God is treating me badly; (He) has made me suffer.

Table 6.3 The four dimensions of suffering

Dimension of suffering	Significant statements
Physical	Death is not important. It is most important to have minimal suffering. I mean, less pain and less dyspnoea. My lung makes me dyspnoeic. Sometimes I have control. I also believe in fate. Sometimes I have urine dripping (incontinence) when I cough ... (9, p.6)
	I feel very painful and suffering, I have severe dyspnoea which make me sleeplessness (22, p.11).
Psycho-social	Do not make me feel emotional (7)
	If I have to die, I would like to die quickly. I live alone and feel very bored at times (9).
Spiritual	I am depressed. I do not want to live any longer. I am suffering. I don't know how to say it, it (my death) should be quick ... I'm really in pain, Miss! (I am) more or less like a lump of rice (stupid fool). I was in good health ... why should I suffer? (22, p.11)

Unresolved pain and suffering

Health care professionals need to be aware that patients may still experience unresolved suffering even if they receive attentive care, since dying is a complex human experience. When the patients could not resolve their pain and suffering, they may have asked their medical practitioners about euthanasia. However, their requests were not considered, as euthanasia is illegal in Asian countries such as Hong Kong.

Euthanasia

Consistent with the findings of Seale and Addington-Hall's [43] research and one local research, [44] when suffering became intense and intolerable a few patients wished to terminate their lives by euthanasia or committing suicide. Three patients initiated a discussion on euthanasia. They were all elderly. One patient considered euthanasia as an issue of resource allocation, while two patients had other reasons. One felt she had no meaning for living, because she felt abandoned by her family. In addition, two patients felt that they had no control over either their physical or social condition.

The first one was a seventy-year-old man. He perceived euthanasia as a social issue. He suggested that the public resources should not be spent on dying people, such as cancer patients.

> I feel that it's best for people with this illness (cancer) to go for euthanasia. I have learnt from the newspapers and television that euthanasia means dying with less pain and quicker. It means that a person can receive an injection to help them die more quickly and with less pain. Like those 'vegetables', they are wasting people's resources. I feel that to live with consciousness is important. Otherwise, it is almost like being a 'vegetable'.

Both the first and second patient raised the issue of euthanasia for discussion during their first interview. The second patient was a woman of eighty. She requested an injection to end her life, as she could no longer tolerate her symptoms and suffering. She used the word 'suffering' ten times in reviewing her life. Her relationship with her only son and his family had deteriorated. Her dying process was unexpectedly prolonged, and she could find no meaning to live. With this sense of uncontrollability and meaningless, she asked the medical practitioner for euthanasia to relieve her intense suffering.

> I called Dr M to give me an injection so that I could go to sleep (and die). He said this was illegal in Hong Kong. I really wanted it because I'm suffering a lot. I asked him during my last admission in June. I was admitted in May/June last year. I suffered a lot: dyspnoea and pain. Early last year, I did not experience such pain. They asked me to go for a follow-up visit on 5th January. I waited until that date and I was in a lot of pain and suffering, so I was admitted for treatment. Another time, I developed dyspnoea in the nursing home. I was suffering a lot (physical symptoms), so they sent me to the hospital. I don't mind where I go (after death). Eh, some people will go to heaven and some will go to hell. I have no fear.

The third patient who requested euthanasia was an eighty-year-old man with cancer of the colon. His reason for having such thoughts was his chronic, unrelieved pain and suffering. Also, he has no family around. His wife had died more than thirty years previously and his children were in mainland China.

> [I have had] pain for over ten years, real pain and severe suffering! It is a lingering experience. I have pain when I have my bowel movement. I think my illness is incurable. I asked the medical practitioner to give me an injection. [I rather] prefer to die...'mercy-killing...' [I feel] helpless, helpless. If the medical practitioner does this, he does not need to tell anyone else that he has offered me 'mercy killing'.

Although hospice research has shown that suffering can be relieved through proper pain and symptom management, some people request euthanasia or wish to commit suicide. These people's points of view are of equal importance, thus one may question why people want to be killed. Hospice care professionals do not generally accept the idea of euthanasia. They argue that the pain and symptoms are under control and the hospice patients should not think of euthanasia.[45] Several researchers have attempted to find out the answer. Seale and Addington-Hall [46] conducted a survey of people who died in 1990 in twenty health authorities in England. They reported that people dying from cancer who received hospice services were twice as likely as others to have requested euthanasia at some point during their last year. This was not significantly different from others who expressed a wish to die sooner. Hospice patients were more likely to feel that an earlier death would be preferable. Therefore, they conclude that 'hospice care appeared not to be associated with any significant reduction in the likelihood of dying people themselves being reported as wanting to die earlier or asking for euthanasia' (p.584). [46]

There are some possible explanations. First, hospice patients and their relatives may have an acceptance of euthanasia. Second, the hospice provides patients with an environment where they are more willing to express their worst fears. Third, hospice care is in fact poor or it reflects a system failure. The legalisation of euthanasia demands our attention to the values of autonomy, personal choice, and maintenance of control over one's fate. Requests for euthanasia may suggest that patients are giving up, and/or they are positively asserting their desire to control events. If this interpretation is true, it intensifies the moral debate about whether to strive to make people who desire euthanasia change their minds, or whether to accept their wishes. Furthermore, it is likely that the more independent dying individuals will be affected. It has been found that dependency is an important determinant of the desire for euthanasia. [43]

Suicide

Suicide is a very complex issue that arouses strong and often conflicting feelings.[33] It is often viewed as the supremely 'bad' death in societies influenced by Judeo-Christian religious traditions, for example, the Americans consider that suicidal persons do not deserve respect or extensive care. [47] Published articles in the medical literature about suicide in the medically ill tend to treat it as an adverse outcome of unrecognised or untreated depression.[48] Under such circumstances, it is often presented as an outcome to be prevented. Health care professionals may assume that people would die from their life-threatening illness if they did not commit suicide. In this way, patients' problems, such as depression, may be oversimplified or under-recognised.

The incidences of pain, depression, and delirium all increase with higher levels of physical decline in advanced stages of illness. In this research, ten patients in the advanced stages of cancer, had become depressed. Four of them mentioned that they had thought of suicide because they were suffering too much. Other patients intended to commit suicide in the following circumstances: when they heard their diagnoses, their cancer relapsed, their body image altered after surgery, and when they could not tolerate any more suffering as they approached death. This finding was consistent with some previous studies on Chinese patients, for example, Cheng [49] reported that three out of five patients in her sample had thought of committing suicide. However, she has not indicated if her patients had actually performed the act. Moreover, one patient in the present research attempted suicide but failed. Another patient committed suicide successfully. Both of them had not mentioned their intentions to commit suicide to me at the time of the interview. The situation of these two patients will be examined in the following section.

Attempted suicide

Mrs Y was fifty-three years old with cancer of the ovaries. She felt she was very smart, as she was able to get a job in a nursing home in her fifties. She had a strong character and had tried everything to cure her illness. She attempted suicide because she felt that she had been defeated in her battle against cancer cells. She considered the defeat to be an ultimate loss, and that she had to accept her imminent death. When her situation was analysed, it was observed that she depended entirely on her physical strength to cope with her life crisis. She performed exercises three times a day and she joined the aerobics class. She conformed to treatment and obeyed medical orders, and felt better. She also changed her diet and even her cooking utensils. Unfortunately, her social connectedness was weak. Her marriage had been an unhappy one and her husband had died a few years before. Her relations with her own siblings and children were not close. Therefore, she did not have any intimate support. In addition, she lost her faith in God when her cancer went into relapse. She was angry with God and felt that nobody could help her. It was clear that she had little social and spiritual connectedness.

> My family was in China. I was the only one who left China. My mother sent me to stay with my grandmother in Hong Kong. My mother wanted me to take care of her. I have one younger brother and one younger sister. Later, they had to stay in China because the Cultural Revolution had started. I had to endure a lot and this makes me unhappy, especially when my daughters are not affectionate. My husband made me angry too. On top of all this, my work has given me stress. I used to keep my feelings to myself when I was angry. May be this is the cause.

> I can say, nobody can really help me. I need to help myself ... . I have to rely on myself. I do not want to say, I don't mean that I don't trust in prayer but I am rather angry. My left lung has pleural effusion and I am suffering a great deal. I feel that God does not treat me well. He has ill-treated me — why do I have to suffer so much? (she showed her anger with God by her repetition of 'Why me?') Every person has some immunity towards cancer. I am unlucky. I often eat those foods (which are not fresh) after the expiry date. I think my disease is related to that. I do not smoke, I do not drink (alcohol), and I behave well. I see some old ladies in Western district. They are very old and they seem to have nobody to care for them. They pick up vegetables and sell them (for a living). They have difficult lives, too, but they do not have cancer.

In addition, her physical symptoms were not under control. She could no longer cope with her situation and wanted to reduce her suffering by terminating her life. Mrs. Y attempted suicide but she was rescued. She was then transferred to a psychiatric unit for special care. One of the hospice nurses visited her once. The nurse had established a good relationship with her and had invited her to pray twice. During the first visit, Mrs. Y cried with the nurse. In the second visit, the patient was less upset and she promised to ask for God's forgiveness. She promised that she would not make another attempt (at suicide) again. The following is the report of the hospice nurse.

A report of a visit to a patient who had attempted suicide

I went to visit her at Queen Mary Hospital; I said 'hello' to her. Her face showed hardly any expression. Several nurses came up to the patient, and she felt good because the nurses were taking care of her. She had mild dyspnoea and she was waiting for an examination. She then addressed her main concern of her attempted suicide. Mrs. Y was quite ready to talk about that. She felt that taking fifty Domicon tablets plus a plastic bag should have made her suffocate. When she woke up, she thought she had died. She did not expect to be alive. I asked if she felt disappointed. She said that since God had not received her that time, she would live 'naturally'. I asked her what I could do for her and Mrs. Y replied that I could pray for her. She said she would not attempt to kill herself again. I had actually prayed twice with her: we asked God to help her. I prayed with her at the hospice unit and also during a home visit. She had asked God to take her 'home' earlier because she was too impatient to wait. Mrs. Y said she was waiting for her daughter to come and said I could leave, if I had something else to do. We spent almost two hours: one hour with the patient and the next hour with her daughter. She felt she needed to talk to her daughter.

Committed suicide

Mr. C was fifty-seven years old with carcinoma of the lung. He was the only patient who committed suicide. I had three interviews with him. During the first interview, he was quite co-operative and willing to talk. He had moderate dyspnoea, anorexia, and muscle wasting of the legs. He felt hopeless when the medical practitioner told him his cancer was inoperable. He had no intimate social relations, since he was a drug addict, and relatives and neighbours rarely visited him. He said he lived alone and had no good friends. His cousin was his next of kin but Mr. C had not informed him about his hospitalisation. He had tried to work in restaurants but had failed to keep a job. During the interview, he had reservations about disclosing his personal feelings. In the second interview, he showed his awareness of his impending death, saying he did not think that he had a chance of returning home. He also indicated that he had experienced very low self-esteem in the past and felt that nobody had offered to help him. He was temporarily transferred to a private nursing home.

This patient was fully aware of his impending death because his general condition deteriorated. In a British research, during the last year of their life, about sixty per cent of dying patients may well have been aware that they were going to die. [50] They could feel death was approaching because of the gradual deterioration of their bodily function.

Unfortunately, this patient was not well accepted by people in the hospice because of his undesirable social behaviour. He was a drug addict and he was discovered selling 'drugs' to other patients in the hospital. He had no social relationships with his family and he had no control over where he stayed and what he wanted to do. His situation resembled closely that of a patient in Glaser and Strauss's [47] study, 'One patient, who had no friends to visit him, felt that he was very alone and that no one in the hospital cared, so he tried to hasten his death by suicide' (p.129). The following is a transcript of part of an interview with Mr. C illustrating his feelings that he was helpless and out of control.

---

r: How are you today? I was told that you would be transferred to the nursing home.

R: Yes. You see that I am still dyspnoeic. They want me to go. What can I do?

r: Perhaps the medical practitioner and nurse wish that you can return home one day.

R: I do not think that I will be going home at all. The medical social worker said that the nursing home was very crowded. Four people live in a small room.

r: The medical practitioner and nurses have said that when you are not feeling well, you will be transferred back to this hospital.

R: Ummm, yes, they have said I could come back.

r: Is there any thing that worries you at all?

R: Nothing (worry me)! Really nothing. I take things easy. I recall the worst time in my life was when I was ill one time. I was almost like a dying dog. Because I went to sleep at the bottom of a staircase.

r: Did you go to see the medical practitioner? Was there anybody around to help you?

R: Nobody. There was nobody around to help me. I struggled along to see the herbalist and I was cured.

r= Researcher R= Patient

At this time, his friend came to say goodbye to him. I stayed on and observed their conversation and interactions. His friend was also a drug addict. They began to share their viewpoints on what a Good Death meant to them, and how they would prefer to die, when they heard that one of their friends had died the day before. Mr. C listed three criteria of his preferred Good Death: 1) the person should die with a full stomach (so that he would not become a hungry ghost); 2) the person should die in spring (the best season to be buried); and 3) the person should die with least pain (physical comfort).

The possible criteria of Good Death from a hospice patient

R: Do you know Mr B? He used to have congee for his breakfast in an open-door restaurant (which was situated) at the corner of the street. He went there as usual. He migrated to heaven (died) after taking congee yesterday. He's already eighty.

F: Migrated? You mean he has died.

R: (He nodded) He was *fortunate to die with a full stomach and no suffering.*

F: Yes, I prefer to *die with a full stomach.*

R: Man has to die one day; the most important thing is to *die without pain.*

F: It is better to die *in spring.*

R: Yes, spring is a good time, summer is good too ...

R= Patient F = Patient's friend

Important patients' cues are often embedded in social conversations. This type of communication can provide useful information about the patients. The above conversation made a strong impression on me and inspired me to explore further what it meant to die a Good Death. Then I determined to find out what a Good Death meant to this group of people who were confronted with death themselves. It was noted that the above patient hesitated to talk about death and dying with health care professionals and their relatives. However, he was more willing to talk openly about these issues with his friend.

The third interview was conducted four days before his suicide. Three volunteers visited him from a charitable agent. He greeted me when I entered the room and was happy to introduce me to his visitors. During the interview, he refused to have the interview taped and also denied that he had any problems that were worrying him. He then showed me his leg, which was in spasm, and his toes were numb. I suspected that there might be some problems in his blood chemistry, then he asked a hospice nurse to explain it to him. His recent blood report showed a lower level of blood albumin and enzymes. He later received some instructions from this hospice nurse. I was surprised to hear the news of his suicide in the following visit. The hospital staff suspected that he had jumped to his death from a height after his evening meal.

In analysing Mr. C's death, his death may not appear to be appropriate or good because he had uncontrolled symptoms and feelings of abandonment. However, it was also noted that he had met the criteria of his preferred Good Death. He died in spring (March), with a full stomach (after mealtime) and the least suffering (a quick release). On the one hand, it is controversial to consider a suicide a Good Death because suicide is normally considered as an undesirable 'bad death' for those who are close to the person (relatives and the hospice staff). They often refuse to accept suicide as a form of good or appropriate death.[51] On the other hand, it is argued that some suicides are rational and represent the person's own wishes. Some patients prefer suicide as 'a way of controlling their dying as they controlled their living, thus wresting this control from the hands of the staff and

---

the rigors imposed by hospital routine' (p.129).[47] Therefore, suicides can also be considered to be their desired Good Death, because they have taken control of their lives.

Table 6.4
Categories and significant statements of being free from pain and suffering (Comfort)

Categories	Significant statements
Being free from pain	Life and death are regulated. It is most important to have no pain (25).
Being free from suffering	Death is not important. It is most important to have minimal suffering. I mean less pain and less dyspnoea. My lung makes me dyspnoeic. Sometimes I have control. Sometimes I have urine dripping (incontinence) when I cough (9, p.6).

Clinical implications

Goal:
Provide patients with comfort from a holistic approach

Effective management of pain and suffering

Pain and suffering must be clearly identified before it can be well managed. Health care professionals have to maintain the standards of clinical competency to help hospice patients be free from pain and suffering. That is, they have to consider the spiritual, psychosocial, and cultural factors that contribute to pain and suffering. A standardised pain assessment form[32] and validated assessment tools for assessing symptoms and suffering [41, 52] can be used. Further, health care professionals should share the meaning of their patients' experiences. Correspondingly, they will evaluate the effectiveness of pain and suffering management at a regular basis. More important, they will facilitate their patients with compassion and understanding.

Pain is personal and individual, no one can ever truly understand another person's pain. What dying people feel may be the tip of the iceberg. The root of pain may lie deep beneath the surface. Therefore, the deep emotions of the patients may not be easily recognised. Health care professionals and caregivers should admit their limitations and possible subjectivity in helping the patients to relieve pain and suffering. Some health care professionals argue that patients may use their complaints of pain as a way of obtaining attention and concern. They may even rely on it as a predictable means of eliciting a response. However, it is important that patients' complaints should always be trusted. A patient's use of such means to attract attention from the hospice staff, indicates that the patient has some unmet needs that require immediate intervention. The hospice staff should not suspect their patients' intentions. Instead, they have a responsibility to perform sensitive and accurate assessment to determine their needs.

Provide intervention to promote comfort

It is important to provide comfort for hospice patients. Despite the importance of comfort in cancer care, the term is often used without definition. Recent efforts to define the concept of comfort and the experiences of patients' comfort [53, 58] have provided an important beginning to understanding this complex concept. Health care professionals can help patients to restore their bodily functions by providing them with physical comfort such as positioning and administration of appropriate medication. In principle, adequate drugs should be given to dying patients to prevent pain from occurring, rather than to control it once it is presented. [16] According to cancer patients, comfort care is a familiar environment, safety, quality of life, normalcy, and a positive mental disposition. [54] The withholding of life support, including nutrition and hydration can also be the treatment of choice in comfort care. [33]

Meanwhile, Bottorff, Gogag and Engelberg-Lotzkar[55] suggest eight comforting interactions which are worthy of consideration. These interventions are 1) gentle humour, 2) physical comfort, 3) providing information, 4) emotionally supportive statements, 5) choices regarding care, 6) social exchange, 7) increasing proximity, and 8) touch. In addition, appropriate use of psychological counselling, psycho-stimulants, antidepressants, anxiolytics, and other drugs may be included.[56] It is essential to involve the patients in this process and work out their care plans individually. In this way, patients are enabled to have a sense of control over their future and their quality of life.

Provide information and education on pain and suffering

Regular patient education programmes on pain and suffering are essential for Chinese patients with terminal cancer. Many Chinese have misconceptions about cancer, pain, and pain management. Thus the aims of these educational programmes are to provide them with appropriate information and assist them to become involved in the care plan. It is important that patients take up the responsibility to report their problems. The content of the programme should also include basic knowledge about Chinese medical treatment. Small group interactive learning methods such as the reflective learning method are recommended because most Chinese patients are not used to active participation. Health educators can provide health information, covering a wide range of topics such as health, illness experiences, and life values, on an individual basis. In this way, the patients are helped to control and modify their environment to promote comfort.

Provide sensitive and compassionate care for patients with spiritual suffering

It is important to provide sensitive and compassionate care for patients who experience spiritual suffering such as depression and loneliness. This is not a time for superficial assessment, or for unrealistic recommendations that are not directly negotiated with the dying patients. Rather, it is a time for in-depth exploration, such as checking

Table 6.5
Summary of Being free from pain and suffering (Comfort)

Related issues	Clinical implications
1. Being free from pain • Cancer pain • Total pain • Ineffective pain management 2. Being free from suffering • Concepts of suffering • The multi-dimensional suffering 3. Unresolved pain and suffering • Euthanasia • Suicide	Goal: Provide patients with comfort from a holistic approach 1. Effective management of pain and suffering 2. Provide interventions to promote comfort. 3. Provide information and education on pain and suffering. 4. Provide sensitive and compassionate care for patients with spiritual suffering.

patients' understanding of their condition, experience of the present, views of the future, and knowledge of the treatment options available. Suicide triggered by a treatable depression, or by misconception about the reality of a patient's condition, should clearly be prevented. [57]

Summary

Findings of previous studies and this research have indicated that a significant proportion of dying patients experience serious pain, despite the availability of effective pharmacological and other opinions for relieving most pain. Consistent with some local studies, such as Yeung,[10] a considerable number of hospice patients in this research experienced pain and suffering. A majority of patients experienced moderate to uncontrollable pain. Meanwhile, all patients presented one or more symptoms and close to half of them had three or more symptoms. Consequently, about half of the patients hoped to be free from pain and fourteen patients preferred not to have any suffering. These findings also reflect the complexities and diversity of these personal experiences. Both pain and suffering should be understood as multi-dimensional phenomena. These patients' pain and suffering were not well controlled, a fact to which immediate attention should be drawn. Further, the research's emphasis on multi-dimensional experiences of pain and suffering has justifiably included other elements of Good Death. These elements are: maintaining social relations, experiencing personal control, and spiritual contentment.

The control of pain (and suffering) has always been an integral and crucial part of the hospice effort. As there have not been any previous studies to understand the experience of pain and suffering of hospice patients, it was not possible to assess the extent of improvement since the commencement of the hospice movement in some Asian countries such as Hong Kong. The findings of this research present a preliminary but pessimistic picture of the experience of the contemporary hospice patients. I also identified the factors that contributed to ineffective pain and suffering management, which could come from the patients, nurses, medical practitioners, and/or their communication. When hospice patients' pain and suffering were unresolved, they might request euthanasia or attempt suicide. These findings present a new challenge and area of debate for health care professionals in end-of-life care.

Thus, the clinical implications aim to provide comfort for hospice patients from a holistic approach. Providing cancer patients with adequate comfort is indeed an imperative attribute of a Good Death. Some interventions are suggested. 1) Accurate and culturally sensitive assessment with validated tools as an essential starting point. 2) Some research-based comfort interventions and evaluation must follow. 3) It is important to teach cancer patients about pain and suffering so that they can take responsibility for reporting their problems promptly. 4) Specific attention and care should be taken with patients experiencing spiritual suffering. This aspect of care needs to be attended to without delay. Likewise, interventions that promote hope, a sense of control, connectedness, and completion will also provide patients with comfort.

7
Maintaining social relations (Connectedness)

Introduction

EVERYONE HAS THE need for connectedness and person-to-person contact. [1-2] Mutual connectedness is characterised by trust, compassion, and shared consciousness within a caring environment. [3] Hence, there must be consistent caring, listening, and focusing on the patients.[4] Supportive social connectedness was important for the hospice patients, because it supported them in facing death, sustained their hope, [5-6] and offered them social and spiritual comfort. [7] Maintaining social relations was a crucial element in achieving a Good Death. Such relationships supported them in sustaining hope and affirming the meaning of life. This chapter presents my findings on maintaining social relations. Since the patients were staying in the hospice unit, they needed to establish good relations with the hospice staff, who assisted them in restoring their health and making adjustments. Undoubtedly, they needed to maintain good relations with their families because they needed to feel that they were valued and loved. I further explore these issues by examining the factors that affected these relations.

Connectedness with the hospice staff: Need for assistance

'Maintaining social relations' refers to the extent to which the dying person is in control of the social self and intimate social relations. Connectedness begins in one's self and is nurtured in relationships. May [8] explains that 'the self is always born and grows in interpersonal relationships'. Interpersonal relationships have the potential to be therapeutic; with meaningful interactions. [4] Therapeutic relationships can facilitate coping and problem solving, and can be existentially nurturing. [9] The hospice patients had to establish relationships with the hospice staff and their families according to this direction. This finding is similar to that of a local research on people with nasopharyngeal cancer. These participants were satisfied with the social support that came from health care professionals, followed by family and friends. [10]

As one approaches death, one's physical condition may deteriorate gradually. Therefore, the patients tended to require a lot of assistance to adjust to their spiritual, physical, and psychosocial changes. Several patients reported that they had received assistance from the hospice staff. Twelve were assisted by health care professionals. Eleven patients had received assistance from health care assistants and their friends. Five patients identified their fellow patients as helping them, and some patients were helped by volunteers and religious visitors. Undoubtedly, they needed to maintain a sense of connectedness with the members of the hospice team, who may have replaced their families as the primary caregivers.

On the other hand, seven patients felt extremely discontented and frustrated because they were not able to maintain supportive social relations. If dying people are constantly abandoned by people around them, they may experience a social death. [11] A typical example of the phenomenon was a drug addict who did not have any contact with his family, while his relationship with the hospice staff was poor. Sadly, he ended his life by committing suicide.

Health care professionals

When the patients became extremely weak and fatigued physically, they needed special assistance in every aspect of their daily activities. Therefore, some patients were most immediately concerned about their relationships with the staff in the hospice unit. Quite often, patients appreciated the assistance they received from medical practitioners who offered them hope for a cure or for physical restoration. Some patients agreed that the nurses had also contributed to the delivery of quality care.

The medical practitioner is good. He tries to keep me comfortable.

The medical practitioners, nurses, and health care assistants all help me. Nurses come to see me often. They help feeding the patients.

They can help to reduce my pain ... .

The medical social worker has helped me most because he found me a place in the nursing home.

Nurses deliver drugs, feed patients, make beds, change patients' clothes, and carry out clerical work. They may talk to the patients for about ten minutes every day.

While some patients expressed their gratitude to the medical practitioners and nurses, some pointed out that they had not received adequate assistance. Consistent with Yeung's [12] findings, the hospice patients were rather disappointed that health care professionals were not always available and were not willing to listen.

The medical practitioners and nurses are busy here. They have no time to talk to me. I wish they could spend time talking to me.
The nurses are young. They have little life experience. I have been sitting out (of my bed) for a long time. Nurses may want to help us. They promised to do something for me, but they might forget about it later.

They have no time (to counsel me). Sometimes I ask but sometimes I do not know what to ask.

Health care assistants

The hospice team is often said to be multidisciplinary. The team consists of medical practitioners, nurses, social workers, clinical psychologists, physiotherapists, and occupational therapists. Of equal importance, hospice patients also require a lot of care from 'non-professionals' such as health care assistants, fellow patients, friends, volunteers, and religious visitors. It is important not to exclude their contributions in maintaining the quality of hospice care. The patients found that their relationship with health care assistants was important.

Today, the health care assistants take up several nurses' clinical duties. These duties include charting patients' fluid intake and output, taking patients' body temperature, lifting patients and changing their position, feeding, and assisting patients in bathing. Significantly, assistance from health care assistants was important as they had frequent and direct contact with the patients. The following is an illustration. Mr. K was seventy- years old with cancer of the lung. He was slim, weak, and dependent. One afternoon, three volunteers from Comfort Care Concern Group visited him, as well as some other hospice patients. Comfort Care Concern Group is a charitable agent that offers hospice and bereavement services to cancer patients and their families. Shortly afterwards, this patient was attended by a student social worker. He was tired from having so many visitors. At that time, Mr. K was in severe pain. He did not inform his visitors that he was in pain, but health care assistant. The following are other examples that emphasise the assistance the patients received from health care assistants.

> Yes, the health care assistants are very helpful.
> Yes, of course, they (health care assistants) lift the patients, feed them, take their temperature, carry out urine testing, bathe them, provide urinals, deliver food, and fill in the intake and output chart.

> I often ask the health care assistant to help me. Some patients do not say thank you to those who help them. Some nurses told me that they were busy ... I do not move a lot because it feels painful. The pain is quite severe. I do not feel the need to tell the nurses. I do not want to give them any trouble. I feel uneasy bothering people and I hope I can

help myself. I feel bad having to ask for people's help to go to the toilet. Today I have had my urine catheter clamped.

Fellow patients

Understandably, fellow patients can offer immediate support to the patients. The patients may be more empathetic with each other because they have had similar experiences. For example, the patient who committed suicide shared his opinions about death and good death only with his fellow patients. Another elderly patient insisted on buying a packet of biscuits for his fellow patient when the food-trolley came round. He said he wanted to express his thanks to his fellow patient who had assisted him when he most needed help.

> Yes, he often comes to my bedside. Sometimes I need somebody to close the windows, for example. Sometimes nobody comes to help us ...

Volunteers

Volunteers are also important members in a hospice care team. Some of them belong to the hospital volunteer group, while some come from charity agencies. Among the patients, a young woman with cancer of the pancreas mentioned that her Christian friends had helped her to change her philosophy of life. She became more accepting of her illness. Another example was a forty-eight-year-old single man who was particularly keen to talk about his help from the volunteers. He was suffering from lung cancer. He developed metastasis of the spine five months after his diagnosis. He shared with me his appreciation of a volunteer who had helped him to accept his illness and explore the meaning of life.

> A volunteer accompanied me to Queen Mary Hospital for radiotherapy for four days. She worked full-time, but she helped me. I was very grateful for her kindness. She did not have anything to eat or drink while I had the radiotherapy treatment. I was moved, and thankful for her help.

Factors affecting connectedness with hospice staff

The two main factors, which affect the maintenance of the hospice patient's connectedness with hospice staff, are namely social and financial status.

Social status

Individual attitudes to and experiences of death are largely affected by society.[13] Traditionally, the Chinese consider the social status of a person to be an important social value. This attitude can be traced back historically. The ancient Chinese government used feudalism to govern the country. People were classified into four social classes: educated people, farmers, manual labourers, and businessmen. The educated people were considered the most intelligent and knowledgeable. Therefore, they were selected (via imperial examinations) to run the country. As a consequence of this differentiation in status, people of different social classes would have different rituals (such as funeral ceremonies). According to Confucianism, one must act according to one's social status (let the prince act the prince, the minister the minister, the father the father, and the son the son). This is called 'establishing one's character'.[14] Chinese communities in Taiwan, Hong Kong, and Singapore have undergone rapid socio-economic changes in recent decades. These changes have influenced some Chinese attitudes towards death and their preparation for death.[15] However, some cultural values, such as rituals and funeral arrangements, are maintained,[16] and the emphasis on social status continues. People from two social categories seemed to have relatively lower social status in the hospice unit. The first category was drug addicts and the second category was people who were involved in 'illegal trade'. The following description is an illustration.

Mr. C was fifty-seven years old with lung cancer. He was a drug addict with no family attachments, and his friends were mostly drug addicts. He was considered a difficult patient and therefore the hospice staff did not generally accept him. The staff discovered that he continued to use 'drugs' in the toilet. Such social behaviour was not acceptable under hospital policy. In addition, he sold 'drugs' to other fellow patients in the hospital. Therefore, most of the hospice staff disliked him. For example, he told me that his requests for assistance were either unattended or delayed. One day, he got dressed ready to join other patients in an outdoor activity. However, his medical practitioner refused to give him permission to go, and Mr. C was upset about this. He experienced social isolation and his feelings of loneliness were intensified. Consequently, his self-esteem and self-image were low and he felt helpless at times. Moreover, he lost a sense of control and hope for his condition.

At the same time, another patient who was a drug addict was perceived as an acceptable, good person by the hospice staff. He was gentle and easy-going. He had social support both from his wife and children. During our interview, he kept crying because he regretted not having fulfilled the duties of a filial son. His mother had recently died and he missed her very much. It was apparent that he had 'an acceptable style of living while dying', [17] hence, the hospice staff accepted him. Thus it can be seen that the social status of hospice patients affects their connectedness with hospice staff.

Financial status

The previous chapter discussed the bearing that patients' financial status had on their chance of alternative therapy and consequently the hope for a cure. Financial status also influenced their preparations for death. Having cancer always has an impact on the patients' relationships with their families. Their relationships can be disrupted by redistribution of roles and social isolation. [18] For example, younger patients had lost their earning power, and this would create some financial consequences. Older patients were often unaware of government social welfare benefits. Some did not know that they were entitled to the benefits and some felt ashamed of receiving government financial assistance. Some patients felt embarrassed about being dependent. Therefore, just a few patients discussed their financial situation openly because most of them were financially dependent. Their financial status had definitely had an effect on their self-image and self-concept. Consequently, they might lose their confidence to maintain social relationships with hospice staff and their families. For example, a few patients felt 'worthless' and 'hopeless' because they were old and poor. Some of them even lost the hope to continue living.

Social isolation and disconnection can create social suffering. [19]

Most of the patients had lived with their families before being admitted to the hospice unit, so they had to rely on them for financial support. Consistent with some previous studies, [12,20-21] a majority of the patients was elderly and the mean age of the sample was sixty-seven. Also, most elderly patients belonged to the socially deprived group. They received a monthly disability allowance of HK$1,200–2,400. Only two patients could afford to seek alternative therapies. However, some patients did not feel comfortable relying on government support. The following are some examples.

A sixty-eight-year-old man refused to apply to the government for financial assistance until he had used up his savings. He had been a businessman but had closed down his shop several years ago. His brothers were wealthy and they could give him financial support if he wanted. He stated that he did not want his brothers to know that he had applied for financial support from the Social Welfare Department. He felt upset at having lost his financial independence.

> I thought I had some (money). Only those who are poor have to rely on government assistance. I have spent a lot of money on alternative treatment because I often consult the private practitioners. I have a flat in Kowloon. Since 1992, I have been supported financially by the government. They help me with several thousand dollars (a month), which is not much. If I need any (financial) help, my brother will help me. My brother does not know that I receive support from the Social Welfare services. The medical social worker will apply for a place in the nursing home for me. I ask myself what I have done to deserve this ...

> My daughter-in-law said to me, 'I have no money, how can I care for you?' They said they have no money. I am useless because I am getting old. The most important thing is money. It's no good to be old and have no money.

Another elderly patient, who had cancer of the colon, worried that his savings might not be enough to live on until he died. He had previously worked in a bank and received a lump sum on his retirement, but he did not expect he would live to be eighty years old. Therefore, he was upset about his financial status and he felt a sense of worthlessness.

> You are right. I feel worthless and pessimistic. In the past, I could

read two newspapers. Now I cannot remember the words. I cannot remember anything. How can I read newspapers if I forget the words? I have lost all my memory. I could read some good things before. Since I have had this illness for the past two or three years, I just follow what people say. Now, I do not have my own opinion. Everything is all right, OK, OK. Also, my handwriting used to be quite good and I used to compose poems. People used to come and ask me to teach them, but everybody is better than me now. I feel that I am useless. My brain cannot function well.

The financial status of the patients certainly affected their social connectedness with hospice staff, their social status, and their perceived capability to control their lives and social relations. It also affected the patients' sense of hope, comfort, completion, and subsequently, the quality of their dying processes.

Connectedness with the family: Feeling valued

Cancer has often been described as a family disease and its impact on all of the individuals surrounding the family member with cancer is recognised. [22] Because the role of family carers in chronic and terminal illness has become more significant, good family relationships are increasingly important. According to Confucian teachings, to maintain harmonious family relationships is a moral obligation. Even today, many Chinese are taught to fulfil this social obligation and value family connectedness. [15] Most Chinese people still maintain the traditional definition of family, that is, 'an individual of blood relationship'. [22] Confucian beliefs encourage an enmeshed family system to perform multiple functions for ideological, social, and economic reasons. According to the Law of Kinship, there are five cardinal relations (ruler (or emperor)-subject, parent-child, spouses, siblings, and friends). In this way, family members are classified into a hierarchical structure according to age, gender, and status. Their interaction patterns are determined during important family occasions such as weddings and the death of a family member. [23]

Therefore, it was not surprising that a majority of patients were mostly concerned about their families. This finding is consistent with some reports on hospice care such as Shum's [24] report. A majority of patients hoped to be valued by their families. More than two-thirds of the patients felt they were valued by their family and had maintained good family relationships.

Strong family connectedness provided psychosocial and spiritual comfort to the hospice patients. For instance, their families showed their hope and affection by visiting the patients regularly and frequently. They also prepared them nutritious food. During the visits, most patients appreciated their families' homemade soup. The preparation of Chinese soup for the patients could have many socio-cultural meanings. First, the family hoped that the patients would recover by drinking the therapeutic soup. The Chinese have traditionally placed a high value on health promotion by way of eating, exercises, massage, and meditation. [25] Second, the preparation was time-consuming and possibly expensive, because some ingredients might be costly. Therefore, preparing soup for one's family was a characteristic way of showing affection and caring in Chinese culture. This finding is consistent with the findings of Lee and Cheung's [26] research, in which over ninety per cent of their participants prepared tonic soup as part of their daily meals.

The hospice patients did not wish to become a burden on their families. They learnt to accept that their families could not visit them regularly. At the same time, they valued family connectedness and hoped their families would visit them frequently and spend more time with them, especially as they approached death. Thus, one-third of the patients clearly indicated that they wished to have company when they died. In this way, they could experience some degree of personal control and hope in their lives ahead.

Relationships with spouses

Studies in oncology related to family care-giving have generally found that approximately seventy per cent of primary family caregivers are spouses, and approximately twenty per cent are children (mainly daughters or daughters-in-law). [27] In this research, forty-nine per cent of the patients were married, twenty-seven per cent were widowed, fifteen per cent were divorced, and nine per cent were single. Some patients were better able to accept their condition because they received support from their spouses. Of the patients, seven men and two women had supportive spouses. Four men specified their wives as their main concern. It was evident that these patients experienced more acceptances during the dying process. The following is an example.

> Cancer is a tumour. I do not know exactly what (a) tumour is. I do not understand it, because cancer is incurable. It will lead to death ... I cried with my husband. They announced it (the 'bad news') in the ward, and there was nobody else around ... Now that he has to do all the housework... I got married at the age of twenty and I am fifty-six now. I have two sons, one daughter, and one grandson. My husband looks after our home well. He just retired last year, so he can help me.

For some families, the period before a patient's death was a time for connection and resolution of outstanding conflict. For others, this time aggravated long-standing family problems that continued to distress the dying person. Some patients were fortunate to maintain connectedness with their families, but some were less fortunate. Several patients reported that their marital relationships were not happy. These patients often suffered emotionally and spiritually. Their sense of hope and control was also relatively low.

A seventy-year-old woman with cancer of the lung angrily criticised her husband's wrongdoing during the interview. According to this patient, her husband was irresponsible. He spent most of his time with other women and did not care for her and their children. Worse still, she had not maintained harmonious relationships with her parents and siblings. Therefore, she had to cope with many problems by herself. She was extremely disappointed with her husband, so she did not allow him to visit her. Her conflict with her husband continued to distress her until she died.

> Those men who sell jade jewellery are not good people (referring to her husband). They like gambling and prostitutes. They are bad! They only spend time with other women. My husband did not care about my son and me. He just spent time with other women. He did not come to sign the consent form for my operation (caesarean section) when I gave birth to my smallest son. His birth weight was over ten pounds... I have no connection with my parents and siblings now because they have gone overseas. They are all wealthy and I am poor. I do not like to be looked down on... I am angry with him (my

husband). I don't want to see him, ever! I saw his back and knew that he had come to visit me. I feel that life is difficult for me. Yes, I cannot forgive him.

Another example was an elderly patient, who felt sad about his poor relationship with his family. He was open and willing to discuss many issues concerning his life and his opinions of death with me. He married twice, but he regretted that he would die without his family members around him although he had two families. He had five adult children with his first wife, but their relationship was poor. He had had a lot of disagreements with his first wife and children. His second wife left him a few years previously, and they did not have any children. He was most upset when his second wife left him, and decided to close down his shop. He said bitterly, 'Basically, I have no children'. The depth of his disappointment was reflected by his preference of where to die and his funeral arrangements. He wanted to stay away from his mother and brothers. Therefore, he hoped to die in the hospice unit or nursing home. Further, he wished to donate his body to the medical school. An alternative was to consider cremation, because he predicted that his children would not attend his grave. His assumption that his descendants would not attend his grave made him very sad. His intense sadness was closely related to his failure to maintain connectedness with his family before and after his death.

Coincidentally, two patients who attempted suicide and three patients who requested euthanasia were either widows or widowers. Apparently, these patients did not receive any support from their spouses. Therefore, they may not have been optimistic about achieving their desirable Good Death if their social connectedness with their children was not particularly strong or they did not have any other source of family support. As a clinical implication, if patients do not maintain harmonious relationships with their families, health care professionals may need to find out if they have other forms of social support. This is important in caring for hospice patients.

Relationships with children

Traditionally, the extended family played a crucial role in Chinese culture.[28] The whole family witnessed death of a family member and accepted death and their responsibility to participate. Some elderly people prepared their coffins and stored them in their houses before they died. The family often surrounded the dying person's bed until he or she died. [17, 29] 'When a Chinese patient is near death, his kinfolk flood the space around his bed and no staff member is surprised by their ritual preparations for his death or by their loud lamentations after death occurs' (p.81).[17]

The cultural value of family connectedness is further reinforced by some traditional Chinese beliefs, such as ancestor worship and filial piety, which originate from the teachings of Confucius. Ancestor worship is widely practised as a way of showing respect to elders who have died and seeking blessings from the deceased. For the Chinese, the line of descendants is treated as an extension of the self and a form of immortality. [30] According to one Chinese idiom, 'Filial piety is the first of the hundred virtues'. This saying reflects the importance of being filial in Chinese communities. According to Confucius, filial piety (*xiao*) does not refer merely to social support for parents. It consists of serving them while they are alive, burying them when they die, and making offerings to them after death, according to the established rules. These established rules are considered rites and rituals in Chinese culture. [31] Confucius further explained: 'We support our dogs and our horses; without reverence, what is there to distinguish one from the other?' Filial piety is a highly virtuous and idealistic representation of Chinese culture. It implies strong devotion to the dying parent. Dying people may bless their descendants with future prosperity and success. [15] 'The attributes of inter-generation relationships governed by filial piety are structural, enduring, and invariable across situations within Chinese culture'. [32] Therefore the older Chinese patients valued filial piety more than the younger ones did.

A majority of patients reported that they were mostly concerned about their children even when they were already adults. About half of the patients indicated that they were loved and cared for by their children. It was also noted that female patients expressed their love to their children more openly.

> I want love and a good relationship with my children. One health care assistant told me that my son was so good to me because he washed my face. My children have paid their filial duty. My son gave me a massage. He washed my face and he prepared soup for me yesterday.

I am feeling much better. They have come to visit me and they have not stopped visiting. My daughter-in-law came in the morning and I feel much better.

An elderly patient valued his children's filial affection **more** than any treasure.

If my children do not show their filial affection when (I am) alive, it will be useless (for them) to prepare me a coffin made of diamonds (when I die).

Nevertheless, some patients also identified that it was difficult to maintain a continuous connectedness with the family when a family member had been ill for a long time. Both parties were likely to feel exhausted and under stress. A common Chinese saying reflects the situation: 'When you have been ill for a long time, you may not find a filial son'. Moreover, there is evidence that filial piety is on the decline and no longer mandates the same degree of absolute practice in contemporary Chinese communities as it once did. [32] Furthermore, with most deaths now occurring in old age, the death of old people is undervalued. [33] Thus, some patients were not satisfied with the support they received from their families, in particular, their children. They complained that they had little contact with their children and that their relationships had become distant. Six patients were unhappy that their children did not care for them enough and some regretted not having an immediate family member in Hong Kong.

Factors affecting connectedness with the family

Gender

The Chinese family is essentially male-dominated. The father-son relationship is the key to the family structure, and the eldest child (preferably the eldest son) is expected to accompany the patient passing through the final stages of life as an expression of filial piety.

[15] Therefore, the death of a man without any surviving sons is regarded as a tragedy. Likewise, a man who dies unmarried or without an heir has a reasonable chance of being worshipped as an ancestor either by his brothers' descendants or by adopted sons. However, the soul of a woman who dies unmarried may not be traditionally treated in this way. Therefore, the social background of a person, including factors such as gender, may influence the quality of his/her dying process.

Field, Hockey, and Small [34] support the theory that there are gender differences in the patterns of care giving. Female relatives (spouses and daughters) often provide the bulk of the 'lay' care of the dying. In addition, since the relationship between mother and daughter is often closer than relationship between mother-in-law and daughter-in-law [35] the patients tended to have closer relationships with their daughters than with their daughters-in-law.

For example, one elderly woman expressed the wish that her son were her daughter so that she could experience more intimate sharing. Therefore, she was very disappointed when her son became impatient with her, and her feeling of social abandonment increased. Because of this, and the progression of her illness, which intensified her pain, the patient asked the medical practitioner for euthanasia.

A few patients continued to maintain traditional Chinese values. Having a son remains an important social value in some Chinese families. A woman recalled her struggle to have a son, and felt that seeing him married was her 'unfinished social obligations'.

> I was over thirty when I got pregnant with my son. I felt embarrassed. I had my son when I was over thirty. My two daughters were over ten years old. The old lady (mother-in-law) teased me for not having a son. She was unkind. She said that I was just like a chicken with 'worms' (so that I could not bear a son). So I was keen to give birth to a son.

Later, when her condition deteriorated, she was keen to see her son marry before she died. She hoped to complete her social obligations as a mother.

Today, social values in Chinese communities may have changed in that having a daughter is as good as having a son, if he or she practices filial piety. Furthermore, there was no observable difference in the needs of the unmarried and married patients.

Effective communication

If the patients maintained connectedness with their families and they felt that they were valued in the family, they might develop a sense of hope, comfort, and reason to live. This connectedness can be facilitated by openness in communication. Openness also allows better preparation for death and spiritual contentment. It further 'prevents poorly considered decisions being made during (a) medical crisis'. [36] Although criticisms have been made that Chinese patients and their family members often express their emotions in subtle and non-verbal ways, [37] a few patients said that the illness experience had substantiated their family relationships. They could communicate and share with more openness than previously. The following is an example.

A thirty-four-year-old woman, recognised the need for her family's support after she developed cancer. She was divorced and worked as an accountant's clerk. I interviewed her five days before her death. She emphasised that she came to know the significance of her family's support after she developed cancer. She had preferred not to express her feelings before, but had now become more willing to share with others. She acknowledged that her family had openly given her tender loving care. She began to accept her condition and to strive for peace of mind. She had clearly changed her philosophy of life. She felt happy and laughed during the interview. Sharing and listening becomes of the utmost importance for the dying person who is struggling to accept his or her own mortality.

It was evident that the hospice patients needed to communicate many things to their loved ones, from simple practical issues to complex emotional and spiritual concerns. [38] Even if the questions and problems could not be resolved, the act of sharing would relieve the patient's inner tension and fear of isolation. This was also a strategy for psychological adjustment, which facilitated the patients' acceptance of changes in their bodies and body image.

The family connectedness of Chinese hospice patients can facilitate spiritual contentment. From the Confucian perspective, death is the continuous remembrance and affection of ancestors. Death does not discontinue the relationship of the departed with the living; but merely changes it to a different level. [39] Intimately connected with ancestral worship is the practice of filial piety. Many Chinese, such as the dying patients, believed that the living and the dying continued

Table 7.1
Categories and significant statements of Maintaining social relations (Connectedness)

Categories	Significant statements
Connectedness with the hospice staff	They can help to reduce my pain ... (13, p.13).
	The medical social worker has helped me most because he found me a place in the nursing home (5, p.3).
	Nurses deliver drugs, feed patients, make beds, change patients' clothes, and carry out clerical work. They may talk to the patients for about ten minutes every day (7, p.9).
	The medical practitioners, nurses, and health care assistants all help me. Nurses come to see me often. They help feeding the patients (8, p.4).
	The medical practitioner is good. He tries to keep me comfortable (12, p.4).
	A volunteer accompanied me to Queen Mary Hospital for radiotherapy for four days... I was very grateful for her kindness. She did not have anything to eat or drink while I had the radiotherapy treatment. I was moved, and thankful for her help (16).
Connectedness with the family	I want love and a good relationship with my children. One health care assistant told me that my son was so good to me because he washed my face. My children have paid their filial duty. My son gave me a massage. He washed my face and he prepared soup for me yesterday (11, p.10).
	Cancer is a tumour. I do not know exactly what (a) tumour is. I do not understand it, because cancer is incurable. It will lead to death ... I cried with my husband. They announced it (the 'bad news') in the ward, and there was nobody else around ... Now that he has to do all the housework... I got married at the age of twenty and I am fifty-six now. I have two sons, one daughter, and one grandson. My husband looks after our home well. He just retired last year, so he can help me (8, p.3-4).

their relationships through the practice of filial piety and ancestor worship. In other words, the function of such caring relationship offers spiritual comfort because it enables transcendence of the present situation for higher meaning and purpose, establishing connectedness and enabling hope.[40] Therefore, patients who maintained social connectedness may also experience a sense of spiritual contentment, thereby achieving their desired Good Death.

Clinical implications

Goal:
Facilitate patients in maintaining connectedness with hospice staff and the family

Identify personal and social resources

Hospice patients often receive emotional and social support from their families and the larger social network. However, the understanding of social support is limited, despite the attempts of some local studies.[10, 41] Nevertheless, some validated instruments can be used to assess hospice patients' social support. [42] The items for assessment include the following: whether the patients have someone to talk to, someone to share hopes and fears with, and someone to have a good time with. It is also essential for health care professionals to conduct a detailed family assessment so that they can facilitate patients' and their families' use of personal and community resources. [12] These patients should also be encouraged to identify their own needs, direct their own care, and seek to engage with other patients who are in similar situations to their own. [43]

Facilitate communication between family members and patients

It may be impossible to care for every dying person in equally satisfactory ways. Hospice professionals may not be aware that they may have prejudices against certain social groups of patients. Therefore, they need to be sensitive and aware of their social and ethical values and attitudes towards dying patients in order to help them die a dignified death. They can maintain openness in communication and willingness to listen. They can also affirm their commitment to support and spend time with patients and their families in the approach to death. [44] The patients should have ultimate control over the involvement of their families, for each family member may have beliefs and expectations about the patient, the disease, and their treatment.

Strengthen the connectedness of the patient, family, and hospice staff

Hospice care aims to achieve a connected relationship.[45] 'Connecting' refers to the rapport between a patient and a health caregiver in which the patient perceives the true caring of the health caregiver who is listening to, understanding, supporting, and encouraging the patient as a human being. [46] In this relationship, health care professionals can intercede for the patients, act as a buffer for them, and act as their advocates.[47] 'Such relationship becomes one of the spirit, of their shared humanity'(p.26). [46] Sharing the hospice philosophy can strengthen the connectedness between the patient, family, and the hospice staff. A typical example is to assist the Chinese family to be present in the final hours. [15] Some families regretted not being able to 'send (their family member) off' on their last journey. Health care professionals need to be sensitive and accurate in assessing the signs of approaching death if they hope to help families be with the patients. For example, nurses can inform the relatives or a person of the patient's choice, in the final hours.

Table 7.2
Summary of Maintaining social relations (connectedness)

Related issues	Clinical implications
1. Connectedness with hospice staff • Health care professionals • Health care assistants • Fellow patients • Volunteers	Goal: Facilitate patients in maintaining connectedness with hospice staff and the family 1. Identify personal and social resources
2. Factors affecting connectedness with hospice staff • Social status • Financial status	2. Facilitate communication between family members and patients 3. Strengthen the connectedness between the family and the hospice staff.
3. Connectedness with the family • Relationship with spouse • Relationship with children	
4. Factors affecting connectedness with the family • Gender • Effective communication	

Summary

Maintaining social relations was an important element in dying a Good Death. There are two main types of relationship. First, patients needed to establish connectedness with the hospice staff. About half of the patients needed assistance from the hospice staff to control their pain and symptoms and to make some adjustments. Most of them acknowledged the help they had received from the medical practitioners. A few thanked the nurses, health care assistants, fellow patients, and volunteers. Several patients specified assistance from health care assistants, who also played an important role in controlling the quality of hospice care for the patients. The social and financial status of the patients had an influence their relationships with the hospice staff. It is essential that health care professionals are sensitive and take care not to have social prejudice against their patients.

Second, the hospice patients felt that they needed family connectedness. The value of the family relationship has long been a characteristic of Chinese culture and no other relationship can replace it. About two-thirds of the patients maintained connectedness with their families. Some patients reported that their filial children supported them, and some were happy with their spouses. Correspondingly, some patients indicated explicitly who they wished to be with when they died. Family relationships may be affected by the gender of the patients or family members. Also, effective communication is significantly important in maintaining family connectedness for the hospice patients interviewed.

Accordingly, the goal of clinical work should focus on facilitating patients to maintain social connectedness by: 1) helping to identify patients' personal and social resources; 2) facilitating their communication with their family, caregivers, and hospice staff; and 3) strengthening the connectedness between the patient, family, and hospice staff. Sharing the hospice philosophy can further strengthen their connectedness. In addition, there is a need for ongoing education for hospice staff, particularly health care assistants, to deepen their understanding of hospice care.

8
Experiencing personal control (Control)

Introduction

CONTROL IS THE ability to make something behave exactly as you want it to behave. Control is the autonomy to make decisions. When individuals who are terminally ill are dependent on others, their personal control is often threatened. Loss of control will produce feelings of fear, anxiety, depression, guilt, hopelessness, loneliness, and confusion. [1-2] From the findings of this research, hospice patients identified that experiencing a sense of personal control is important for a Good Death. This chapter presents my findings on experiencing personal control. The patients identified two important decisions in which they hoped to participate. First, they hoped to have a choice where to live. Second, they hoped not to die alone.

The concepts of personal control

Control is the ability to regulate or influence intended outcomes through selective responding. 'Perceived control refers to expectations of being able to participate in making decisions and engaging in actions in order to obtain desirable consequences and avoid unfavourable ones'.[3] Therefore, personal control involves an attitudinal component (belief in the right of others to personal control), and a behavioural component (freedom from constraints on their capacity to act).[4] Some caregivers suggest that dying persons should have the right to define their needs and choices.[5] They may have a sense of participation in physical care [5-6] or a sense of having control, [5] which is essential for dying a Good Death. They 'preferred to have as much control as possible in making decisions concerning care rather than its opposite of having others make decisions' (p.26).[5] In this way, the autonomy of dying people is respected. [7-8] Dying people maintain a similar view of personal control. Weisman [9-10] stresses repeatedly that dying individuals must not lose control.

The dying person does, as much as possible, choose to set conditions on what kind of death is wanted. Implicit is the imperative for the person to retain a sense of control until the very end. [9-15] Several researchers[16-17] agree that a Good Death is one in which the person experiences some degree of mastery or control. The shift to the palliative mode has moved the power base in the relationship between health care professionals and patients, from professional domination to increased personal control by patients. The emphasis on patients' personal control as the priority is clear.

Thus, experiencing personal control refers to the state where the dying person is in control of his or her life journey, including the environment where he or she will die. That is, the individual will decide where and with whom he or she will die. For example, they may have a peaceful death at home [18] and they may have significant others (family and/ or friends) around them[5, 18] when they die. For the hospice patient, the nature of the setting and the experiences of fellow patients are also relevant to achieving a Good Death. [19] Some hospice patients in this research may not have verbalised their wish to have a sense of control explicitly, but may have used other ways to express the need for control.

Several patients had asserted their right to be involved in making decisions on various aspect of their care. They frequently said they hoped to make decisions on how, where, and with whom they died[19] when they were given an opportunity to express their needs. Some of them had not shared their hopes and wishes with their families or hospice staff, because they felt that their decisions would not be considered.

Having a choice about where to live

People live with the consequences of where they choose to die. Those who choose the hospice have a different set of challenges from those who choose to die at home, although neither route is easy. Similar to findings in other countries, the hospice patients in this research were expected to have an average life span of six to twelve months. [20-21] They would either return home or they would be transferred to a nursing home when their symptoms and pain were under control. Patients may commonly die in institutions, which can be hospitals, independent hospices, or nursing homes. A few may die at home. Some patients emphasised that they did not always have the opportunity to decide where they wanted to stay until they died. 'I have not discussed with my family about where I should stay'. Some health care professionals and relatives did not want the patients to have an open awareness of their condition, and such caregivers would avoid discussion of death-related issues with the patients.

Dying in an institution

For some people, the hospice movement appears to provide a more acceptable option for dying patients than the typical institutional setting. Patients prefer to stay in a restful and quiet environment[14, 22-23] which the hospice can provide. In addition, a positive experience of a fellow patient's death was typically helpful. Johnston and his colleagues[24] point out that hospice patients who have witnessed a death are found to be significantly less depressed on standardised measures of emotional distress.

Three patients in this research complained that there was nobody around to help them. Staff seemed to have no time for communication, as they were too busy. A few patients did not feel comfortable with seeing their fellow patients dying and they preferred to avoid the scene of death. While some patients expressed rather negative feelings about hospice care, some patients had contradictory opinions on the hospice services.

Most of the patients considered that staying in a hospice unit would be more convenient for the rest of the family. Therefore, about half of the patients preferred to stay in the hospice unit until they died. Five patients stated their wishes eagerly. A few said they were not willing to return to the nursing home because it had poor facilities. Patients who did not have a good connectedness with their families also preferred to die in the hospital. Not every patient had the courage to voice his or her wishes. Several patients indicated that they were not frequently involved in deciding where they lived (and died). The following is one example.

> Now that I do not like to die at home. Somebody said that I could go to a nursing home or hospital. I'd like to stay in the hospital because I would be happier here, it is air-conditioned. I'd like to stay away from home (in the last days). I do not feel like going back to see them (the relatives), because some of them may talk about me and make me feel bad. I do not like this. I don't want to see them. I don't want to trouble my family. I don't like people playing 'mah-jong' (a kind of gambling game). I prefer to die in a quiet place.

Most families preferred the patients to die in the hospice unit where they could have better health care. For example, they had no oxygen supply at home. Either the families could not satisfy their needs at home or the patients did not want to place an extra burden on their families. The other reason was that there was nobody to take care of the patients at home. In addition, some Chinese families may believe that if death occurred in hospital or in a hospice, the family was less likely to be disturbed by the patient's spirit. [25] Some of them were reluctant to be transferred or discharged from the hospice unit. For example, a seventy-four-year-old woman was waiting to be transferred to a nursing home. The patient and her family did not want to leave the hospice unit, and hoped to stay for a longer period. Unfortunately, their requests were rejected. The woman returned to the hospice unit after two days because her condition had deteriorated. She died a few days later.

A fifty-seven-year-old man, who was a drug addict, highlighted his feeling of powerlessness during his second interview. He expressed his frustration at being asked to leave the hospice unit when his condition started to show some stability. He insisted that he was not well but he had to leave the unit. His negative feelings were further aggravated by his awareness of his imminent death.

> Yes, you see that I am still dyspnoeic. They (the hospice staff) want me to leave. What can I do? I don't think that I will be going home at all. Mr. P (the medical social worker) said that the nursing home is lousy because it is crowded. Four people have to live in a small room ... Yes, they said I could come back.

According to the hospice staff, there were several difficulties in allowing the hospice patients to stay until they die. First, the health service aims to balance the cost and effectiveness of hospice services. Therefore, health administrators encouraged the patients to discharge themselves home or to a nursing home when their symptoms were under control. This may also improve hospice patients' morale and hope that they could 'recover'. Second, it is difficult to assess the progress of a dying person because it can change rapidly, with physical changes occurring almost daily. [26] Third, some patients did not welcome a return home.

The data regarding where the patients died was traced retrospectively from the hospital records. It was reported that thirty patients died in institutions. Two patients were still alive; one patient had returned to his hometown in mainland China to die. He did not regard Hong Kong as his 'home town' because he was not born there, so he returned to China and lived there until he died. I do not know whether this patient died at home or in the hospital. Several patients had clearly demonstrated their sense of control over where they died.

Dying at home

Traditionally, the Chinese prefer to die at home with family members around them. [18] Similarly, Hindu villagers (Pandits) stress the importance of the place of death and of culture. [13] Madan[13] points out that a Good Death is a great 'passing on', which does not just happen, but is achieved if one can let go of the life-breath in full consciousness, at a time and place of one's choosing. In general, Pandits prefer to die at home, in the house in which they have lived, because they regard their house as a microcosm of the universe. In this way, dying persons will experience a sense of control and dignity. In their view, hospice home services seem to be particularly suitable for supporting a person towards a Good Death.

Other studies, such as Catalan-Fernandez's [27] study on the Spanish, also emphasise that people should die at home because the quality of life is much better at home. Catalan-Fernandez[27] argues that hospitals are not the best places to die, as the technical assistance provided in the institution will increase the family's distress. He explains that if patients and relatives are to be provided with adequate care and support facilities, the experience of caring for patients at home will be more positive. Therefore, the provision of adequate social support facilities and care services is recommended.[15] In his personal experience with his father, Byock [26] asserts that confirming the place where he would die was an important decision for his father before his death. Once his father had decided to die at home, he knew there was nothing left undone. His life was in order. Love had been expressed and good-byes had been said.

Six patients said they hoped to die at home. Mr. W, a married man with several adult children, much preferred the idea of dying at home. However, he worried that his family did not like his preference.

> Home is my home. Those who have homes should stay at home (to die). It must be the case. It should be like that. Some have homes while some may not have homes. How can they go home? Nowadays, the environment at home is very complicated, for example, young people like to smoke. I mean, the youngsters smoke a lot. Some family members do not like it. If you want to go home, they may not like it ...

Several hospice patients expressed their wish to have a choice about where they died. Such behaviour may be considered as evidence of experiencing personal control. For example, a middle-aged patient made 'an unexpected preparation' a few days before his death. He packed up all his belongings and said that he was ready to go home. He prepared himself to die at home because he seemed to know that he would die very soon. Another elderly patient asked his children to take him home one week before his death. These patients exhibited some observable behaviours, described by Callahan and Kelly[28] as experiences of 'near-death awareness'. [28] This elderly patient died very unwillingly as he appeared restless and anxious in his last days. He seemed to have unfinished business. Clearly, some dying people could feel their imminent death and some wanted to die at home. Unfortunately, their requests to die at home were not always approved. The following are some examples of patients who were not welcome to die at home.

A sixty-one-year-old man with cancer of the lung, who developed dyspnoea and pleural infusion, was admitted several times for symptom control. His wife stated that she did not want him to die at home because she did not know how to do resuscitation. Therefore, he was admitted repeatedly. He described the phenomenon of moving in and out of the hospice unit by comparing the situation of the hospice patients to illegal hawkers. He said that the hospice patients had to be transferred here and there, like those hawkers who had to be alert because they had to run away from the hawker patrol inspectors. They found it difficult to find a place to settle (selling their goods illegally here and there for a living). Although the illegal hawkers were not welcome by the inspectors, they wanted to stay in the streets. He emphasised that changes in the places of residence for the hospice patients had made them felt unsettled and unwelcome. Eventually, this patient returned to Mainland China and died in his home town.

Another patient experienced a similar situation. A seventy-year-old woman with cancer of the parotid glands was not encouraged to stay home by her children, because she had an unhealed wound that produced a foul-smelling discharge. She was then left with a strong feeling of rejection.

The wish to die at home has been an ethical dilemma in some Asian countries. On one hand, some hospice patients in this research hoped to die at home: familiar surroundings where they could see the familiar faces of their families. They could experience strongly the intimacy of family connectedness, which would offer them hope, as well as psychosocial and spiritual comfort. On the other hand, they were afraid of being a burden on their families. Consequently, their family connectedness may be challenged or altered. If they stayed in hospital, they would have better access to medical and nursing care but they needed to adapt to a new environment in the hospice unit. Therefore, dying people should be helped to decide the place to stay in their final days, so that they may have peace of mind before they die.[26] Health care professional could attend to this aspect of patients' need.

Having company

'True presence'

It has been documented that most dying persons fear abandonment.[29] A presence will ease any sense of abandonment that the dying may be experiencing.[30] Thus, it is important to let the dying person know that he or she will not die alone. 'Being truly present means that the carer is with the person physically, emotionally, and spiritually, focusing his or her attention on the present time, in the present place, with the present person' (p.70).[19] Thus, a true presence can be felt on many levels. Sensitive individuals, especially those who are dying, can perceive and relate to a true and complete presence by relaxing physically and emotionally and feeling free to express themselves. For example, sitting silently with a dying person may be a moment of the most meaningful communication. It is a matter of just touching their hands — whatever is natural — to make them feel that someone understands and cares.[31]

From the Chinese perspective, 'a good death is regarded as one in old age, passing away in the presence of family members with no unfinished family responsibility, with pain well controlled and with a clear conscience' (p.793).[18] The emphasis on dying a Good Death in the presence of family members is clear. Therefore, most hospice patients in this research did not want to die alone. When they were asked if they wanted any company in their final days, the answer was always positive. However, most patients did not let their desires and wishes be known to their families. They explained that their children were busy with their work. Nevertheless, one-third of the patients asserted that they wanted to have company when they died, and all preferred their immediate family member(s) to stay with them. The presence of company could reflect the social connectedness of the patients, because their families valued them.

The following is an example. A woman stated that she needed someone to be with her when she died. She was seventy years old with cancer of the lung. She was very dyspnoeic and could not talk for a long time. She felt anxious because she could not communicate her needs. Her communication was further blocked by the fact she spoke the Shanghainese dialect, which most health care professionals did not understand. She expressed to the nurse that she wanted her children to come more often but she also considered that they were at work. Her daughter was a housewife who lived quite far away from the hospice unit. Her son was in the UK. He had come back to Hong Kong twice to visit her and was willing to return if his mother's condition deteriorated. The patient's daughter managed to spend a few hours with her just before her mother passed away. However, her son was not present when his mother died and there is no further record on what happened to the patient's children after the death of this patient.

From the caregivers' perspective, 'true presence' can be an equally invaluable experience. 'Accompanying someone at the moment of death could be a powerful source of learning and of growth towards self-actualisation and valuable experience' (p.72). [32] Spending time and being present with patients was the basis of acknowledging humanity. [33] Both caregivers and care receivers benefited from this shared and growing experience of dying.

Dying alone

Some patients may wish to avoid dying in a lonely way. However, it is equally important to respect the views of those who prefer to die alone. Three patients in this research preferred disengagement. 'Disengagement' is to leave the world quietly. [22-23] One sign of impending death is an increasing disengagement from the world of the living. [30] The dying person will gradually disengage or separate from the world of the living in the last days or weeks. There are some indications for such disengagement: less verbalisation, rejection of others, and increased sleep. They prefer not to be disturbed, but would rather have the opportunity to continue their separation. In both situations: having company or being alone, the will of the dying person need to be respected. [27] In this research, one patient asserted that he did not want to see anybody at his final hours. He expressed to me that he wanted to detach himself from the rest of the family when the time came. This appeared to be a preference for disengagement.

In a strict sense, all people die alone. No matter how much care the dying person is receiving, he or she has to complete his or her own journey. Above all, dying is the loneliest journey[34] and dying alone is not easy. Loneliness was a recurring theme that several nurses associated with death. 'No one goes with you. It's a solo act' (p.70). [32] An eighty-four-year-old man with cancer of the colon expressed his loneliness after death of his wife and son. Then he had migrated to Hong Kong to live with his relatives. He was left alone and therefore felt that he had no family members to look after, although he had some supportive relatives. He regretted not having his family around, because to him, family connectedness represented something quite different from that of relatives. This perception of connectedness seemed to be particularly true for older Chinese. Therefore, health care professionals might acknowledge patients' personal control, and accommodate their wishes to allow them more control over the dying trajectory by establishing a partnership in decision making.

Factors affecting the strength to control

To maintain one's personal control depends largely on one's strength. Self-judgement of efficacy determines the choice of behaviour and which activities will be attempted and which avoided. It also affects the amount of effort devoted to a task and the length of persistence when difficulties are encountered. [35] When the patients perceived themselves as having the strength to control, they may have less anxiety. Based on the findings of this research, the strength of an individual's personal control is related to one's psychosocial (age and financial status), physical, and spiritual status.

Psychosocial status

In this research, the Chinese family contributed predominantly to the decision as to where a patient died. Chao [14] observes that when a Chinese person is sick, he or she may authorise the family and health care professionals to make decisions for him/her... 'The Chinese are unlike their Western counterparts in that they do not stress free choice' (p.146). Direct communication with the patient may be neglected as health care professionals often consult the family members about the patient's needs and desires. [36] Hence, Chinese patients may lack personal control in the decision-making process.

Further, when adults become classified as elderly, there is a tendency to reject the principle of respect for personal control. It is generally assumed that the elderly are incompetent and inauthentic in making decisions. They are often stereotyped as not wanting to make any decisions or having no capacity to do so. [37] In this research, many patients were over sixty and they were seldom involved in making decisions for their care plans. As mentioned in the previous section on maintaining social relations, the financial and social status of the patients could influence their strength to control. Some patients, who were financially independent, were able to make their decisions related to their treatment plans and their preparations for death more autonomously, as compared with the less wealthy patients.

The social situation of hospice patients did not seem to be confined to Chinese patients. In Mesler's[4] study, his participants also described vividly the difficulty of hospice patients in asserting their personal control. The author further recommends patient education to assist hospice patients.

> People don't live with control. A lot of people don't have the educational base, and the sense of personal responsibility for their own health and their own bodies, just because they're not trained to do that generally in society, in this kind of society, where that's kind of contracted out to the medical world. But then suddenly, people are dying: they're at the lowest point, in many cases, of their lives … And all of a sudden people are looking to them to take control and responsibility of how they want to live the rest of their life with this terminal disease. That makes hospice very complicated; you have to start right away with education (p.176).[4]

Even if the hospice patients preferred to die at home, their suggestions were not likely to be supported by their families. The following conversation illustrated some viewpoints of the families. During a field visit, the wives of two patients exchanged their ideas on where the patients should stay. They talked about it in the presence of their husbands, but did not involve them in discussing the issue. They exchanged their worries and anxiety about caring for their husbands at home. They explained that they were frightened because their medical knowledge was inadequate. Therefore, they preferred their family members (the patients) to stay in the hospice unit.

The concept of personal control seems to be assimilated better by younger Chinese, because they have the chance to study it both at school and from the mass media. Certain socio-demographic characteristics have been reported to have an impact on the preferred role in decision-making for the hospice patients. The majority of patients in this research, being old and less educated, always preferred the medical practitioners to make treatment decisions for them. [38]

Physical status

In this research, the patients' preference to stay at home or in an institution depended largely on their physical condition and their family relationships. For example, the experience of pain and suffering definitely affected the patients' strength to control. The patients could also change their minds from staying at home to staying in the hospice unit as their conditions deteriorated. The following is an example. A fifty-six-year-old patient with lung cancer stated that she hoped to go home when she was reasonably well (she was speaking nine months before death). Then, she changed her mind, preferring to stay in hospice when her condition deteriorated, approximately one month before her death.

As the patients' illnesses progressed, they would gradually lose their physical abilities, social identities, social status, and strength to handle difficult situations. They became dependent and vulnerable. Therefore, some patients might live with 'paternalism' and overprotection. Yeung [39] in his personal experience as a patient with nasopharyngeal carcinoma, points out that 'there is a strong sense of powerlessness among Chinese when they are facing death'. Equally, hospice care professionals should be aware that the hospice patients may 'give up' their control and transfer responsibility for decision-making to others.

Spiritual status

Patients were often unclear about Buddhist or Taoist teachings. For example, some of them were not sure if they would be reborn after this life. Although they may not have thought deeply about the teachings of Taoism or Buddhism, they sought spiritual blessings through praying to the Buddhist and Taoist deities. 'It is important never to forget that the effect of our actions depends entirely upon the intention or motivation behind them, and not upon their scale'. [40] Confucians and

Taoists consider that everything follows the cosmic way (Tao). In this way, people may misunderstand that they should act passively. They should not change things around them and they should not escape from death. They cannot fight against the power of the universe; otherwise, they may experience fear and suffering. [41]

On the contrary, ancient scholars such as Confucius and Mencius also taught people to cultivate their spirit. The emphasised that 'the reasonable spirit ought to decide for itself, and not permit itself to be taken captive. That is the appropriate gift of heaven to man; it is the law of humanity; it is the special dignity of man, conferred by heaven. Therefore, a person must fight to preserve that dignity for heaven prepares those whom it destines for great things, through suffering and labour' (p.106). [42] These ancient Chinese teachings encourage people to cultivate their personal power. Maintaining personal power is maintaining one's dignity.

Thus according to such teachings, dying individuals need to maintain their personal power in order to preserve themselves. Accordingly, health care professionals need to help patients build up their personal power (Te) through their awareness and knowledge of the physical laws as they operate both in the universe and in the minds of others (Tao). 'We need the power to direct events, without resorting to force' (p.11). [43] From the above discussion, it can be tentatively concluded that the hospice patients in this research hoped to be given opportunities to make decisions. Ultimately, they hoped to have a choice about where they died.

Table 8.1
Categories and significant statements of Experiencing personal control
(Control)

Categories	Significant statements
Having a choice about where to live	Can I stay here and not move around? They said the medical practitioner wanted me to be discharged. I felt very upset (25).
Having company	(I want) my sons (to be with me at the end). I am not afraid of being alone (6). Wife and daughter (at the dying bed) (19). Son and daughter -in- law (20).

Clinical implications

Goal:
Facilitate patients in maintaining their personal control as they wish

Assess the patients' willingness to control and plan their care accordingly

Hospice patients may have different views on participating in and making decisions about their care. First, some patients prefer to be passive and have no control over their future, such as their care plan. These patients usually rely on their family members to make decisions for them. They believe their family will do the best for them. Their wishes to delegate their decision-making power to their family members should be respected. Arranging meeting(s) with the family might help them.

At the same time, however, some patients are happy to take an active role in making decisions for their future. They may prefer to have a sense of control over their future. Health care professionals need to recognise their responsibilities to help these patients to identify their abilities and capacities to make treatment decisions. [51] To feel a sense of control, patients must be encouraged to focus on goals in which progress can be seen. In addition, the patients need to receive information concerning treatment options, [38] and be given a choice of different interventions, which aim at increasing their sense of control, self-confidence, and the ability to cope. [44-45] Meanwhile, some patients may prefer to have a participatory role with the carers (either health care professionals or family members). They prefer to make decisions in a combined effort with the caregivers. These patients should be assisted accordingly.

Maximise resources

The mobilisation of resources is important in maintaining personal control. Physical, psychological, social, and material assets are evaluated with respect to the demands of the situation. Examples of physical resources are the person's health and energy. Psychological sources refer to beliefs that can be drawn upon to sustain hope, skills of problem solving, self-esteem, and morale. Social resources represent the social network and support system from which the patients may obtain information, tangible assistance, and emotional support. Material resources include money, tools, and equipment. Nurses and social workers can help the patients and their families to make best use of the available resources. [46]

Involve the patient in participating in decision-making on his or her care plan

Since an important element of hope is a choice, patients should be encouraged to make their own health decisions. Nurses can maximise opportunities for patients to participate in decisions affecting living and dying. Patients can be facilitated to identify areas that are controllable and which are less controllable and to accept their limitations. Other interventions to encourage their participation in making their own decisions include symptom relief, emotional support, promoting autonomy and independence through education, encouragement and counselling, and provision of team approach to care. [37] Thus patients can realise a measure of self-respect and can live through the dying process in a more meaningful and dignified way. [1, 47]

Provide specific liaison services for the patient and the family when patient is near death

Health care professionals should be knowledgeable and skilful in reporting the signs of dying and near-death. In this way, dying persons may have company when they die and as they wish. A person experiences many changes during his or her dying process. Physically, the body is shutting down. 'The dying person may be sleepy but able to be awakened and have awareness of the surroundings. Or, the senses may be dulled, and there may be little awareness of what is happening in the environment. Sleep may be so deep that the dying person cannot be awakened and is unresponsive' (p.14). [48] Other signs of dying are: dyspnoea, blurred vision, dryness of mouth, profuse sweating, and unrelieved oedema. Emotionally, the dying person may gradually detach from the outside world and pull inwards. Mentally, a person may decrease or lose clarity during the dying process. Periods of restlessness, confusion, unresponsiveness, and incontinence are among the common changes. [48] Near-death awareness often includes visions of loved ones although the dying people do not necessarily signal the imminence of death. Some review their lives and come to a more complete understanding of the meaning of their lives. They do not feel fear but they express concern for those who will be left behind.

Table 8.2
Summary of Experiencing personal control (Control)

Related issues	Clinical implications
1. The concepts of personal control	Goal: Facilitate patients in maintaining their personal control as they wish
2. Having a choice about where to live	
• Dying in an institution	1. Assess the patient's willingness to control and plan his or care accordingly.
• Dying at home	
3. Having company	2. Maximise resources.
• True presence	
• Dying alone	3. Involve the patient in participating in decision-making about his or her care plan.
4. Factors affecting the strength to control	
• Psychosocial status	4. Provide specific liaison services for patient and family when patient is near death.
• Physical status	
• Spiritual status	

Summary

A core element of dying a Good Death which emerges from this research revolves around the dying patient's exertion of personal control, rather than leaving control to the medical experts to cure the disease. The personal capacity of patients directly affected the extent of personal control. This includes psychosocial status: age and financial status, physical status and spiritual status.

The patients in this research had preferences about the type of environment they wanted to be in as they approached their death. The two major preferences were having a choice of where to stay and whom they wanted to be present at the time of death. Two-thirds of the patients indicated where they wanted to die. About half of the patients hoped to die in the hospice units and some patients preferred to die at home. It was clear that the element of control for hospice patients has not been seriously attended. The findings of this research showed that nearly all patients died in the institutions and none died at home, when more than one-fifth had hoped to die at home. In addition, the hospice patients did not seem to have adequate personal capacity to maintain personal control; perhaps because the family found it difficult to look after the patient when he or she was dying. Without more social support and resources in the community and a change of attitude towards dying at home, the dying person's wish to die at home can hardly be achieved. Similarly, the traditional Chinese value of dying with company needs to be reconsidered.

The decision to have company was more difficult. In this research, ten patients had asserted their wishes. This aspect of need was seldom attended to because the patients may discuss their needs neither with health care professionals nor their families. In wishing to die at home or in an institution, ten patients made it clear that they desired company when they were dying. This notion supported the other element of dying a Good Death: maintaining social relations. In the final hours, they may want at least one close family member to be present [49] — parent, spouse, children, siblings, or friends. From the Chinese viewpoint, having the presence of some family members before one's death is important. [18] It is believed that 'those who die alone will have no descendants after their transmigration' (p.91). [50] Due to changing values, younger hospice staff may not recognise that having company is valuable and essential for Chinese dying persons.

If health care professionals are to help patients to be accompanied when they die, they have to be skilful in detecting the signs of dying and near-death and report them promptly.[48] From one patient's point of view, 'They used to lose their consciousness two to three days before death and they could keep their eyes closed all day'. In principle, the hospice patients should have the right to know their condition and make decisions about their care plan according to their needs. In reality, it may be difficult to measure the extent of their control over their daily lives. First, many elderly Chinese hospice patients did not know their rights or might not understand the concept of human rights. Second, they may be stereotyped as having no or little capacity to make decisions. Third, they lost their physical abilities to handle difficult situations. Fourth, they may believe that heaven had taken control of all aspects of their lives that made them feel powerless.

Most hospice patients valued the opportunity to discuss death-related issues such as choosing where to live and with whom they died, because these were major concerns for them. In some Asian countries, health care professionals and the families, but not the patients, made most of these decisions for the patients. To improve the current situation, it is essential to involve the patients in the decision-making for their care plan. Most important, the hospice patients can be encouraged to verbalise their needs and maximise the available resources. They can be encouraged to make decisions about their care plan. The hospice professionals need to be sensitive to the signs of dying and near-death awareness so they can provide specific liaison services for the patient and the family whenever needed.

9
Preparing to depart and bidding farewells (Preparations)

Preparing to depart

GOOD PREPARATIONS BEFORE death are always helpful. Several authors emphasise the importance of preparations for death, noting that bidding farewell to staff, friends, and family is an essential element in a person's quest for a final resolution. [1-2] People take time to prepare themselves emotionally for dying. [1,3] They need to fulfil their wishes, say good-bye and give messages, and arrange their funerals as a preparation of farewells. [4] Some dying persons are concerned with their personal cleanliness and appearance. [1, 5] Preparing to depart (preparations) was identified as the sixth element of dying a Good Death from the perspective of the Chinese hospice patients in this research. This chapter presents my findings on preparing for departure. The preparations of the patients included personal preparations such as bidding farewell, organising material affairs, leaving instructions, and giving gifts, and public preparation of funeral arrangements. As compared with some previous studies in Western societies, [2] there were differences in the meaning of 'farewell' and consequently their preparations for death.

'Preparation' refers to a state in which a dying person may have accepted his or her death and had made preparations for departure. The patients may have shown their readiness in this context. Some patients did not prepare for their death personally as they had delegated the responsibility to their next of kin, such as their spouses and children. There were other reasons too. First, the dying individuals had to rely on their families for financial support, so they may have felt inadequate at verbalising what they wanted to prepare. Second, death remains a taboo subject in Asian cultures. Some families did not feel comfortable talking about issues related to death with the dying persons themselves. Therefore, these patients did not reveal their views on preparations. Third, if the patients regarded death as a personal matter, they may not feel comfortable talking about their funerals. Therefore, four patients specified that they did not want to bid farewell to their families because they had no property left to give to their children. The findings on preparations in this research were preliminary because there were no previous studies on this topic in Asian countries for comparison. Implications of the present findings suggest future studies to focus on this area of concern of the dying persons.

Personal preparations

To achieve a Good Death, a person needs to complete his or her unfinished business, resolves his or her residual conflicts, and make all the necessary preparations. Other main activities include informal willing; talks about death and dying and talks about role reorganisation for illness.[2] In this research, the hospice patients made their personal preparations for death by leaving instructions and/or giving gifts. Most of them had instructed their children to care for their spouses after they died. Five patients said that they had made financial arrangements with their families. A few patients had left some instructions to their children, while a few patients had given gifts to their relatives (Table 9.1).

Table 9.1
Summary of preparations

Type of preparation	Frequency
1.Organising material affairs	5
2. Leaving instructions	3
3. Giving gifts	3
4. Preparing for funeral	13
5. Bidding farewell	5

Organising material affairs

When the patients were asked if they had bid farewell to their families, they often related it to organising material affairs, including the money in their bank accounts. Five patients mentioned that they had to make arrangements for their money and properties but they did not describe the details. One patient specified that she would be able to prepare herself better if her physical condition was better. She was a young woman with cancer of the pancreas. She had arranged for the ownership of her flat to be transferred to her sister and she died three days after the interview. Some patients had transferred their money to their family members. The following is an example.

> I have done all my preparations. I have transferred my money to my daughter's bank account. My husband is good. He helps me to do a lot of work and we have talked about everything. The hospice nurse always comforts me, and visited me when I returned home. If anything happens, I can be admitted here immediately .

Financial status seemed to have a great deal of influence on the patients' preparations. Patients with better financial status would make better or more preparations. As mentioned in previous chapters, most patients were financially dependent elderly people. Several patients did not want to bid farewell to their children because they had no property left for them. The following is a typical example. A 68-year-old musician with lung cancer claimed that he did not bid farewell to his children because he had nothing left to give his children. He worked for a funeral company, and since he was paid on a daily basis his income was not high. He had no retirement fund or any other funding to support him after his retirement. Nor was he covered by any health insurance. He indicated that his wife was his main concern because she had lost her eyesight last year and was very dependent on him. He felt upset at leaving his wife soon when she needed his assistance most. When I visited him the second time, his wife was with him and cried during the interview. They both experienced some degree of anticipatory grief.

> I have discussed it with my children. My concern was to have somebody to look after my wife. I have not discussed any further arrangements. My children will be in charge of the funeral arrangements. I would not mind either cremation or burial. I have nothing much to think about. I have no property because I used to be paid daily. I have no retirement pension and I have not taken out any health insurance.

Leaving instructions

In contrast with the West, Chinese moral tradition originates from human-to-human relationship, instead of God-to-human relationship. Chinese morality is essentially socially oriented. [6] Therefore, education is an important part of life in Chinese culture. Children receive moral education first from the family before they go to formal school. The continuous educational and socialising effects are obviously important. [7] Therefore, a few patients bid farewell to their families by leaving them some instructions. These patients were mothers, and their instructions concerned maintaining harmonious relationships with family members and being morally good people. Such patients perceived leaving instructions and blessings to their children to be their social roles and obligations before they finally left their families. The following are some examples.

An example is a 70-year-old woman with cancer of the lung. She was a single parent whose main concern was her children. She had been separated from her husband for many years. She was angry with him because he did not care about his family. As she approached death, she left her three adult children with some instructions. The instructions concerned the relationship among the siblings, which is one of the Five relationships in Confucianism. [8] She encouraged her children to love one another and support each other to build up their strengths when they had difficulties. She illustrated her instructions by using the example of Chinese chopsticks.

I have instructed my children to love one another. Just like chopsticks: a bunch (of chopsticks) is much stronger than a single one. I did not know what to say, (and) what to teach. They have to share and help each other when they have difficulties. Nothing much, this is what I have told them.

Another example was an elderly patient with cancer of the kidney who was too ill to walk. Her husband was also ill and hospitalised. She wept that she had worked very hard while she was young. She told me that she had left her adult children some instructions because she knew she had to pass away soon. She also emphasised the importance of maintaining good sibling relations in the family.

We made bean curd and sold it for a living. We (and her husband) have raised our four children together. Our lives were tough. I am not stupid. I teach them and advise them that brothers and sisters should not quarrel... when mother is away (passes away).

Will

The above pattern of public preparation suggests a pattern of social priorities which put the welfare of survivors above that of the self. With reference to the findings of some previous studies, people in the West make a will even before they are aware of their deaths. [2] Some people took out life insurance too. On the other hand, many Chinese are reluctant to make wills. This finding is supported by several studies on Chinese views of wills. The patients included Chinese in Singapore, [9] some Chinese Americans [10] and some Chinese Australians. [11] Some Taiwan Chinese families would comply with the patients' will, while some would not. [5] Some patients thought that talking about death might bring bad luck. Consistent with some previous studies, [11] none of the hospice patients in the present research mentioned that they had life insurance or had made a will.

Giving gifts

It was quite a common practice for older Chinese people to pass some pieces of jade on to their children. Jade symbolised that their blessings would continue after they died. In Chinese culture, jade means 'good fortune'. [12] Jade is regarded as something precious, pure, and supremely excellent. For example, in the Shang and Zhou Dynasties, people regarded jade as a supreme thing. The nature of jade represents good manners, humanity, wisdom, happiness, loyalty, trust, and justice. Jade is highly respected in Chinese communities.[13] Therefore, the patients in this research gave their children some pieces of jade as the best of their blessings so that they would be remembered in the future. Some people hope to 'live on in the minds of those whom he or she has loved' (p.41). [14]

Jade is also a symbol of resistance to decay. Clearly death and decay of the body often go together. Therefore, it is logical for the Chinese to assume that if bodily decay can be arrested then life can go on. Hence, great attention has traditionally been paid to finding decay-resistant wood for coffins, and wealthy people place pieces of jade in the mouths of the dead. In ancient Chinese dynasties such as the Han, some rich people were buried with jewellery, especially jade, [10] or wearing clothes which was made up of small pieces of jade. [15] A few patients gave their children or next of kin; several pieces of old jade. 'I have given my sons some of my jade jewellery'. Some patients gave their immediate families and relatives furniture, plants, and pets as gifts before they died.

Public preparations: Arranging funerals

Preparing funerals has also been identified as an essential public preparation. [2, 16-17] It has been an important part of dying according to some US studies in the 1960s and 1970s. Some are studies by Lipman and Marden,[18] Glaser and Strauss,[19] and Kalish and Reynolds. [20] Similar to the findings of two previous American studies, [20-21] the Australian sample had made funeral arrangements. However, the percentage of Australians who had made funeral arrangements was less than that of the Americans. More Australian patients had made funeral arrangements before their illness (twenty-nine per cent) than those who made them after awareness of dying (thirteen per cent). Funeral arrangements included the patient's talking to a funeral director about costs and procedures. [2] In Taiwan, Chao[5] indicates that planning for one's remains and funeral is important for some Taiwan Chinese patients and indifferent for others.

Most patients in this research, considered public preparations for death to be a significant life event. Historically, the Chinese family arranged the funeral properly in order to comfort the dying. Funeral arrangements are often the last wishes of dying people. It was also part of the practice of filial piety to one's parents. In Chinese culture the descendants would feel good about the existence of 'social ties' between them and their ancestors . People in the West appear to have similar ideas. The places of death and means of disposal of the body are complementary to the Good Death model. [22] Today in mainland China, despite decades of campaigns under Mao that aimed to erase anti-progressive feudal practices from Chinese memory, Feng Shui, festivals, and rituals that have framed rural life for centuries are as important as they ever were. As suggested by the Chinese Community Party, cremation and simple armbands are standard ceremonies in cities like Beijing. However, in the countryside, more than 80 per cent of the dead still receive a coffin burial despite decades of official discouragement. [23]

In some Chinese communities, a funeral ceremony remains an important social event. The details of the rituals may only be carried out in some parts of Hong Kong, such as the New Territories. [23] Some elderly patients considered preparing their funerals as a public way of bidding farewell to the living. This would be the last chance to show the dying respect and to grieve. There were several areas in which the patients had shown concerns while they prepared for their funerals: the budget for the ceremony and their beliefs about death and life after death. Hence, arranging one's funeral can be perceived as social as well as spiritual preparation.

The funeral is often regarded as a person's last journey in the physical world before he or she is buried. Making arrangements for the funeral should be the last, but not the least thing one can do for oneself. Despite the private nature of the topic, about half of the patients gave me information about their preparations for deaths. Arrangements included the place of burial, type of coffin, and means of disposal. Chinese generally see the choice of appropriate place for burial as important, especially for those who believe in Feng Shui. Three elderly patients asserted that having a grand funeral ceremony was important for them, their families, and friends (Table 9.2).

Social preparations

James Watson, a Harvard anthropologist who has conducted extensive studies in Chinese culture, called traditional funeral rituals a cornerstone of the Chinese identity or 'cultural cement'. [23] 'To be Chinese is to understand, and to accept the view that there is a correct way to perform rites associated with the life cycle, the most important being weddings and funerals'. [23] According to Watson, these ancient rituals serve as fundamental proof of Chinese identity. Rituals such as funerals often help families and their members. Rituals mark the loss, help family members express their grief, and give the family a sense of continuity. [24] Therefore, the Chinese were traditionally under a great deal of social pressure — funeral rituals were performed under the critical eye of the community, and approval and acceptance hinged on them. Funeral rituals also publicly reflect the achievements and social status of the dead.

Most Chinese stress the importance of their social status in both living and dying. People make different funeral arrangements depending on their social class and financial status. For some families, funerals continue to be seen as an indicator of an individual's social respectability, and they may spend extravagantly for fear of public censure or supernatural retribution. [25] For example, it is expensive to buy a piece of land with good Feng Shui for a burial. Therefore, funeral arrangements can be an expensive social event.

If the hospice patient was financially independent, he or she may have had an opportunity to communicate his or her needs to the family. However, financially dependent patients may not have this privilege or may not be so willing to talk about their funerals. This practice is still observed in contemporary Chinese societies. In this research, two-thirds of the patients were elderly and working class. Some patients were not involved in making decisions about how to dispose of their bodies and where they were to be buried. For example, an eighty-three-year-old lady stated that she wished to have a grand funeral ceremony. However, she was not optimistic about her wish because her son would not do as she wanted, partly because of his financial situation. Therefore, she did not tell him her wishes.

On the other hand, an 80-year-old male patient had demonstrated more control over his future. He was a wealthy businessman and could afford to spend money on his funeral. Therefore, he could decide every detail of his funeral according to his wishes and he felt contented about the arrangements. For example, he had many relatives and business friends, so he had arranged a big hall to accommodate his family members and guests for this occasion. He felt contented to be able to do some preparatory work for his personal funeral and the burial place. He considered his funeral an important event for himself, his family and his friends.

> I look at myself (sighing)... I have the coffin and place for burial in Junk Bay. I have paid HK$120,000 for this. I have made all the arrangements. I have also arranged for some money for my wife.

Religious preparations

Religious rituals

For some people, arrangement of a funeral is a social event. For others, it is likely to be a religious preparation. According to Confucius,

> Man is composed of two parts; the substance of one is aerial, that of the other is spermatic. To bring together these separate parts, morally reconstituting the deceased for a moment by the offerings; that is the great thing. Everyone dies. The corpse and the inferior soul go into the earth and decompose; the aerial soul rises and becomes glorified, if there is a reason for it (i.e. becomes one with Tien, Heaven). [26]

Confucius believed that a person's aerial soul continued to live. Meanwhile, the Taoists believe in immortality and some people can escape from death. By the fourth century BC, a set of beliefs had developed in which there were ways for human beings to escape death, either by living for a very long time, or by being reborn in a new form after what only appeared to be death. Meanwhile, most Chinese may not be sure of what happened after death [27] and if they could escape from death. Buddhists believe that all humans live for many life times, not just one, with the form of each life shaped by how one lived in their previous existence. Good life will lead to happy rebirth (i.e. a Good Death) as a person or even a god. Evil deeds lead to rebirth as a beggar or an animal. This is one concept of reincarnation. [27-28]

Many Chinese believe a proper funeral will make the dead ancestor happy in the after life and it is more than a moral obligation. [23]

Therefore, the prospect of creating a 'hungry ghost' — the result of a neglectful burial — is considered dangerous. [29] The rituals and mourning also symbolise the respect and affection of the descendants. The details of the funeral ceremony reflect the faith and beliefs of the dying person: his or her beliefs of death and life after death. For example, Buddhists believe that when a person dies, his or her body should not be touched for at least eight hours. [10] This is because the spirit will undergo a painful process while leaving the body. Therefore, it needs a quiet and undisturbed environment after physical death.

Disposal of the body

The way patients organised their funeral plans reflected their beliefs on death and life after death. When they were asked about their preferred means of disposal, about half of them preferred a traditional burial in a cemetery while only one-fifth of the patients considered cremation. This finding corresponds with the traditional Chinese thought that people should be buried, rather than cremated, to keep the body intact. [10] Otherwise, people would have died a bad death if they could not keep the body intact (the body was separated into pieces). A bad death is perceived as a punishment from heaven. [30] Examples of people who could not be buried 'intact' were prisoners and those who died in accidents. 'To die in pieces' was considered a great source of shame to the dead, the family, and their ancestors.

These social concepts need to be adjusted with the contemporary social changes. For example, the Hong Kong Government encourages people to have cremations rather than burials because of a shortage of land. During 1997, over eighty per cent of the dead were cremated, a ten per cent rise over the figure of seventy per cent in 1996. Human remains buried in public cemeteries have to be exhumed after six years and are either cremated or re-interred in an urn cemetery.

Feng Shui

Taoists also believe in the effect of Feng Shui (geomancy) when they bury the dead. If the funeral is not carried out properly, it may cause illness and accidents. [23] Funeral preparations are often regarded as a private matter. In this research, none of the Chinese hospice patients specified the need to be buried in a place with good Feng

Shui. Some primary residents of New Territories in Hong Kong may be more concerned about Feng Shui, because their ancestors had been assigned land for the burial of their families. Land with good Feng Shui is usually expensive; again, this factor would be considered by the patients.

Examples of cultural preparations

Rituals are important both for the dying person and the family. Rituals acknowledge the loss and help family members express their grief. It further gives the family a sense of continuity. [24] For example in Chao's [5] findings, planning for one's remains and funeral is important for some Taiwan Chinese patients and indifferent for others. Some were concerned about the performance of religious rites of passage. Similarly, the hospice nurses reported that some hospice patients in this research had made culturally relevant preparations. The following are some examples. First, an old man with lung cancer wore a special costume, which was worn by the dead person, during the funeral ceremony, before his or her death. Some Chinese beliefs claim that a person must wear new clothes while he or she is still alive as a preparation for transcending to the afterlife. Such preparation will be 'effective' only if the person wears the new clothes before he or she dies. This type of clothing is called 'clothes of longevity'. [15] This patient did not have any religious faith but he practised ancestor worship. The relatives and the dying person thought that it was important to lead a good life in the next world (death). The Chinese popular belief considers two indicators of good life and good death. First, they need to have enough clothes to keep them warm. Second, they need to have enough food so as not to become a hungry ghost. These beliefs are reflected in Chinese funeral ceremonies and festivals such as Ching Ming and the Ghost Festival.

A seventy-two-year-old man with cancer of the lung was a typical example. When this patient's condition deteriorated his children gave him a bowl of sweetened Chinese tea, symbolising that they wished their father to have a 'sweet and good' journey to the next world and sent him off with good blessings. As mentioned in Chapter Two, most Chinese believe that there is a world after death and that they will meet their family member(s) again. Third, three patients gave out several pieces of old jade to their close family members. The hospice patients in this research believed they would continue blessing their descendants after they died. This belief underlies the practice of ancestor worship. The strength of such belief is the continuation of a 'social tie' and a family's obligation to their ancestors. [31]

Farewells

Some dying persons will bid farewell formally or informally in their last days. Farewells can have four mutual components: affection, regard, reassurance, and acceptance, and these will often be interspersed in conversations about other things. [2] Farewells can be completed in several ways: a family conference chaired by the dying person, individual conferences between the dying person and his or her significant others, letters, journals, audiocassettes, or videotapes.[1] Therefore, it may be hard to notice if any farewells take place or not and the phenomenon has not been reported by researchers in more recent studies. [16, 32]

The patients in this research were not eager to express their opinions on their preparations before they died. About half of them reported that they had made some form of farewell to their families. Five patients did not elaborate on what they had done. They seldom bade farewell to the people they wanted. As compared with the findings of some studies in the West, such as Kellehear, [2] less Chinese patients in this research had made their preparations for death. A majority of Australian patients bid farewell to their families and friends, while only half of the Chinese hospice patients in the present research had done so. Consistent with the findings of a research on Taiwan Chinese, a majority of the patients (85 per cent) did not bid a formal farewell to their loved ones. [5] They may do this informally, but Chao has not explained clearly what she meant by formal and informal farewells. The concept of 'farewells' may be interpreted differently by people from different cultures. Farewell means saying good-bye for people in Western cultures while for the hospice patients in this research it often meant 'leaving instructions' or 'distribution of their properties'.

In a traditional Chinese family, the father was the head of the family. He took charge of the administration of all family properties.

The family properties would be distributed among children before or after he died. The perseverance of Confucian ethics on the solidarity of the family is maintained by avoiding family partition. Therefore, several patients relegated the act of 'bidding farewell' to 'distribution of their properties' to their surviving relatives. Four patients showed that they did not bid farewells to their families because they had left no property or money to them, although they had no obligation to do so. Consistent with a recent research on Australian Chinese, [11] preparing a will is uncommon in Chinese communities. The wealthy person may have made a will before he or she died, to indicate clearly the distribution of his or her properties.

Factors affecting the patients' preparations

When the patients in this research were aware of their impending death, they also had an awareness of the limitation of time. Their personal and public preparations for their own deaths could be regarded as evidence that they were able to regain some sort of control over their future. There were two main factors, which affected the patients' preparations for departure: communication of death and dying in the Chinese context and acceptance and preparations.

Communication of death and dying in the Chinese context

In this research, the hospice patients' reluctance to bid farewell to their loved ones may relate to Chinese communication behaviour. The Chinese are relatively less expressive and most of them prefer to keep their feelings and ideas to themselves rather than share their feelings with others. Many hospice patients in this research had felt it was difficult to find a good listener. One important preparation for the listener is to be familiar with the patient's culture if he or she hopes to communicate with sensitivity and empathy. One needs to be familiar with the person's terms of reference. Otherwise, the information disclosed by the patients may not be interpreted and understood correctly.

A majority of health care professionals in Asian countries receive Western education. For example, Hong Kong was a British colony for 100 years until 1997. Their knowledge about Chinese culture is relatively limited.[33] Although there may be informal sessions about Chinese culture in general education classes at university, the level of knowledge may be elementary. The knowledge obtained will not be sufficient to help health care professionals understand the complex world of dying people in the Chinese community. Future incorporation of Chinese culture into formal education programmes to strengthen this aspect of knowledge for all health care professionals is crucial. Another important quality of the listener is non-judgement. Very often, health care professionals think that they know far more than the dying person does. The attitude of superiority may prevent effective communication.

Despite cultural differences, communicating with the dying people is an important aspect of hospice care. Both medical practitioners and nurses agree that talking with a dying person about what will happen can create tremendous discomfort and difficulty. Very often, family and friends talk about everything except the fact that someone is dying.[34] Health care professionals may be afraid that what they say will be either too threatening or too trivial. Some patients were unwilling to discuss their preparations for death, including their funeral arrangements, because the discussion was death-related. As discussed in Chapter Four, making preparations could be considered as a consequence of death awareness. Some patients did not feel comfortable talking about preparations for death because they may have felt that these issues were private matters. They may also have felt that they were taboo subjects, or did not want to reveal their financial situations.

The experience of interviewing hospice patients has given me new insights into communication in Chinese communities. A majority of hospice patients were comfortable and willing to communicate their needs to me. They were happy to talk and share their experiences, including reviews of their lives and preparations for death but I had to establish mutual trust by demonstrating my understanding and concern during the interviews.

Acceptance and preparations

Because of the nature of the topic, most patients did not want to disclose too much about their opinions on preparations for departure. They often had mixed feelings of sadness and acceptance, which affected their openness in discussion. They were sad that they had to leave their loved ones, and some of them may have had no idea about their life after death. Some patients accepted the timing of their death because of their old age, beliefs, religious faith, and/or completion of their social obligations. Therefore, they either talked about it briefly or diverted the discussion to other topics. Quite frequently, patients left the decisions to their families. Some reported that they had made all their preparations but they were reluctant to elaborate. Nevertheless, some patients felt that when they had finished their 'business' or preparations for their death, they had shown their acceptance of death and would die a Good Death.

Table 9.2
Categories and significant statements of Preparing to depart and **bidding farewells (Preparations)**

Categories	Significant statements
Personal preparations	
Organising material affairs	There is not much to say (about preparations). I have some savings and I have added my daughter's name. I ask them to be happier (12).
	I will talk to them and the money will be given to my family (13, p.17).
Leaving instructions	I have instructed my children to love one another. Just like chopsticks: a bunch (of chopsticks) is much stronger than a single one. I did not know what to say, (and) what to teach. They will have to share and help each other when they have difficulties. Nothing much, this is what I told them (11, p.25).
	I teach them and advise them that brothers and sisters should not quarrel... when mother is away (passes away) (27).
Giving gifts	I have four or five pieces of old jade. I have given them to my relatives. My main concern is my dog. My subordinate will look after it (7).
Public preparations	
Preparing the funeral	This old lady (my mother-in-law) died at the age of over 100. She died in old age. She was buried at Butterfly Hill. We bought a place for her in Guangdong province, near Hong Kong. This is a good piece of land. Yes, my daughter has bought one for me as well (11, p.9).
Bidding farewell	I have discussed it with my children, now I have nothing to say (23).

Clinical implications

Goal:
Facilitate patients to make preparations for death

Initiate discussion of 'death' and relevant preparations

Since preparations is one of the essential element of dying a Good Death, health care professionals have to make more effort in this aspect of care. They can initiate and encourage discussion of 'death' issues with Chinese hospice patients using the terms and descriptions they prefer. It is hoped that such patients may gradually gain an acceptance of their death and make their preparations. Nurses can also encourage the patients to communicate their needs to their families and arrange for visits by religious representatives according to the patients' wishes.

Provide information and resources on funeral services

Most hospice patients have thought about their funerals. Some would share their ideas with health care professionals while some refused to do so. It is important that health care professionals understand the patients' preferences and identify their needs sensitively. The social workers can help them with financial assistance. They can also give them appropriate advice on information and resources about funeral arrangements. Both the patients and their families need to be aware of the availability of the services so that they can consult the relevant services when they need to.

Provide information about bereavement services

All dying people anticipate their imminent death and they grieve for themselves before they die. 'Grieving in each other's arms can raise us to new heights of intimacy and love' (p.19).[34] This intense personal experience can be very frustrating. At present, most hospice services in the hospitals include bereavement care. There are also two community-based bereavement centres in Hong Kong: Comfort Care Concern Group and Bereavement Centre and Jessie and Thomas Tam Centre of The Society for Promotion of Hospice Care Limited. These organisations are self-supported and not government funded.

Introduce advance-care planning

Advance care directives, which are short statements by patients wishing to avoid 'heroic measures'.[35] Having 'advanced directives' when a patient is admitted to hospital are common practices in the West. Two types of advance directives are worth considering: 1) wills in which patients specify their preferences for or refuse specific medical treatments; 2) the patients appoint a surrogate who has the authority to make medical decisions for them if they become incompetent. Both wills and advance-care directives can be introduced to patients who are more willing to make autonomous decisions and take an active part in their care planning. In this way, the patients who desire to experience a sense of personal control will be assisted in making their decisions.

Table 9.3
Summary of Preparing to depart and bidding farewells (Preparations)

Related issues	Clinical implications
1. Personal preparations • Organising material affairs • Leaving instructions • Giving gifts 2. Public preparations: arranging funerals • Social preparations • Religious preparations • Examples of cultural preparations 3. Farewells 4. Factors affecting the patients' preparations • Communication of death and dying in the Chinese context • Acceptance and preparations	Goal: Facilitate patient to make preparations for death 1. Initiate discussion of 'death' and relevant preparations. 2. Provide information and resources on funeral services. 3. Provide information about bereavement services. 4. Introduce advance-care planning.

Summary

People who were able to talk about death and preparations for death seemed to have better acceptances of their imminent death. Therefore, preparation was identified as an important element for dying a Good Death. The personal preparations fell into three main categories: leaving instructions, giving gifts, and organising material affairs. In this research, about half of the patients had performed these activities to bid farewell to their families. Thirteen patients had discussed issues related to their funerals. Some had carried out both the personal and public preparations of funeral arrangements and bidding farewell. Altogether, more than half of the patients shared their viewpoints on their preparations for death and a majority of these patients also mentioned the word 'death' and related issues in the interviews. These hospice patients considered death less taboo, so they were willing to share their opinions.

As some Chinese people believe that talking about death would bring them bad luck, less hospice patients in this research bade farewell to their relatives, or had their life insurance and wills prepared, which were relatively common practices in the West. Further, the hospice patients in this research seemed to emphasise spiritual preparations more than material preparations as they hoped to maintain a social tie with their families after death. Funerals are regarded as significant social and spiritual events for the Chinese. Preparing a funeral means preparing a public farewell to family and friends. It also reflects the social status of the dying person. Therefore, few patients were interested in discussing the ceremony in detail because they could not afford to prepare a funeral ceremony according to their wishes. Meanwhile, some patients considered preparations for death as personal matters and did not describe the preparations in details. They may only have discussed it with their families. Therefore, some patients did not verbalise their needs to health care professionals. Other patients had delegated the responsibility for the funeral arrangements to their families. It is important to respect dying persons' privacy and wishes when they do not want to discuss their preparations in details. Just as important, health care professionals need to find out what best they can offer to dying persons in preparing for a Good Death. Appropriate preparations for death often strengthen social connectedness between patients and their families, consequently affirming their social identify. This may further bring the dying person a sense of control and hope for a future after death.

In practice, the hospice patients who wish to prepare for departure should be assisted. The first essential element is sensitive and compassionate communication to initiate and encourage the discussion of preparations. Second, health care professionals can provide information and various resources on funeral services, which will facilitate their funeral arrangements. Third, bereavement care should be offered whenever necessary. Finally, advance-care directives, which have been practised in some Western countries, can be introduced for those patients who wish to have more autonomy in making decisions for their care planning and future.

10
Accepting the timing of one's death (Completion)

Introduction

BOTH NURSES [1-4] and dying people [5-6] argue that a Good Death is allied with a sense of acceptance and of appreciation for having lived according to the best standards possible. From the findings of this research, accepting the timing of one's death (completion) was an important element of dying a Good Death for hospice patients. In this chapter, I discuss the findings of accepting the timing of one's death and some related issues. These issues include completing social obligations; dying in old age; accepting death as a natural part of life; and experiencing a meaningful life.

Accepting the timing of one's death

Some authors argue that death is essentially 'good' only when it occurs 'on time' [6-7] 'To die at the right time in the right way— those are the hallmarks of a sterling death' [8] However, when is the appropriate time to die?

A common view is that a timely death is one that occurs 'when a person has completed his [sic] span of life, his powers wane, and the eventual increasing decline suggests that it is time for the individual to depart this life'. [9] It is also widely believed that death is timely if it is appropriate to one's time of life. [8] Furthermore, as people approach death, they may possess a sense of readiness related to their style of life, to their situation in life, and to their mission (aspiration, goals, wishes) in life. [8]

Kearl[7] has pointed out that the time at which death normally occurs in the life span and how long it typically takes people to die shape both cultural beliefs about death and individual fears. Furthermore, he explains that the quality of the relationship between the dying person and the family is an important element in Good Death because death is a dual process that simultaneously involves the dying and those they will leave behind.

Therefore, a person usually refers to having a Good Death when they have completed their life tasks, when they are about to die in old age [7-11] and have completed all their unfinished business. [11] In dying a Good Death people recognise and resolve possible residual conflicts and satisfy whatever personal wishes remain.[12] Consistent with the findings of these studies,[7-9, 11] some hospice patients were observed to have better acceptance of death. There were several circumstances that facilitated the patients' acceptance 1) having completed their social obligations; 2) dying in old age; 3) accepting death as a natural part of life and 4) having experienced meaningful lives.

Guessing the timing of death

Most of the patients were conscious of how long they would live. Some of them accepted the timing of their death and developed a sense of readiness while others did not. Understandably, most patients were cautious about the limited time they had left once they were aware of their imminent deaths. [13] Part of the uncertainty of timing may be due to differences in the nature of cancer, especially terminal cancer. Most patients guessed the amount of time that was left for them. Some had referred to their experiences with their relatives who died of cancer. The following is an example.

Mrs. Y was a fifty-three-year-old woman with ovarian cancer. She wished to live longer because she was not ready to retire and therefore not ready to die. When her cancer relapsed, she lost hope for recovery and trust in God. She estimated the 'time which was left for her' by relating the death experiences of her husband and mother.

> My husband had nasopharyngeal cancer. Later it spread to his lungs and he died. I recall that it took almost one year from the time of metastasis to death. Therefore, I think I am in a similar situation. I was diagnosed in January, and then I had metastasis in August. Now it is September/October. The symptoms are showing. I tell myself I should have nothing to regret. There is nothing to regret. God has given me several months from the time I discovered that I had cancer until the time of metastasis.

> My mother died during the years of the Cultural Revolution. [I am] over fifty years old. She died from cancer but she was not hospitalised. I was in Hong Kong at that time. My family told me that she had severe abdominal distension. She probably died from intestinal carcinoma. She was over fifty years old as well. Yes, I have thought of that. Is my disease hereditary? It's possible.

Meanwhile, hospital staff also had their expectancies of when the patients would die. [14] For example, a few patients were informed by medical practitioners that they would probably live for a few more months. There are always pros and cons of 'knowing when' one will die. The advantage is one can schedule one's timetable and complete one's preparations before the 'deadline'. Patients may spend some time resolving possible residual conflicts and satisfying whatever personal wishes remain. [12] It seems that a person can have better control over his or her future, in particular, the timing of his or her life and death. However, some patients were understandably anxious as they approached the 'assigned date' of death.

Accepting the timing of one's death

People tend to act on behalf of the elderly without consulting them. Therefore, the elderly seldom assert their own needs and values.[15] In this research, some patients stated that people often assumed they were ready to die and nobody would miss them much after they died. Ten patients indicated their readiness to die. The reasons for their readiness include, first, their cancer had metastasised. Second, they were old and third, their religious faith helped them to develop readiness.

> I am old enough, I will not mind dying. This is not a problem (for me). It is almost time to complete (my) life... I do not want to live any longer. I tell God that it is almost time. I would like to have a good ending.

Not accepting the timing of one's death

Five patients did not seem to accept that it was the right time for them to die. Some patients between the ages of thirty and fifty experienced some emotional disturbance, such as anger and depression. They did not accept the timing of their death because they felt they were too young to die. A few patients had unfulfilled wishes such as: touring and seeing other parts of the world or seeing their grand-child or child gets married, and spending time with the family. Therefore, they were unhappy, angry, and frustrated as they recognised their lives would end soon. The following is a reflection by an eighty-four-year-old patient who had cancer of the kidney.

> I have worked hard my whole life. I have raised seven children. I really want to enjoy my retirement. I have closed my shop and I do not want to have any more money. It is useless to have more money.

Quick death Vs lingering death

Most people perceive cancer death as a lingering death.[16] A lingering death means a 'delayed' death that is painful and full of suffering. Unrelieved physical pain and non-acceptance of death often attribute as the causes of psychological pain. [17]

Therefore, eleven patients preferred to have quick death and avoided lingering death because they did not want to suffer and linger on. They perceived that the timing of their death was unnecessarily prolonged. This was more obvious in patients who had dyspnoea.

> This illness (cancer) is definitely worse. This (illness), I have to wait, I have to wait.

> I am feeling depressed. I have lived long enough, I do not want to live any longer...I am suffering ... I don't know how to say, it (my death) should be quick... I do not want to suffer like that... I do not have much feeling now...

Because of the uncontrolled pain and suffering, some hospice patients felt that it was meaningless to live longer. They might perceive their dying as 'lingering'. Eight patients felt anxious as they approached death. For example, an elderly woman with cancer of the lung, experienced fear of dying as she approached death.

> (I am) afraid that my condition will deteriorate, (I) am afraid of death... (It is) incurable... I have to experience death myself .

Suicidal death

A few patients were very frustrated with the inappropriate timing of their death. They could not tolerate their pain and suffering any longer and/or might want to experience a sense of control over their future. They did not want to wait for their natural death to come but decided to appoint a date for their death, which would be most appropriate for them. Therefore four patients had thought of attempting suicide. Two made the actual attempt: one was unsuccessful but the other was successful. The issues of attempted suicide and suicide have been discussed in Chapter Six.

In reality, it is not easy to be sure of patients' acceptance of the timing of their death because acceptance is a complex and subjective experience of the hospice patients. Based on the findings of this research, the degree of acceptance varied from individual to individual and it also changed periodically during the illness. Accepting the timing of one's death seemed to be closely related to patients' spirituality and their sense of hope. An example is a patient who was informed by the medical practitioner that he had six months to live. He seemed to accept the timing of his death and he stated that he had completed his preparations several years ago. After six months had passed, the patient felt helpless and hopeless. He refused to talk to people and became increasingly withdrawn. This example represents the complexity of the phenomenon of accepting the timing of one's own death. Although the dying person may have indicated his or her initial acceptance of death, such acceptance may not last until the end of his or her life. Five patients were observed to have similar experiences.

Completing social obligations

Maslow has described his personal feelings about a meaningful (timely) death following a serious heart attack that occurred soon after he completed writing a book that was important to him. 'This is what David Levy called the 'completion of the act' ... I think actors and dramatists have that sense of the right moment for a good ending, with a phenomenological sense of good completion — that there is nothing more that you could add'. [18]

In Chinese culture, although traditional Chinese beliefs have not identified the meaning of Good Death explicitly, to die for righteousness and/or to complete one's social roles seems to give a sense of completion and would be a form of Good Death. Many Chinese people today, particularly elderly people, still hold the value of completing their social obligations as one of their goals in life. Therefore, a majority of the hospice patients in this research accepted that they would die soon because they had accomplished their social obligations. According to the Law of Kinship, there are five cardinal relations: emperor (or government) -people, parent-child, spouses, siblings, and friends. [19-20] In order to judge one's value, one can be assessed whether in his relationship to the government, he is a loyal citizen; in his relations to his father, he is filial; in his relations towards brothers, he is honest and sincere. The moral obligations that the *Analects* of Confucius had developed can be summarised as 'Jen'. 'Jen' is benevolence and the fulfilment of appropriate interpersonal relationship as the supreme ideal theme for the conceptions and conduct of human life.

Completing parental role

An ancient Chinese idiom says, 'If you raise your children without giving them instructions, it will be the fault of the father.' Needless to say, a mother has similar social obligations. Therefore, parents have important moral and social obligations to educate their children. Traditionally, most Chinese families have many children. In this research, several patients had to raise between seven and nine children, and it could be difficult for them. Close to half of the patients who had completed their parental responsibilities were observed to be more accepting of their impending death. Some informed me of this with an expression of satisfaction. This was because they were able to see their children holding down proper and stable jobs and leading reasonable lives. In addition, they were able to see their children having families and grandchildren. Five single parents among the patients were proud that they managed to raise their children on their own. Completion of parental roles had certainly helped some patients to accept the timing of their death better. The following are some examples.

A seventy-year-old patient with cancer of the lung indicated that he had fulfilled his obligations as father and husband. His family consisted of his wife and two adult children's families, but he did not consider his children filial to him. He had retired from his job. He was diagnosed two months prior to the time of the interview and he was informed that he had six months to live. He made all possible preparations for departure and he stated during the interview that he was ready to die.

> Yes, frankly speaking, (I) only (have) six months to live. I have nothing to complete. My medical practitioner asked me to complete my unfinished business the first time I saw him. I completed everything seven years ago. Now my children have grown up, they have jobs, and they are married. I have left nothing undone. I have done what I can. Yes, I have instructed (my children) about everything and I have completed everything. I also have grandchildren.

Another example was an eighty-four-year-old man with cancer of the colon. He was happy to talk about his obligations as father and his acceptance of the timing of his death. All his children had good jobs and properties such as flats or houses. He remembered and described them clearly one by one. To have one's own flat or house can be an indicator of one's social achievements.

> I have worked hard my whole life and I have raised seven children. I came to Hong Kong at the age of twenty-six with only forty dollars. I feel that my children are all right. They are financially independent and they have their own flats.

Consequently, some patients might feel angry and upset if they could not fulfil their social obligations. The following is an example. A seventy-year-old woman showed self-pity that she could not resume her duties as a mother. She had two filial adult sons. As she was hospitalised, she could not look after her family. Instead, she needed others' assistance.

> I have to leave my home unattended. I need people to help. I have a home and yet I cannot go home....

Another example was a fifty-six-year-old woman with cancer of the lung. She was also unhappy that she could not look after her teenage son who was a form five student. He would sit for a public examination in a few months' time. She was worried for him because he was not doing well in his school work. She was also anxious about leaving him when she died.

> My child may give me some worries (she sighed for a while). I married at the age of twenty. Now I am fifty-six. I need to cook for them (the family). My last son does not work hard. He studies in Ho Chuen Yiu Secondary School. He is now in form five but he just plays ball games and does not enjoy his studies. I do not know what he is doing. I cannot follow him all the time. He does not listen to anybody because he thinks he is big enough. He is quite tall now. I am a bit worried about him.

Traditionally, Chinese parents arranged marriages for their children but this is no longer a contemporary practice. Nevertheless, some patients still considered seeing their children married to be another major parental obligation. Therefore, nine hospice patients indicated better acceptance of the timing of their death as their children had their own families and/or children. At the same time, some patients hoped that they could live longer so that they might be able to see their children or grandchildren get married. The following are two examples.

The first example is Mr. L, a forty-five-year-old man with cancer of the lung. He knew that his condition was deteriorating, so he brought forward the date of his son's wedding. In this way, he could attend his son's wedding. A wedding was regarded as an important family event and the patient was very pleased with the re-arrangement. Although he was angry about having cancer he seemed to have better acceptance of his imminent death after he had fulfilled his obligations as father. He died about a month after his son's wedding.

The second example is an elderly female woman, Mrs. L, who hoped to live longer so that she might see his son getting married. When she attended the outpatient clinic, she requested the medical practitioner to inform her son that her illness was serious, in the hope that her son would get married sooner, but the medical practitioner refused to assist her. Her son refused to get married, too. He explained to his mother that his marriage was important to him and he could not get married in such a hurry. The following is her report of her conversation with the medical practitioner.

> I told the medical practitioner that I really want to see my son getting married. I asked him to tell my son that I just have a few more months to live, so my son may get married sooner. The medical practitioner and the nurse laughed. I do not want to die now. I want to wait and see my son getting married. Then I will die in peace. This is my worry. My son has a girlfriend; however, he has not made up his mind yet. I am going to die. I hope to live for another two to three years. I really want to have 'a cup of tea' from my daughter-in-law (part of the wedding ceremony). My son replied, 'Please do not care about me too much, Mother. You are happy to have that 'cup of tea' from your daughter-in-law, but what happens afterwards? He asked me what would happen after his wedding. Yes, he may have a hard time because this may not be a good marriage.

Completing children's roles

As mentioned in Chapter Six, many Chinese practised filial piety in parent-child relationship, which is based on mutual expectations of caring and love. [21] Filial piety is a highly virtuous and ideal representation of Chinese culture. It implies strong devotion to the dying parent. One has to treat one's parents with respect (filial piety) and take care of the older generation. [22] Since the majority of the patients were elderly, most of them were either parents or grandparents. They were more concerned about their relationships with their children than with their own parents. However, their parents might have influenced their social conduct as 'responsible parents'. Just three patients referred to their obligations to their parents. The following is an example. A forty-six-year-old patient, who was a drug addict, reflected on his affection towards his mother. He regretted that he had not fulfilled his obligation as a 'filial son' and this was probably his unfinished business before he died.

> (For) Six to seven years, I wept whenever people mentioned my mother's death because she was precious (to me). Hey... (He smiled bitterly). She has four sons and I am the least useful (child) among her children. Hey, this is true! This is true! If she were alive, she would have given me some instructions. No matter whether she scolded me or not, I would feel happy. No, (I have not fulfilled my role as a son). I am not eager to earn money. I am rather playful. They (his siblings) have earned good livings. They have cars, for instance.

Based on some traditional cultural values, several hospice patients in this research indicated the importance of completing their obligations as parents even though their children were adults. They might consider fulfilment of their obligations as their main purpose in life. Therefore, most of them showed better acceptance of the timing of their death when their children were able to live independently and well. Some of them were happy to see their children have their own families and children.

Although some patients did not emphasise what they had contributed to their children, they shared with me the outcomes of their obligations. For example, five indicated that their families valued them and nine indicated that their children paid regular visits. Hence, they did not have any unfinished business and they were ready to die. In this research, completion of their social obligations, whether they indicated it explicitly or implicitly, certainly strengthened some of the patients' social connectedness and gave them socio-cultural spiritual comfort.

On the other hand, some patients did not stress their fulfilment of social obligations. There were many reasons for this. First, they had no children or their children stayed overseas. Second, six did not reveal their acceptance of the timing of their death because they might not expect a reciprocal commitment from their children, even though they had completed their parental obligations. Consequently, they might have little contact with their children and/or feel that their children were not caring enough. Further, a few patients might not have regarded their parental obligations as important. Their acceptance of the timing of their death was associated more with their illness and age than completion of their social obligations.

Dying in old age

Death of the elderly is often perceived as appropriate, simple, and gradual relinquishment of a life that has reached its assigned span.[23] Therefore, dying in old age is generally accepted as Good Death by many researchers in both Western cultures [7,10] and Chinese culture.[24] Since the Zhou Dynasty, before Confucius' time, dying in old age has been regarded as 'good' in China because it was a natural death. However, with the current social and cultural changes, the meanings of old age are changing accordingly. Based on the findings of this research, the hospice patients may place personal meanings and socio-cultural meanings on 'dying in old age'.

Personal meaning

Seven patients believed that death was a natural process. Nine patients accepted their imminent death because they were old: six of them were over seventy. Consequently, older patients were more ready to accept that they were going to die. 'I do not want to live any longer, I speak to God that it is almost time (for me to die), I would like to have a good ending'.

Four patients appeared to gain an acceptance of the timing of their death when they compared their age with their parents' age when they died. It was interesting to note that male patients compared their age with that of their fathers and a female patient had compared her age with that of her mother when she died. The following are some examples.

> My father was just over thirty. Therefore, I am quite happy with myself. At one time, some people said I would not live up to fifty because I was too busy with my work. Also, I liked coffee.

> My father was worse (than me). He died when he was around fifty. I am older than him (the patient was seventy). I am luckier, as I have lived twenty years more. It looks as if I am in a better position. This is life that (we) must walk along. We can have a long or short (life span). My life (span) is neither long nor short. That is OK. By short (life span), I mean forty to fifty. By long (life span), I mean eighty. Not everyone can reach the age of 100.

Socio-cultural meaning

An ancient Chinese saying states that it is rare for people to live up to the age of seventy. Therefore, dying in old age is a blessing rather than a sad event. The family should celebrate for their family member who can live up to the age of seventy or beyond. [22] In this way, the age of seventy can be an indicator of longevity. 'Living up to the age of seventy or over is longevity'. Consequently, the funeral of a person of age over seventy is called a 'laughing funeral', which means a happy event.

However, the term 'old age' may carry some ambiguous meanings today. At what age should a person be considered 'old'? With the current advancement of medical treatment and improvement of the health care system, many people can live up to the age of seventy or eighty. On one hand, it is encouraging to see more people achieving the state of 'longevity'. Most Chinese, if not all, hope for 'longevity'. On the other hand, the ageing problem has become a social problem in many countries. As discussed in Chapter Seven, many elderly patients were financially dependent on others and some were not able to maintain good quality of life socially and physically. Therefore, some elderly people have chosen suicide as their final exit.

The following is an example of an eighty-four-year-old patient, Mr. L, who felt he was too old to stay alive. The uncertainty of how long he would live had given him many problems. He had received a lump sum of money as his retirement fund more than twenty years ago. He did not want to live longer because his financial situation did not allow him to live well. Also, he became dependent, for example, his vision and memory deteriorated, his legs were weak, and he had had several falls. In addition, his wife had died many years before and his children were in China. He felt lonely at times even though he maintained social connectedness with his relatives. It was clear that he did not accept the timing of his death even though he had lived to the age of eighty-four.

> The best time to die is seventy to eighty, not beyond eighty years old. I think one should not live too long. There would be too much suffering, just like with me. To live up to seventy is good, eighty is maximum. (One) should not live longer than that.

Historically, Chinese considered dying in old age a natural and good death. Justice [25] extends the meaning of Good Death in Indian culture: death without any illness. Therefore, people dying of cancer would not be considered to have a Good Death in Indian cultures. Age also influences the extent of control the patient has over the situation[26] and how relatives, health care professionals, and others respond to the dying person. Therefore, several other factors may determine whether dying in old age is good or not. These factors include the dying person's goals in life, comfort, social connectedness, and sense of control and hope.

Accepting death as a natural part of life

In the present research, more than two-thirds of the hospice patients had some kind of spiritual support, which enabled them to accept the timing of their death. 'Spiritual' means seeking for meaning in existence, experience of God, purpose, and value in life, non-material aspects of life, and trust in the transcendent. [27-28] Spirituality is the state or quality of being concerned with spiritual matters and is 'our aid and comfort in the face of death'. [29] Many patients were eager to cling onto some kind of 'religion' or 'belief' that would provide them with a sense of hope and peace of mind. Some of them might have 'turned to religion' since becoming aware of their prognosis. Their spiritual resources mainly came from Chinese traditional and popular beliefs and Christianity. Some patients had no religious beliefs.

Traditional Chinese beliefs

Taoism and Buddhism are the two most common traditional religions in Chinese culture. Taoism encourages people to maintain a harmonious relationship with the universe. That is, to live and die with peace of mind according to the law of nature. Therefore, people need to accept death as a natural part of life and they should not be afraid or anxious about death. Buddhists consider that all life is suffering. They believe that people are anxious and fearful because they are egocentric and can only see everything from their own perspective . Buddhism teaches people to stop denying the inevitable, ever-changing character of life and death, and invites them to reach a state of perfect peace or to have a better rebirth. Such acceptance will eventually bring people a new peace of mind. Both Taoism and Buddhism encourage people to maintain peace of mind and to accept death.

Close to half of the patients believed in Chinese religions. Some followed their parents and worshipped multiple gods such as the God of Heaven and God of Earth. Most Chinese worship Taoist and Buddhist gods and they perform religious practices as required by these beliefs. For example, Wong Tai Sin and Che Kung are significant examples of Taoist deities in Hong Kong. Many Chinese attend the Temple of Wong Tai Sin and ask for blessings on the first day of the Chinese New Year. Very often, they pray for good health and peace (of mind) for every member of the family. Many Chinese also visit the Temple of Che Kung on the third day of the Chinese New Year for similar reasons.

The following description is a significant example of a Buddhist patient who demonstrated her acceptance of the timing of her death when she died. Mrs Y was a sixty-three-year-old woman with cancer of the colon. She told me about her family, social background, and her tough life. She had looked after her family well and maintained an intimate family relationship. She felt peaceful because she had completed her social obligations. Her children were good to her and they all had jobs. She had some grandchildren too. She had had cancer for about two-and-a-half years at the time of the first interview. She had made the necessary preparations as she had discussed the related issues with her children and bade farewell to them. More importantly, she had faith in Buddhism.

She listened to Buddhist music at all times with her earphones and she was able to maintain peace of mind. She believed she would go to a bright and happy world after she died. Finally, she requested the company of her daughter, who was also a Buddhist, for her last few days. In addition, her religious friends visited and prayed for her. She died peacefully in the company of her daughter in the hospice unit.

Meanwhile, it is noted that some patients' ideas about the teachings of different traditional Chinese beliefs were rather unclear. For instance, their understanding about death and life after-death had some variations.

> I am a Buddhist. I believe in the existence of Buddha but I do not believe in reincarnation. Sometimes I go to the Buddhist temple. Sometimes I follow a friend. I'd rather consider fate.

> I am a Buddhist. I believe I will go to heaven.

These patients did not believe in reincarnation or they thought they would go to heaven.

> I believe in Buddhism but I seldom worship gods in the Buddhist temple. My family worships multiple gods. I simply take one religion. I feel that if I have not done anything bad, I should be able to go to heaven.

This patient did not attend the temple regularly and he might not be a practising Buddhist.

One clinical implication suggested by the above accounts is that hospice staff should assess the religious background of their patients carefully. They cannot assume that patients who believe in Buddhism or Taoism will always be able to maintain peace of mind and accept the timing of their death.

Chinese popular beliefs

Today, many contemporary Chinese also practise one or more popular belief systems, which have their origins in Taoism, Buddhism, or Confucianism. In this research, ten patients practised ancestor worship. Seven patients believed in fate and a few worshipped multiple gods such as Kuan Yum, Wong Tai Sin, Che Kung, God of Heaven, and God of the Earth. Confucius emphasised belief in 'Tien Ming' which consists of meanings of fate and mission.[30] Therefore, some Chinese people believe in heavenly fate that decides the time of birth, the hour of death, the manner of death, and the experiences between life and death. [31] This explained why some patients could endure whatever happened to them with few complaints. The beliefs in fate, ancestor worship, and/or multiple gods may have facilitated some hospice patients to accept the timing of their death.

> Yes, this is my fate. I do not want to think further. I believe in fate. Fate means that when one's time comes, one will leave (die).

Christianity

Cancer patients who are church attendees can cope better and have lower levels of stress. [5] They may have a higher level of life satisfaction than those who do not go to church services. Although several patients believed in Buddhism, Taoism, or Chinese popular beliefs, some patients were Christians. However, not every Christian patient died with his or her faith. A few of them who believed in God also experienced intense depression. For example, a Catholic patient attempted suicide, but she was unsuccessful. She was angry with God because He had not cured her. She thought that God was not helping her although she had adjusted her life by going to church and praying more often.

On the other hand, some Christians believed that there must be something more 'powerful' than cancer. They believed that there was something keeping them living — the belief in a 'God' who could strengthen them with eternal hope.[32] Consequently, these Christian patients would accept death as a part of God's eternal plan.

Mrs. A was a typical example of a Christian who had demonstrated strong faith, hope, and love of God. Her family and friends valued her and visited her regularly. They were present when she died in the hospice unit. Therefore, her spiritual connectedness with God and the family and her psychosocial-spiritual comfort contributed largely to her acceptance of the timing of her death. She could endure the suffering of having cancer and approach death with peace of mind and acceptance. She also possessed the strength to communicate her needs to the people around her and she maintained her hope by communicating with and thanking God. Therefore, she experienced a sense of control over her life and her future.

During one field visit, I approached her and asked her if I could interview her. She replied that she was thirsty. Therefore, I helped her with several spoonfuls of water. She was contented and asked if I was a Christian because I was kind to her. I asked her how she felt about being ill and staying in the hospital. I also asked her if she had any problems. She shook her head (no problems) and thanked God for keeping her in the hospice unit. She accepted what had happened to her and responded to me with a grateful demeanour. She said her hope for eternity had given her a greater capacity to endure her present suffering.

The interview did not last long because Mrs. A was tired and sleepy. I helped the patient to get comfortable and left her. She was aware of her impending death but her words were gentle and tender and she did not have any negative feelings about her situation. Although the interview with Mrs. A was relatively short (about thirty minutes), it was significant because she experienced serenity and acceptance.

Non-believers

Four patients had no particular religious beliefs and some of them were uncertain about life after death. Seven patients hoped that they would go to heaven after they died. Four patients indicated that they felt they accepted death although they did not have a particular religious faith. A sixty-six-year-old man with cancer of the lung was an example. He worked as a musician for a funeral company and he was familiar with different funeral ceremonies. His mother was a Christian but he had not followed her.

> I believe all religions are good. They all teach you to become a good person. I do not believe that there is only one religion which directs people to eternity. Some visitors (volunteers from some religious organisations) were not sure if they were paying me a visit or they were

preaching the gospel. I have no worries at all. I trust myself and I do not believe in any god or ghost. I trust myself most. My wife is afraid of the ghosts in the hospital. She said she was frightened of meeting the ghost(s) in the evening, so she always comes in the daytime.

Based on the findings of this research, several hospice patients showed better acceptance of the timing of their death because they accepted death as a natural part of their lives. Faith in god(s) of either Chinese or Western religions may give patients a sense of hope and a source of unconditional acceptance. Just as important, health care professionals have to recognise that religious faith and beliefs may not be adequate to predict or explain what dying people experience as they approach death. Little is known about the relationship between religious faith and practice and the individual's personal orientation towards death. [15] Therefore, health care professionals cannot assume that every patient with religious faith can accept death as a natural part of life and die peacefully. At the same time, non-believers might accept the timing of their death without apparent religious support.

Experiencing meaningful lives

As life draws to an end, people like to review their lives and ask themselves questions such as what will come next. 'What purpose was my life? My illness and my death?'[33] Erikson [34] suggests that the aim of the last stage of life is to have reached a state of ego integrity where the individual has found meaning in life as it comes to its end. 'Integrity simply means a willingness not to violate one's identity, in the many ways in which such violation is possible'. [35] Thus, some elderly patients reminisced about their past lives, a process called life review. Life review is thought to be therapeutic as it enables people to reflect on their past events and reintegrate their past conflicts. In this research, several patients made life reviews during the interviews.

In the process of life review, these patients were searching for the meaning of their lives. Most of them related their meanings of life to Confucian and Buddhist teachings on being a morally good and accountable person. Both Confucianism and Buddhism encourage people to keep moral principles and self-control, but with different intentions. They teach people to live a morally good life and have faith in self-improvement, which will eventually allow them to reach a state of spiritual contentment and acceptance of one's death. [36] Therefore, four hospice patients in this research showed better acceptance of the timing of their death because they had experienced meaningful lives with their families.

The following are descriptions of two patients who had experienced meaningful lives according to Confucian teachings. In addition, both of them had completed their parental roles and they accepted that they would die soon. An eighty-four-year-old patient claimed that he had maintained Confucian moral teachings throughout his life. He did not think that his wealth could make him accept the timing of his death, but the fact that he had been a good person did.

> To me, the values of life are to be a good person who would not hurt people and not act against his conscientious heart. Money is useless when you have no time to enjoy life. Even you were the most brilliant person, you become worthless if you have a terminal illness. It is important not to be ashamed of your conscientious heart (mind). It is important not to hurt others for the sake of yourself. I have not done anything harmful to other people.

Another patient, who had cancer of the lung, also considered that living with traditional moral values had been most important for him. He stated that his life was meaningful because he had kept his moral responsibilities as a father and husband. Although he had gone through the Cultural Revolution in China, he continued to uphold traditional Confucian moral values. Therefore, he instructed his children to be good persons and he was contented that he had led a morally correct life. He stressed repeatedly that his social obligations were not just towards himself and his family but also towards his ancestors. He said he would not feel ashamed when he met his ancestors after he died, which influenced his acceptance of the timing of his death.

> I have been very devoted to my family because the family is most important to me. We must be good people although we are poor. Otherwise, we would bring shame to our ancestors.

Meanwhile, several patients had modified their philosophy of life after recognising that they had terminal cancer. Some began to value living a more meaningful life. An example was a forty-six-year-old clerk who used to work diligently, even after office hours. He had spent most of his life earning more money for a better living. However, he changed his philosophy of life after he had cancer. Some volunteers who gave him support and assistance influenced this change. He also showed better acceptance of his imminent death.

> Positively, this illness has changed my philosophy of life. I have come to know a group of volunteers. At the beginning, I did not believe there could be a group of such good people. Before this, I felt that people did not often care for each other. The volunteers often visit me and keep me company. This makes me feel that the meaning of life is important... Now, I don't mind so much about life and death. I have earned many days. In the past, I used to enjoy eating and playing, like everybody else. My goal of life was to earn more money. Now I feel I have wasted a lot of time. There are many things that cannot be bought by money.

Another example was a young female patient. She was an accountant clerk. She had been exploring the meaning of her life after she found she had cancer (for nine months). She was divorced. She began to accept what had happened to her because her sisters' affection and care had given her a meaning to live. Further, her Christian faith also provided her with the meaning of life. She began to accept the timing of her death.

> In the past, I would not speak about it (the affection of my sisters) to other people. I did not know how to talk about it. I feel that my family loves me very much. Now I do not feel shy to tell them that I love them too! I have learnt to have better acceptance, now that I do not have any unfinished business... Everyone has to leave (die) once. I believe I will have another life.

Based on the finding of this research, some hospice patients showed better acceptance of the timing of their death when they had experienced meaningful lives or when they began to find some meaning in their lives. Very often, these patients' life purpose was to fulfil their social obligations to their families and the community. Some patients also emphasised the importance of showing affection to people they had loved before they died.

Table 10.1
Categories and significant statements of Accepting the timing of one's own death (Completion)

Categories	Significant statements
Accepting the timing of one's own death	My main concern is that my body would not suffer too much. I would not mind going (dying) anytime. It could be tomorrow, may be tomorrow (10, p.7).
	I am old enough, I will not mind dying, this is not a problem (for me). It is time to complete (my) life... I do not want to live any longer. I tell God that it is almost time (for me to die). I would like to have a good ending (26).
Completing social obligations	I made bean curd and sold it for a living. I have raised my four children (27).
	I do not want to die now. I want to see my son get married. Then I will die in peace (11, p.12).
Dying in old age	I have come across cancer because my brother-in-law died of cancer of the lung as well. He had lived for six months... I am not fear, I am already seventy years old and (I do) not have to fear! (7).
Accepting death as a natural part of life	I believe in God: Buddha and Christianity... they all teach people to be good persons. Confucius was the best man. I do not think about it (life after death). I believe in Tao (25).
	I thank God for sending me there. My hope for eternity will give me a greater capacity to endure the present suffering (14).
Experiencing meaningful lives	In the past, I would not speak about it (the affection of my sisters) to other people. I did not know how to talk about it. I feel that my family loves me very much. Now I do not feel shy to tell them that I love them too! I have learnt to have better acceptance, now that I do not have any unfinished business... Everyone has to leave (die) once. I believe I will have another life (33, p.2).

Clinical implications

Goal:
Facilitate patients in achieving better acceptance of the timing of their death as they wish

Identify spiritual needs and concerns

One of the roles of health care professionals is to assist dying people to identify, develop, or reaffirm sources of spiritual energy and to foster hope. [37] They can also help them to give meaning to their lives.[38] Therefore, it may be easier to approach spiritual assessment by asking whether they are happy and if they have peace of mind. Next, it is important to identify the resources to meet their spiritual needs. According to Shelly, [39] the first resource is the nurse (or health care professional) in the provision of time spent in communicating with the patient. The other resources can be their social obligations, traditional cultural religions/beliefs, Chinese popular beliefs, and other religions such as Christianity. Health care professionals should not predetermine that religious believers may have better acceptance of the timing of their death than unbelievers may. Similarly, they cannot assume people of older age have more readiness to die.

Meanwhile, other validated assessment tools may be used. For instance, the McGill Quality of Life Questionnaire has incorporated questions about personal meaning, achieving life goals, and finding life worthwhile. [40-42, 47-48] This may be useful for assessing the spiritual needs of the Chinese hospice patients.

Provide spiritual care

'Health professionals may not cure the disease, erase the pain or quiet their fears, but they can listen. Being heard sometimes relieves both pain and anger'. [43] From the findings of the research, it was clear that the hospice patients needed spiritual care as soon as they knew the diagnosis. Provision of spiritual care to the hospice patients should not be considered as a 'luxury' service. Instead, it is an essential duty of health care professionals. [44]

Spiritual care becomes more obvious as the patients prepare for their departure. Being willing to be empathetically part of the experience and meaning of the dying person's world is the most caring social act health care professionals can offer. [45] Unless the person is in a state of denying death, he or she often has had some time to consider his or her beliefs about death and come to relatively peaceful terms with them. Health care professionals may not provide meanings of life to the person who is suffering and dying. Nevertheless, they can encourage the person and listen carefully to his or her own inner spiritual voice. Furthermore, they can spend more time listening to those patients who cannot maintain connectedness with the family and hospice staff.

To maintain peace of mind, health care professionals can help the family and the dying person to let go and die peacefully. Christine Longaker[46] discovers that for such a person to be able to let go, 'he or she needs to hear two explicit verbal assurances from loved ones'. First, they must give the person permission to die. Second, they must reassure the person they will be all right after he or she has gone and that there is no need to worry about them. Finally, the effectiveness of spiritual interventions needs to be evaluated.

Table 10.2
Summary of accepting the timing of one's death (Completion)

Related issues	Clinical implications
1. Accepting the timing of one's death	Goal: Facilitate patients in achieving better acceptance of the timing of their death as they wish
2. Completing social obligations	
3. Dying in old age	1. Identify spiritual needs and concerns.
4. Accepting death as a natural part of life	2. Provide spiritual care.
5. Experiencing meaningful lives	

Summary

The findings presented in this chapter indicate that accepting the timing of one's death is an important element of dying a Good Death. Accepting the timing of death is a state in which a person often has peace of mind and calmness. He or she may be satisfied with his or her life, thus may indicate a sense of readiness to die. Consistent with some previous studies, some patients in this research indicated that it was the right time to depart [7-9] and to die without despair, depression, or suicidal ideas. Some claimed to have experienced meaningful lives. [8] Others have expressed the feeling of a good ending, of a willingness [18] and readiness to die. [8]

These patients tended to show better acceptance under the following circumstances: when they 1) completed their social obligations; 2) died in old age; 3) accepted death as a natural part of life; and 4) experienced meaningful lives. First, they may have fulfilled their social obligations as parents, spouses, and/or children. Completion of one's social roles often represents one's emphasis on maintaining family connectedness. Accomplishment of these obligations could also indicate substantiation of a meaningful and responsible life for a majority of patients in this research. This could also bring the patients spiritual comfort.

Second, most patients were elderly and therefore may have accepted the timing of their death better. Hospice patients found their personal meaning of 'old age' when they compared their age with that of their parents who had died. They may also refer to the socio-cultural meaning of 'old age'. Dying in old age, living up to the age of seventy, has long been considered as Good Death in Chinese culture. Today, many people can live to this age but they may not be happy. Therefore, people have to consider other factors that make 'dying in old age' an important element of Good Death.

Third, several patients experienced a sense of acceptance because they had religious faith. They believed that the gods they worshipped would bless their lives and death. Their religious faith or beliefs facilitated them to maintain an eternal hope of a better life after death. Nevertheless, some non-believers might have developed a similar acceptance of their death. Fourth, affirmation of the meaning of life would further sustain one's hope and control for a future. It could also offer the patients feelings of spiritual comfort and acceptance.

At the same time, some patients did not accept the timing of their death. Therefore, they might perceive dying as prolonged and lingering. A few of them even determined to control the timing of their death by attempting suicide. It was observed that patients' acceptance of the timing of their death was a unique experience. It could vary from individual to individual and from time to time during the course of their illness. For example, some patients perceived dying in old age was good, while some elderly patients considered their impending deaths were prolonged. Therefore, health care professionals have to be sensitive and careful when they carry out spiritual assessment and interventions.

It is also noted that most of the contributing factors to the patients' acceptance of the timing of their death are spiritual in nature. Therefore, some implications are suggested to assist those patients who want to develop better acceptance of the timing of their death. These interventions include identification of patients' individual spiritual needs and concerns and provision of spiritual care for hospice patients.

11
A Harmonious Death

Introduction

THIS CHAPTER PRESENTS a theory of Chinese dying behaviour based on the description of the seven elements. The discussion begins with a brief summary of the seven elements, followed by a presentation of the theoretical framework. The seven elements are further categorised into three main relationships that the patients considered valuable. According to the patients, to die a Harmonious Death meant to live in harmony with their caregivers until they died. In Chinese culture, Confucianism, Taoism, and Buddhism all agree that a good death emerges from a good life. This idea is familiar to dying persons in Western cultures, such as East Londoners. [1] Three groups of caregivers were of particular importance to them: ancestors, heaven/gods; medical practitioners, and their families. Finally, the present theoretical framework of Harmonious Death will be compared with the existing models of Good Death in order to highlight the significance of the present framework.

Summary of findings

There are seven important elements to facilitate a Harmonious Death. These seven elements include death awareness, hope, comfort, connectedness, control, preparations, and completion. These elements constructively unite the dying person and his or her caregivers (health care professionals and family) and the universe (ancestors, heaven/ gods),[2] in a beneficial hierarchical and socio-cultural relationship.

Consistent with some previous research, [1,3] Having an *awareness of dying* is an essential first step into achieving a Harmonious Death. Accordingly, the episode of breaking/ receiving bad news could be regarded as the first crucial reference point in the patients' illness. The patients developed an awareness of dying when they knew their diagnosis, because they often associated cancer with death. As death remains a topic of social taboo in most Asian communities, the patients may discuss their illness and future using terms and expressions with which they felt comfortable. Alternatively, they may talk about cancer and death with openness and acceptance; therefore, this social behaviour could be considered quite specific evidence of death awareness in Chinese communities. Despite the apparent differences in presentation, both groups of patients might die with a positive experience.

At the time when patients developed their awareness of dying, they might lose hope and sense of control for a future. Naturally, people hope for longevity, hence, the immediate *hope* for patients was to seek medical treatment that offered them a cure or prolonged their lives. Traditional Chinese medical treatment was a popular choice of alternative therapy. The patients also made adjustments, which included adjusting to the hospice environment, changing their lifestyles, and psychological adjustments. The outcome of these adjustments also reinforced their social connectedness with their caregivers and spiritual connectedness with their ancestors and heaven/ gods.

Patients also hoped to die with *minimal pain and suffering*. They frequently referred to pain as a physical painful experience and suffering as an emotional feeling. It is important to recognise that both pain and suffering are multi-dimensional experiences. Patients often experienced moderate or severe pain together with several symptoms. Consistent with the findings of Brallier[4] and Benoliel,[5] patients felt that if they had a sense of control and *social connectedness* with their caregivers, they would experience psychological and social comfort respectively. Likewise, they needed to be given spiritual comfort and care from their ancestors and/or heaven/ gods.

The fifth element of dying a Good Death was control. The hospice patients needed to experience a sense of *personal control* as soon as they developed death awareness. For example, they required information about their condition, which was often controlled by medical practitioners and their families. When they were more ready for the timing of their death, they needed the opportunity to discuss about the preferred environment where they would die. They were concerned about two choices: the place where they stayed and the person(s) accompanying them when they died. In reality, they were not always involved in making decisions about their care plans.

The hospice patients often made one or more *preparations*. These preparations could be classified as personal and public preparations. Personal preparations included the following: organising material affairs, leaving moral instructions and giving gifts. Giving jade as a gift, which symbolised lasting blessings and goodness, was quite common. The patients were also concerned with their funeral arrangements, which may include good 'Feng Shui' to comfort both the dead and the survivors. Meanwhile, patients would bid farewell to their families and friends in preparation for death. They interpreted the meaning of farewell differently. Farewell means saying goodbye in the Western culture, while it often meant 'leaving instructions' or 'organising material affairs' to the Chinese patients. Also, funerals always mean a public farewell to family and friends. On the whole, the dying patients placed more emphasis on spiritual preparations than material preparations and they hoped to continue the 'social ties' after they died.

Finally, patients would show better *acceptance of the timing of their death* under four circumstances. First, they had completed their social roles, which often represented their emphasis on maintaining family connectedness. Accomplishment of these obligations could also mean substantiation of a meaningful and responsible life. Second, they died in old age, therefore their deaths were perceived as good and natural. Third, patients had religious faith. Their faith or beliefs helped them to maintain eternal hope of a better life after death. Fourth, patients experienced meaningful lives that further sustained their hope and control for a better future. In this way, patients may also feel spiritual comfort and acceptance.

A Harmonious Death

In reviewing the seven important elements for a desirable good death, I observed that the dying patients were concerned with maintaining harmony in their relationships. Thus the theory which derives from the present research is entitled a Harmonious Death. Literally, a harmony means a balance maintained between interrelated aspects of a continuum; or a dynamic equilibrium between two 'opposite' components. [14-15] My observations agree with sociologist King's [6] comments on the Chinese social system. 'What constitutes proper human relationships is the central problem in Chinese projects.... Liang Sou-ming compares the Chinese social system with Western ones, asserts that Chinese society is neither individual-based nor society-based, but relation-based' (p.111). [6] Liang writes, 'The focus is not fixed on any particular individual, but on the particular nature of the relations between individuals who interact with each other. The focus is placed upon the relationship' (p.94).

The Chinese hospice patients hoped to establish a peaceful and comfortable relationship with their caregivers and heaven. Patients were particularly concerned about their relationships with three groups of caregivers, namely, their ancestors and/or heaven/gods, their medical practitioners, and their families. The seven elements are grouped under these three relationships as follows (Fig.1). First, the patients' awareness of dying and hope have close associations with their concepts and beliefs about heaven, life, and death, so these two elements were important in their relationship with heaven. Second, medical practitioners occupied a dominant position in determining patients' comfort and experience of personal control. Therefore, these two elements are discussed in terms of their relationship with medical practitioners. Third, connectedness, preparations, and completion are topics, which concern family relationships. The following section will examine the structure and function of each relationship, and its contribution to achieving a Harmonious Death (Fig. 2).

Fig. 1. Core elements of Harmonious Death

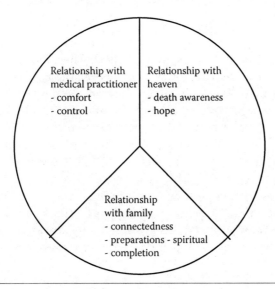

Fig. 2. Harmonious Death

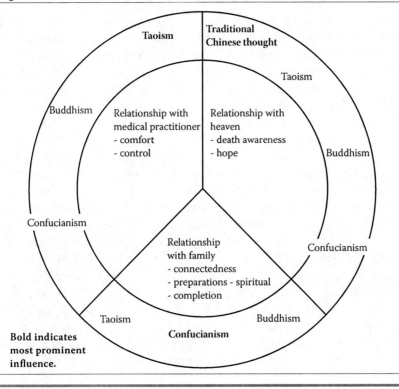

Relationship with heaven

According to the hospice patients in this research, a Harmonious Death meant maintaining harmonious relationships with heaven, their medical practitioners, and families. The following discussion will follow this order of priority. The relationship between people and heaven is clearly a hierarchical one: heaven is superior and people are inferior. [7] Heaven governs human life and death. The patients had great respect for heaven and they believed in the rule of heaven or heavenly fate. Therefore, some patients did not complain about having cancer and facing death. They accepted their situation because they believed this was their fate. Many Chinese maintain their harmonious relationships with heaven by worshipping 'heavenly gods' and their ancestors at home. [8] Twice a year on Ching Ming Festival (in spring) and Chung Yeung Festival (in autumn), many descendants visit their ancestors' graves to worship and remember their ancestors. [9]

Being aware of dying

Patients often developed an awareness of dying when they discovered their diagnoses. Therefore, the episode of breaking/ receiving bad news has been regarded as an important reference point of patients' illness. Both medical practitioners' and the patients' perceptions of death were important. Their perception of death would definitely affect their behaviours during the process of breaking/receiving bad news, which were predominantly 'bad' as the name implies. Therefore, patients tended to respond to having cancer with intense emotions because they were confronted with a premature death. [10-12] They often associated a premature death with punishment, which was one of the fundamentals of traditional Chinese beliefs. [13]

Traditional Chinese thoughts about heavenly blessings and suffering were based on an ancient official document, *The Book of History* (*Shang Shu*). In this book, some moral principles to guide the emperor were recorded. People would be granted Five Blessings if their emperors had ruled the country based on these moral principles. The Five Blessings were longevity, wealth, health and harmony, love of virtues, and a natural death. If they went against these principles, people would be punished by the Six Sufferings, including death and illness. [13] Today, many contemporary Chinese views of life and death are rooted in these traditional beliefs. [14] Patients might believe that they would receive a reward if they had maintained harmonious relationships with heaven/gods and their ancestors. On the other hand, patients might perceive illness and death as curses or punishments from heaven/gods and/or ancestors. In this way, patients' perceptions of death frequently carried moral-spiritual meanings, which affected their subsequent behaviours. They might avoid any discussion of death and continue to maintain it as social taboo. They may also indicate the need to know the 'truth' of their diagnosis, so that they could do something to restore these relationships in harmony.

For a similar reason, patients might believe that they had done nothing harmful to others or they had behaved morally well before they had cancer. Patients may relate their meanings of life to Confucian and Buddhist teachings of being a morally good and accountable person.[16] Accordingly, patients' openness and willingness to discuss death-related issues varied. Some patients were more open and willing to talk about these issues than others. Consequently, some presented evidence of death awareness more explicitly by mentioning the word 'death' in their conversations, while some did not do so. However, both groups of patients made adjustments and preparations and improved their family relations.

Confucius encouraged people to spend time solving problems of the present life and working towards righteousness and goodness until they died, rather than discussing the unknown future or afterlife. The Confucian view of death was one of continuous remembrance and affection instead of fear. Taoists believe life and death are complementary to each other and they suggest that one should not fear the natural control of one's life and death because one cannot reject or escape the natural law of the universe. [17] Both Confucianism and Taoism believe that people's lives and deaths are largely under the control of heaven. That means people have relatively little power to influence the decision of heaven. Therefore, patients who would die in old age and had experienced meaningful lives presented better acceptance of the timing of their death. To the patients, meaning of life often referred to the moral principles, which were taught in Confucianism or Buddhism.

Despite the fact that both Confucianism and Taoism encourage people not to fear death, the dying patients generally had this fear. Buddhism explains that people fear death because they are egocentric. Therefore, it advises people to accept the inevitable, ever-changing character of life and death and to build up good karma for a better rebirth. Chinese traditional thoughts on heavenly blessings and suffering seem to exert more influence on patients' awareness of dying and acceptance of death than the three traditional schools of thought.

Hope

When the patients developed an awareness of dying, they naturally hoped for a cure and physical restoration.[18] They hoped to have a long life and die naturally (whatever they may understand by this phrase). Longevity usually means dying at the age of seventy or above and it also carries a positive religious meaning of divine gift or reward. [13] People who achieve longevity will usually honour their families as well as their ancestors. This also explains why patients earnestly sought medical assistance to prolong their life span.

Traditional Chinese medical treatment was a popular choice for the dying patients. The main reason for this popularity is obvious. Chinese medical treatment, which is based on the Taoist Yin-Yang philosophy of health, is widely accepted by Chinese people. [19-20] Taoists perceive health as a state of equilibrium or harmony within the bodily organs and an integration of mind-body-soul. Homeostasis within the body reflects the balanced changes of the body to the external (cosmic) environment. For example, sleeping and waking are tied to the earth's rotation. Life is sustained in the presence of such harmonious balance within the body. Illness or death can result if this homeostasis is seriously affected. [21] Therefore, patients made adjustments to restore their bodies to harmony and prolong their lives. Patients' harmonious relationships with heaven and family would enhance the harmony within their body-mind-spirit. Their hope largely depended on their beliefs of Taoist philosophy of holistic health — the Yin-Yang harmony. Their hope might also have foundations on Buddhism or Taoism.

Relationship with medical practitioners

As death becomes an institutional event, health care professionals have replaced family members as witnesses of death and carers for dying persons as well. [22-24] Consequently, patients made adjustments to the hospice environment to obtain the best possible health services. Hence, their relationships with hospice staff, in particular medical practitioners, were significantly important. Their relationships with medical practitioners seemed to have a tremendous effect on their dying behaviours and consequently, may contribute to the success of a desirable Harmonious Death. People generally respect and obey authority figures. When people are sick, health care professionals are regarded as professional authorities that have obligations to restore their health. Medical practitioners are highly respected by people in Asian countries such as China and Japan [25] and they have an exceptionally superior status. Needless to say, all patients maintained distinct hierarchical relationships with medical practitioners. Therefore, patients and their families seldom challenged medical practitioners at the time of the disclosure of bad news. Very occasionally, patients might ask for some clarification of their diagnoses when medical practitioner withheld information.

Medical practitioners have replaced the family as the key decision makers for the dying patients. They contributed primarily to the quality of the patients' end stage of life. According to the accounts of the patients, medical practitioners had full control over information on the patients' condition[1, 3, 26-27] including their diagnosis and treatment plans. Second, they influenced patients' sense of hope if they disclosed the 'bad news' with a hopeful and empathetic attitude.[28] Third, medical practitioners could contribute to patients' comfort as they planned their treatments, including where patients died. Occasionally, they were able to estimate the timing of the patients' death and informed them of their life expectancy. It is not an exaggeration to say that the quality of patients' lives rested predominantly on their relationships with the medical practitioners. The following discussion will focus on patients' possible outcomes in maintaining a harmonious relationship with medical practitioners: comfort and control.

Comfort

During the episode of breaking/receiving bad news, medical practitioners might try to soften the 'painful truth' of patients' diagnoses by using other words or phrases instead of the word 'cancer'. They might also withhold the truth of a patient's diagnosis. As a result, patients might not develop the awareness of dying which is essential for their preparations for death and/or adjustments. In this context, patients and their families always listened to the medical practitioners' announcement with little doubt and initiated a harmonious relationship with medical practitioners.

During the course of illness, patients often experienced pain and suffering. Effective control of patients' pain and suffering relied on effective communication between patients and hospice staff. The possible barriers included differences in socio-economic backgrounds and poor communication. Dunlop[29] observes that medical practitioners tend to come from higher socio-economic groups and might have limited personal experiences of suffering. Meanwhile, poor communication was due to either under-reporting by the patient or under-assessing by nurses or medical practitioners.[30]

Meanwhile, patients did not want to be a burden on the hospice staff.[31-32] They did not want to draw attention to their own individual needs,[25] and therefore endured pain. This was the main reason for under-reporting. Other patients endured pain because they did not want to take Western medicine frequently. Western drugs were thought to be 'Yin', which would have a 'cold' or harmful effect on their bodies. On the other hand, patients who held to the Buddhist belief that suffering was inevitable[14, 33-34] may have less guilty feelings that they were being punished and cursed as perceived by traditional Chinese beliefs. Buddhism does not condemn people who contract illness, that they might have done something morally or spiritually wrong to others or their ancestors. In particular, the Buddhist notion of karma has brought comfort to patients who have experienced hardship in their lives.[14] Therefore, the Buddhist view of illness and suffering seemed to be more acceptable to the hospice patients. For this reason, some patients, even though they knew little about Buddhism and or they may not have carried out any Buddhist practices, still claimed that they were Buddhists.

Patients needed to show their faithfulness to medical practitioners who often objected to them 'shopping around' for impossible cures.[35] Consequently, patients may refuse to disclose the truth that they had taken Chinese medical treatment as an alternative. In addition, they did not want to report that they had received non-pharmacological interventions. In reality, reports of some local self-help groups indicate that complementary treatment such as Qigong, massage, meditation, and aromatherapy have become popular in caring for dying people[20, 27, 36] Just as important, when patients had harmonious family relationships, it also strengthened their sense of comfort. In short, the Buddhist view on illness and suffering seemed to be more acceptable to the hospice patients. These patients were able to 'clarify' the meaning of one's own death and not to feel stigmatised for any moral wrongdoing. Consequently, they might have more confidence in maintaining harmonious relationships with others.

Control

As mentioned previously, some patients maintained their harmonious relationships with the medical practitioners by leaving the decisions of their care plan to them. They did not mind whether they were given the choice to decide or participate in the care planning. Therefore, they were mostly passive and obedient. Doyle (p.2) [37] reflects the contemporary social status of the elderly patients precisely. 'I feel passionately that we live in an age when human life and people's lives are less and less seen as having value except in economic terms. People are made to feel needed and valued only when they can earn and contribute to society. When they are unemployed or old or diseased and dying, no one speaks of value'. Mesler's [38] work describes similar phenomena. More importantly, the traditional Chinese belief in divine control had a profound influence on the dying patients. Confucianism and Taoism also support this belief.

In the hospice setting, medical practitioners resembled the ruler of the clinical unit, as described in Confucius's five cardinal relationships. They controlled many aspects of the patients' lives as discussed previously. In addition, changes in social systems and social values have strengthened the medical practitioner's role as 'ruler'.

The Chinese used to die in their homes in the presence of their families. [24, 39] The family accepted the dying person and took up their responsibilities to participate in this social event. With such reinforcement of harmonious family relationships, dying people were likely to die with peace of mind because they were surrounded by loved ones in their own homes. Death has now become an institutional event that people seldom talk about. Therefore, some hospice patients may have preferred to die in the hospice unit for several reasons. First, the hospice unit provided medical facilities for treatment and resuscitation procedures. Patients and family members might still want to have resuscitation when patients lost their vital signs. Second, they might believe that if death occurred in a hospital or in a hospice, the family was less likely to be disturbed by the patient's spirit. [29] This was a popular belief. Third, the families may not welcome the patients dying at home because they may have unpleasant wound discharges, for example. In this way, patients had to die in the institution and they needed to maintain harmonious relationships with medical practitioners who were their key decision makers.

At the same time, some patients did want to be involved in making decisions related to their future. They hoped to have a choice about where and with whom they died. Two patients determined to maintain their personal control over their own death. They did not violate their harmonious relationships with medical practitioners because they had respect for authority. [40] The first one had poor social relationships with the hospice staff, as he was a drug addict. His relationship with heaven was unclear because he did not mention his religious faith or ancestors. He experienced personal control of his death by determining the date, time, and place according to his wishes: he committed suicide. Another patient, who was frustrated with the policy of the hospice unit, felt unsettled and unwelcome in the unit. He finally settled his own problems and fulfilled his wishes by returning to his hometown in China, where he died with peace of mind.

People's determination to make decisions for themselves may relate to some ancient thoughts too. 'The reasonable spirit ought to decide for itself, and not permit itself to be taken captive. That is the appropriate gift of heaven to man; it is the law of humanity; it is the special dignity of man, conferred by heaven'. [41] According to Confucius and Mencius, people needed to cultivate their spirit until they internalised virtues such as altruism and righteousness. Only after achieving this state of mind, should people seek chances to make their own decisions and be independent. [41] The traditional dying social behaviours of the Chinese people have changed dramatically with the current changes of social values and social systems. The hospice patients respected medical practitioner to such an extent that they viewed them as became 'rulers' of their lives as described in Confucius's ideal social system. Therefore, they often adopted an obedient and compliant attitude in order to maintain a harmonious relationship with medical practitioners. In doing so, they might die comfortably in the institution as they wished.

Relationship with the family

Several ancient Chinese scholars pointed out that the true meaning of human existence should be sought in the context of human relations (quoted by Wang Yang-ming,). [15] 'Fundamental to the experience of life are to exist, to enjoy life and to search for life's meaning; none of these can be realised without the involvement of others' (p.187). [21] According to Confucianism, a person's virtue and value can only be assessed through his or her performance in relation to others and his or her impact upon human society. Therefore, Confucius categorised people into Five Relationships: ruler and people, father and son, husband and wife, elder brother and younger brother, and friends [39,42] Family relationship or kinship is most important because three of the five cardinal relationships occur within the family. People are aware of their obligations, which derive from this essential notion. In their relations with the government, they should be loyal citizens. In their relations with their fathers, they should be filial. In their relations towards brothers, they should be honest and sincere. They can also achieve some communication and harmony with heaven through ancestral worship but they have no access to the controlling power of heaven, except through the medium of the ruler. The ruler performs the state sacrifices on behalf of all his people. [7]

According to the five cardinal relationships, family members are classified according to age, gender, and status into hierarchical structure. [39] Confucianism considers that three of the Five Relationships — ruler and people, father and son, and husband and wife — must be governed by the principle of super-ordination and subordination. [7] Yet until recent decades, few Chinese had not heard of the proverb, 'What is of utmost importance to a family is harmony'.[43] Most Chinese are aware that harmony within a household can be attained only when its members are willing to accept and to maintain the hierarchical status differentiation existing within the family.[43] Accordingly, patients' family connectedness, preparations for death, and sense of completion depended largely on their relationships with their family members.

Connectedness

Among Confucius's Five Relationships, the relationship between parents and children was regarded as the most important [15] and was emphasised frequently by the hospice patients. Therefore, the patients referred to their family relationships mainly in the context of their children and spouse. The value of a harmonious family relationship has traditionally been a characteristic of Chinese culture and there is no other relation that can possibly replace it. Similar to relationships with medical practitioners, effective communication was significantly important in maintaining a harmonious family relationship.

Patients' family connectedness always possessed moral-spiritual meanings because their 'social ties' continued even after they died. They believed that the living and the dying continued their harmonious relationships through the practice of ancestor worship and filial piety. [44] That is, they would be worshipped as 'ancestors' who reserved the duty to bless their descendants. Meanwhile, both Buddhism and Taoism do not challenge the ancestral rites but often assist in family-centred ceremonies and sacrifices. Filial piety is the root of all virtues and is given the highest priority among all virtues in Chinese moral culture. According to Confucius, filial piety did not refer merely to social support for parents. It did consist in serving them while alive, in burying them when dead, and in making offerings to them after death according to the established rules. [41,] [44] Filial piety also implies strong devotion to dying parents. Such a caring and harmonious relationship offers people moral-spiritual comfort because it facilitates transcendence of the present situation for higher meaning and purpose, establishing connectedness and enabling hope.[45] Patients may have experienced spiritual contentment and readiness to die because they felt their families valued them. Therefore, patients who were parents may leave moral instructions to their children as preparations for death. They may also leave the funeral arrangements to their children. Finally, they may wish for the company of the family at the dying bed. It is clear that a continuous 'social tie' of the living and dying is maintained through the practice of ancestor worship and filial piety.

Preparations

Patients' personal and public preparations for death offered further evidence of their harmonious family relationships. They regarded funeral arrangements as significant life events. There are several functions of proper arrangement of funerals. First, patients would feel respected and loved by their families. They believed a proper funeral would make the dead ancestor happy in his or her afterlife, and saw this as more than a moral obligation. In this way, patients were enabled to maintain an extended harmonious family relationship with their ancestors in the world beyond. Second, funeral arrangements are also practices of filial piety towards the parents. The rituals and mourning can symbolise the respect and affection of the descendants. They also serve as fundamental proofs of Chinese identify.[46] The descendants will feel gratified by the existence of 'family social ties' between the ancestors and the descendants. Further, Confucians view rites as a way of pleasing or influencing heaven, gods, or ancestors.[14] Such practices as ancestor worship and funeral ceremonies serve to reinforce the Five Relationships between people, and are looked upon as important elements for dying a Harmonious Death.

Patients who believed in an afterlife claimed that they would meet their family members again. Therefore, they might have other cultural preparations. For example, they were dressed in new clothes or they were given sweetened tea before they died. The details of funeral ceremonies also reflected patients' traditional or religious beliefs about death and the afterlife. More patients preferred a traditional burial in a cemetery than cremation. These findings reinforce the continuation of the traditional Chinese belief that people should be buried rather than cremated in order to keep their bodies intact.

Meanwhile, patients may make some personal preparations such as organising material affairs, leaving moral instructions, and giving gifts. As mentioned previously, Chinese parents always carried out their moral and social obligations to educate their children. Therefore, the patients may be eager to leave some moral instructions to their children before they died. They may also bid farewell to their families by organising material affairs such as bank accounts. In a traditional Chinese family, the father was the head of the family and took charge of organising the material affairs of the family. This social behaviour may reflect the effect of devotion to Confucian ethics on the solidarity of the family by avoiding family partition.

Completion

The hospice patients might experience a sense of completion before they died. They had shown better acceptance of the timing of death under the following circumstances: when they 1) completed their social obligations; 2) died in old age; 3) accepted death as a natural part of life; and 4) experienced meaningful lives. These circumstances always reflect the existence of harmonious family relationships. As patients accepted their death, they maintained peace of mind, which further facilitated harmonious relationships with their families.

Completion of one's social roles often represents an emphasis on maintaining family relationships. Accomplishment of these obligations could also mean substantiation of a meaningful and responsible life for the dying patients. It could also bring patients social and spiritual comfort that they may meet their ancestors in the next world. Patients who would die in old age might also indicate that they had maintained harmonious family relationships and they had most likely led a happy life. Longevity has long been considered a heavenly reward as documented in *The Book of History*. This traditional Chinese thought has been valued by many Chinese people since that time.[13] Therefore, dying in old age would always give honour to the family and ancestors. Taoism also considers dying in old age an appropriate form of natural death. [17, 34, 47] Meanwhile, an individual's religious faith could further enhance a feeling of personal acceptance. Therefore, patients who held religious faiths could accept death as a natural part of life. Non-believers might also develop a similar acceptance.

The dying patients reminisced about their past life through life reviews. They often reflected upon the meaning of life with respect to Confucian and Buddhist teachings on morality and harmonious family relationships. Affirmation of the meaning of life would also sustain patients' hope for and control over their future. One example was a patient who stated that his life was meaningful because he had kept his moral responsibilities as a father and husband. Although he had gone through the Cultural Revolution in China in the 1960s, he continued to uphold Confucian moral values. He stressed repeatedly that his social obligations were not just for himself and his family, but also for his ancestors. He would not feel ashamed when he met his ancestors. Similarly, a female patient began to accept what had happened to her because her sisters' affection and care had given her meaning to live. Her relationship with her family improved greatly.

From the above accounts, it is clear that traditional Chinese beliefs and religions have exerted a powerful influence on contemporary Chinese views on life and death. The Chinese social system is, indeed, neither individual-based nor society-based, but relationship-based. The ancient beliefs of the Five Blessings and Six Sufferings have offered people some moral principles to follow. This underlies the fundamental relationship between heaven and the people. Consequently, people build their hope on the promises of the Five Blessings, which include longevity. Taoism also advocates longevity. Taoism derives the philosophy of health and promotes health and longevity by various methods, based on the theory of Yin-Yang equilibrium. This culture-specific philosophy of health has been widely accepted by Chinese and even people of other cultures today. In addition, Taoism, Buddhism, and Confucianism encourage people to lead independent lives, as they become morally mature. Therefore, participants may review their lives at times. If they had led a morally good life, they would have the confidence to maintain harmonious relationships with heaven, including their ancestors and their families. They needed to create and maintain harmonious relationships with medical practitioners, as they required the assistance of the health services.

Confucius laid out a simple but practical framework to guide people reaching a happy and moral life. The proposal of the Five Relationships forms the cornerstone of his teachings. In exploring the ideas or theoretical frameworks that may affect the patients' views of Harmonious Death, it was noted that Confucian teachings were significant. First, patients felt that death would be 'good' if they maintained a harmonious relationship with their ancestors or heaven/gods. They would not shame their descendants and ancestors or they might have a better afterlife. The goodness of their lives (and deaths) was also judged on the basis of their social obligations. Needless to say, death would be 'good' if they maintained a harmonious relationship with the family. The evidence of such goodness included the following: the presence of filial children and supportive spouse; proper funeral arrangements to bid farewell to their families and friends; and a sense of spiritual contentment and completion. Overall, among the traditional schools of thoughts, Confucianism appears to be most influential in guiding the Chinese people's thoughts and behaviours, in their relationships with people and heaven.

Accordingly, the following section will further examine the relationship between Chinese moral tradition and Harmonious Death. The discussion begins with a brief review of the origin of the nature of moral tradition with Confucianism at its core. I follow with a further examination of the nature of Chinese moral theory and its application to living and dying with heaven, medical practitioners, and family. This will enhance a better understanding of the relationship-based theory of Harmonious Death.

Chinese moral tradition and Harmonious Death

The Chinese patients' views of their present life and future death and or afterlife were deeply rooted in ancient traditional beliefs and religions. These beliefs and religions have profound influences on Chinese thoughts and behaviours, and may be further internalised and perpetuated. It might be due to their moral education began formally and informally in their childhood. People were urged to revise family ethics and pursue a morally acceptable life. [15] As indicated in the previous discussion, Confucianism seems to have an overwhelming impact on contemporary Chinese moral ideals. Such moral tradition informs people how they should live and consequently, how they can die harmoniously.

Chinese moral tradition

Origin of Chinese moral culture

Morality is the system of beliefs about how we ought to live (and die), in other words, what we should do and should not do. Such beliefs about one's character and conduct are generally referred to as moral beliefs. In Western countries, traditionally, morality has had a very close relationship with Judeo-Christianity; moral education is particularly emphasised in religious studies. [48-49] Chinese culture with the humanistic philosophy of Confucius at its core, has enjoyed a similarly lengthy history of almost 4,500 years since the time of Yao and Shang (1766 BC–1111 BC). [42] Confucius has been the most influential person in the Chinese moral tradition. 'Confucius has been able to shape a civilisation for so long in the landscape of East Asia'. [50] He lived during the Zhou period and felt that he experienced a world of chaos. People then, as now, asked the questions, 'What is life about?' 'How can I lead a happy life?'. It was believed that every person wanted happiness, which could be achieved through the development of a good character and the practice of good conduct. Confucius therefore sought to revive the values of what he considered to be a Golden Age of peace and harmony at the beginning of the Zhou Dynasty (1027–256

BC). [14, 51] He greatly appreciated the early Zhou emperors who had ordered the feudal hierarchy and devised the rites and music that he venerated. In other words, Confucius attempted to re-establish human order by developing a set of moral teachings that served as a practical system of human values at a time when Chinese society had fallen into social disorder. [42] Thus, in contrast with the West, Chinese moral tradition emphasises human-and-human relationship, instead of god-and-human relationship. Chinese morality is essentially social. [52]

Confucius repeatedly stressed the importance of moral practice. Confucius did not only preach in words, he also reinforced his teachings and principles by example and by his achievements with his disciples. Likewise, the hospice patients frequently evaluated their moral practice during their course of illness. First, they might relate it to having cancer and confronting death. Then, they might relate it to pain and suffering experiences. Therefore, patients may increase their religious activities or cling to one religion. Finally, they might achieve peace of mind as they completed their obligations and headed for a possible rebirth or afterlife.

Other philosophers such as Mencius and Hsun Tzu also made a considerable contribution to the growth and development of Chinese ethical and moral theory. Both philosophers emphasised the importance of moral education, which started at home, and mothers were always the most influential persons. Therefore, the mother's role was well presented by the female patients. They felt 'good' when their filial children valued them. Therefore, they might leave them with moral instructions before they died. A male patient had reflected what his deceased mother had instructed him before she died.

Meanwhile, the introduction of various philosophies and religions such as Taoism and Buddhism has had a significant influence on Chinese moral culture. Taoism has its origins between the fourth and third centuries BC, when some thinkers tried a non-interference approach. Similar to the Confucian, Taoists believe that everything in the world was produced by the cosmic Way (Tao), which provided harmony and balance. They believe that humans unite with the Tao, and share its creativity and harmony. In the beginning of the universe, there was the unity of Yin-Yang (life and death, light-darkness, heat-cold). [53] Buddhism has existed in China for more than 1,800 years. The ideas of retribution in the next life, compassion for others, and so on, clearly lie in the notion of an afterlife; of the relation with one's act in this life to one's future life. [33] Nevertheless, Chinese moral has remained Confucius-centred.

The nature of Chinese moral theory

There are several aspects of moral life. First, it refers to particular action and activities, such as killing others, sexual relations, and promise-keeping. Second, it expresses itself in terms of virtues and personal qualities such as honesty and generosity. Third, it may be described as patterns of expected behaviour and character built into the social culture, in any complex society.[49] As a moral philosopher, Confucius has also covered these aspects of moral life in his teachings. Confucius further described clearly his expectations of a moral life, which he expressed in terms of virtues and personal qualities. The supreme virtue was 'Jen' (benevolence or goodness). In practice, 'Jen' simply means loving people. Another virtue Confucius emphasised was righteousness (Yi). 'Yi' does not have any religious connotation. It means doing what is morally right and proper in any situation with special regard to the Five Relationships upon which society is believed to be based.[14] To summarise these personal qualities, 'Jen' is the inner quality of goodness in a good person; 'Yi' is its outward manifestation in action, by which his or her character may be judged.

As Confucius has stressed the importance of moral practice, the following section will examine how the hospice patients related Chinese moral theories to their living and dying. The discussion will explore the extent of influence of Chinese moral tradition on the patients' harmonious relationships with heaven, medical practitioners, and family respectively during their course of illness.

Harmonious death: Living and dying with heaven, medical practitioners, and family

Confucian's world-view can be summarised into two main ideas. First, all people on earth form are one universal community organised under the ideal of 'all-under-heaven in one family'. Second, all people have an inner linkage with heaven, an awareness of inward transcendence. Such inner unity exists not only between each person and heaven, but also between all the people on the earth.[7, 14] Confucius's moral philosophy focuses mostly on human relationships that unite to be under the control of heaven. The ultimate aim of these relationships is to maintain a harmony. A harmonious relationship implies a dynamic equilibrium between two 'opposite' or interrelated components. The two components appear to be opposite to each other because they are governed by a super-ordination and subordination hierarchical structure. Therefore, all categories such as heaven and people, life and death, good and evil, are not opposites but rather interrelated aspects of a continuum. Everything in heaven is assigned its specific quality, function, status, and value, all contributing to the grand cosmic harmony. [15] This is the concept of Yin-Yang equilibrium or harmony. The idea of such symbiotic relationship between human beings and nature is basic to the Confucian-Taoist philosophical idea. [21]

Both Confucianism and Buddhism emphasise that a Good or Harmonious Death emerges from a good life. In particular, Confucius advocated the Five Relationships, which taught people how to live harmoniously with other people. [14, 54] Therefore, the ideas of Harmonious Death expressed by the Chinese hospice patients were based on their beliefs in Confucius's Five Relationships and cosmology: living and dying with heaven, medical practitioners, and the family.

Living and dying with heaven

In ancient China, people had considered the existence of heaven well before the time of Confucius. Chinese emperors were considered to be as appointed by mandate of heaven. The people had high respect for the emperors or authorities at large, whose supreme governor was heaven. People had no access to the controlling power of the cosmos or heaven except through the emperor; this is the concept of kingship. [7, 14] Heaven regulated the social order of the earth and monitored the performance of the emperor because it cared about its people. Heaven would grant people with the Five Blessings or Six Sufferings depending on the emperor's performance. [13, 14, 54] These traditional beliefs remained popular and well considered by the hospice patients in this research.

Confucius did not spend a great deal of time discussing the apparent uncertain matter of death and life after death but he did not deny the existence of spirits.[14,17] Similar to Confucianists, Taoists believe that everything in the world is produced by the cosmos (Tao), which provides harmony and balance: human unites with heaven, life unites with death. Taoism seems to have exerted a powerful influence on the Chinese people's concepts about heaven and its relationship with people, such as control over people's lives and deaths. Buddhism does not use the word 'heaven' but the Buddhist beliefs of Cause and Effects as a regulating mechanism of people's behaviour are quite similar to those found in Confucianism and Taoism. The idea of a moral universe has persisted from Confucianism to modern times. The challenge to the individual is to comprehend heaven's way. [14] The hospice patients' acceptance of their illness and imminent death depended largely on their beliefs about life and death and the control of both. If they believed in the divine control, they may have better acceptance and openness about death. Subsequently, they could redefine their hope for a better rebirth or life after death, and endure their pain and suffering.

Chinese also have long believed in the existence of the soul after death along with their belief in heaven. Ancestors are to watch over the living, but they must be given love and respect by the descendants in order to ensure their attention. [14] Clearly, ancestor worship can strengthen 'family ties' and play an important role in ensuring the continuity of the family. [33] People who died in old age may bring honour to their ancestors by achieving longevity. Patients who had fulfilled their social obligations might have a sense of completion and spiritual integrity because they believed that they would meet their ancestors in the next world. They might hope that they could receive a reciprocal relationship from their descendants after they died. Their concerns about funeral arrangements and ancestor worship also reflected the value they placed on maintaining a continuous harmonious family relationship.

Living and dying with medical practitioners

Since dying has become an institutional event, patients needed to establish a harmonious relationship with medical practitioners who could offer them a cure and hope to live longer. As discussed before, such a relationship represented that of ruler and people in Confucius ideology. According to the hospice patients, medical practitioners generally expected them to perform absolute 'loyalty' with total respect and obedience. In order to maintain a harmonious relationship, the patients played an active role in this context. For example, they accepted whatever the medical practitioners told them with little or no doubt. They showed trust in their treatment plans, which were mainly Western medicine. They would not disclose the fact that they sought alternative treatments, such as Traditional Chinese therapy, based on the Taoist model of health. They made several adjustments but they made minimal complaints about their illness. Further, they learnt to accept that they were not involved in most of the decisions about their care plan.

Meanwhile, patients may pray for blessings from their Buddhist or Taoist gods or ancestors, which may provide them with spiritual energy to play the role successfully. Buddhist conceptual meanings of illness and death could create psychosocial and spiritual comfort and appeared to be more acceptable by Chinese people, such as the hospice patients in this research.

Living and dying with the family

Confucius explained one's duty in the family. 'At home, a young man (person) should be dutiful towards his parents; going outside, he should be respectful towards his elders; he should be cautious in deeds and trustworthy in words; he should love everyone yet make close friends only with those of benevolence' (p.4). [55] To practise these traditional duties or obligations, patients maintained the practice of filial piety and ancestor worship, which are the core values of family relationships. [44] Hence, both personal and public preparations for death were important for the hospice patients in this research.

In the family, parents have been the most influential persons in terms of moral education, which starts at home. [14] Accordingly, patients were happy to talk about their filial children and some even left them with moral instructions before they died. For a similar reason, they demonstrated their readiness to die when they had completed their social-moral duties.

Only if patients could maintain harmonious relationships with their families, would their wishes to die a desirable death become possible. First, patients may be given more information about their condition. They may receive more emotional support to accept the bad news and make adjustments. Second, patients may have a better chance to undergo Chinese medical therapy, which may help them to redefine and maintain hope. Third, they may be given permission to die at home surrounded by their family members. Fourth, they may be given the opportunity to discuss and arrange their funerals or other personal and cultural preparations for death according to their wishes. Last but not least, they may experience a sense of spiritual comfort and integrity if they were loved and valued by their families.

The Chinese hospice patients conceptualised their Harmonious Death as harmonious relationships with heaven, medical practitioners, and the family. Their emphasis on relationships was based on Chinese moral tradition, which has persisted over 4,500 years, with Confucianism as its core.

The Good Death models

It should be noted that the Harmonious Death of Chinese people is not a linear process of dying, such as those proposed by Kubler-Ross, [56] Weisman, [10] and Pattison. [57] People who are confronted with their imminent death need not achieve all the elements of dying a good death, or necessarily in that order. Rather, it is a dynamic process. From the review of literature in Chapter Two, both caregivers and patients seem to agree on several elements contributing to a Good Death. These elements are: controlling pain and symptoms; accepting death; making one's own decisions; maintaining hope; receiving family and social support; preparing for death; and bidding farewell. The findings of this research have included all these elements. Therefore, the present theory will provide an integrated framework, which addresses the needs of dying person from a holistic approach.

I will compare the present theoretical framework of Harmonious Death with the existing models of Good Death, based on three studies: Kellehear,[3] Young and Cullen[1] and Chao,[27] whose patients were dying persons. I will not include other studies on Good Death such as Lee[58] or Byock,[59] for example, for comparison because they are not empirical studies. The purpose of the comparison is to highlight the significance of the present framework (Fig. 3).

Fig. 3 Comparison of Harmonious Death and other models of Good Death

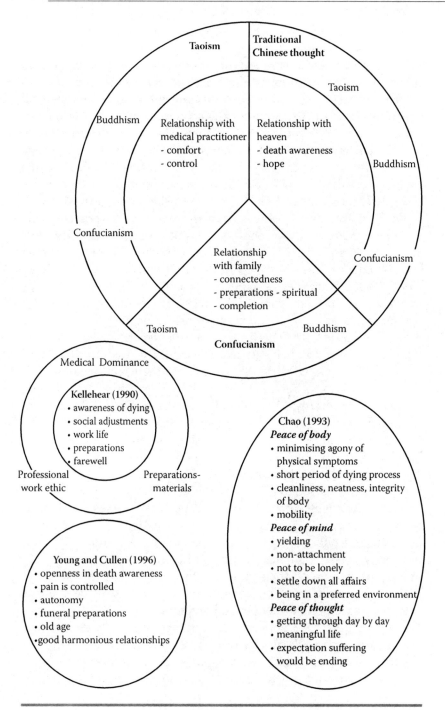

Kellehear's study (1990)

Kellehear's[3] pioneering quantitative research of Good Death focused on the social conduct of dying people in Australia. The five features in his model are: awareness of dying, social adjustments and personal preparations, public preparations, work, and farewells. According to Kellehear,[3] an ideal Good Death 'finds one in old age, under medical care and materially prepared for the economic and social welfare of survivors' (p.185). In addition, there should be minimal disruption to one's social life and working life. That is, the individual should continue working for as long as possible. These were three culture-specific social practices of Good Death. Social adjustments and farewells are two other features that Kellehear argued to be cross-cultural.

Both Australian and Chinese patients agreed on several elements of dying a good death: awareness of dying, adjustments, preparations, and farewells. First, both the Australian and Chinese patients considered awareness of dying an essential first step in achieving a Good Death. Awareness of dying used to be self-detected, but it has mostly been replaced by medical detection. Second, both groups of patients made some adjustments to improve their health but with a different emphasis. They both sought alternative therapy to maintain their hope in recovery or lengthened life span. The Australian patients' social adjustments were mainly centred on their relationships with spouse, children, other relatives, and friends, while the Chinese patients were interested in adjusting to the hospice environment, changing lifestyles and psychological adjustments. This may be because only ten per cent of Kellehear's patients were staying in a hospice. Third, both groups of patients stressed the importance of preparations for death, although the nature of their preparations showed some variations. In this research, less Chinese patients prepared their wills and bade farewell to their families and friends than Australian patients did. Also, Chinese patients presented both personal and public preparations that might have moral-spiritual meanings. Some examples include giving gifts of jade and leaving moral instructions to their children. In general, Australian cancer patients were concerned with material preparations, while Chinese patients focused on moral-spiritual preparations.

A major difference between the findings of Kellehear[3] and the present research is the social feature of work life. The Australian patients considered their relations to work an important feature of Good Death, while the Chinese patients did not. Nevertheless, the Chinese patients have repeatedly stressed the importance of financial status in achieving their desirable good death. For example, their financial status would affect their hope for a future, their connectedness with hospice staff, and the extent of their personal control.

Young and Cullen's study (1996)

Young and Cullen's[1] recent research focused on East Londoners in Britain. They identify six elements of Good Death: openness in death awareness, control of pain, good harmonious relationships with kin, autonomy, funeral arrangements, and old age (Fig. 3). First, the findings of both studies agree that death awareness is essential to die a good death. The patients hoped that their medical practitioners would be honest with them. Second, both British and Chinese patients stressed that pain should be controlled, but the British patients did not place emphasis on their experience of suffering. Third, both groups of patients pointed out that a harmonious relationship with their kin was significant. Fourth, these patients needed to experience a sense of 'autonomy, freedom, liberty for maintaining control... it has a particular relevance for people who are seriously ill, or those whose independence is under threat from infirmity or age' (p.48). [1] Lastly, both British and Chinese patients emphasised that funeral arrangements and dying in old age were important elements of dying a good death.

However, the British patients in Young and Cullen's research did not address the need of hope as clearly and explicitly as the Chinese patients. This is the major difference between the two studies. There may be several reasons for this. First, the East Londoners might not have raised the issue of hope as an element of Good Death during the interview. Second, they might have thought about hope privately but they did not think the researcher was the right person with whom to share these thoughts. Third, the researcher might not have picked up on the cues given by their patients because of a preoccupation with the fact that only the medical practitioners could provide the patients with hope. 'The duty of the doctor is to keep hope alive, and thence to keep intact the presumption that death can be held off for at least a bit longer' (p.99).[1] Nevertheless, Young and Cullen [1] comment briefly that both patients and caregivers have difficulty in keeping hope alive, and this is perhaps more so for the bereaved. They also point out that medical practitioners have a duty to keep patients' hope alive.

Chao's study (1993)

Chao's [27] studied the meaning of good dying among Chinese patients in Taiwan (or Taiwan-Chinese patients) with terminal cancer. She identifies three patterns of good dying: peace of body, peace of mind and peace of thought (Fig. 3). The first pattern is peace of body. It has four themes which include: minimising the agony of physical symptoms, a short period of dying process without lingering death, cleanliness, neatness, and integrity of the body, and mobility. The second pattern is peace of mind. This pattern consists of five themes: yielding, non-attachment, not to be lonely, settling all affairs, being in a preferred environment, and enjoying nature. The third pattern is peace of thought. The three themes in this pattern are getting through day by day without thinking, having a meaningful life, and having the expectation that the suffering would end.

The findings of Chao's [27] research and the present one have consensus on the following five elements of Good Death: comfort, control, connectedness, preparations, and completion. First, both Taiwan Chinese and Hong Kong Chinese patients considered a control of pain and suffering would give them comfort. Both groups of patients addressed the physical and spiritual dimensions of suffering, which were related to their beliefs about an afterlife. The Hong Kong Chinese patients extended their view of suffering to the psychological and social dimensions as well. The Taiwan Chinese patients were also concerned about their mobility but the patients in this research were not.

Second, both Taiwan Chinese and Hong Kong Chinese patients hoped to experience a sense of personal control over the environment when they died. The Taiwan Chinese patients specified the need to stay in a restful and quiet environment. The Hong Kong Chinese patients did not mention this preference, but they indicated the need of company when they died. Third, both groups of patients supported that social connectedness with health care professionals and family was important. The Taiwan Chinese patients hoped to have the company of their loved ones and not to be lonely (at all times), while the Hong Kong patients stressed that they needed to be loved and valued. The need for family affection and connectedness in Chinese culture is significant.

Fourth, both groups of patients emphasised the importance of preparations for death, including funeral arrangements and farewells. Nevertheless, there were some minor variations. The Taiwan Chinese patients indicated the need for cleanliness, neatness, and integrity of body before they died, while the Hong Kong patients did not. Chao [27] explains that her patients had not received adequate nursing care to maintain their personal hygiene. Also, there may be different facilities in their clinical settings. Taiwan Chinese stayed in oncology wards, while Hong Kong Chinese patients stayed in palliative care units. The palliative care unit always has better spacing and is air-conditioned. Lastly, both groups of patients stressed the importance of a sense of completion. They preferred to have a short period of dying, yielding, and experiencing a meaningful life, and they would have better acceptance of death with spiritual faiths, such as Buddhism and Taoism.

There are some important differences in Chao's [27] study and this one. The present research has identified death awareness and hope as important elements for a Harmonious Death. Chao [27] has not addressed these two elements explicitly in her three patterns of Good Dying. Taiwan Chinese patients might be kept in the context of closed awareness. Therefore, they did not have the opportunity to discuss their views on death and hope with the researcher. However, the Taiwan Chinese patients, who had faith in the afterlife, maintained peace of thought by 'getting through day by day without thinking'. She also reports that the Taiwan Chinese patients hoped to know the 'truth'.

In these comparisons, it is noted that dying persons, regardless of socio-cultural background, shared a common need for social and family support. In other words, their relationships with their family or kin contributed predominantly to the achievement of a Good or Harmonious Death. Therefore, the dying persons also addressed the importance of funeral arrangements, whether they were materially or spiritually oriented. With the exception of the British research, [1] the patients of the three other studies included farewells as elements of dying a good death. Meanwhile, the patients in the four studies also addressed the importance of their relationships with medical practitioners. For example, in the context of death awareness, the Australian patients affirmed medical dominance. [3] Young and Cullen [1] and the present research support this finding. However, Taiwan

Chinese patients seemed to place more emphasis on the inadequacy of nursing care in Taiwan. As a result, they stressed the need to be kept clean and tidy. Apart from the Australian study, the patients of the three other studies hoped to have minimal pain when they died. Further, the Chinese patients in Chao's [27] and the present research described their emotional experiences in terms of 'suffering'.

The main difference among these four studies is their emphasis of moral-spiritual needs or 'relationship with heaven', in achieving a good death. The Australian patients perceived death solely as a social phenomenon [3] while the British patients expressed their spiritual needs rather vaguely. [1] However, the British patients briefly mentioned the need for ancestor worship and hope for an afterlife. On the other hand, both groups of Chinese patients seemed to make clearer indications of their moral-spiritual needs. Both Taiwan Chinese [27] and Hong Kong Chinese patients agreed that they needed to accept death as a natural part of life. They may also have experienced a meaningful life. In addition, the Hong Kong Chinese patients placed more emphasis on their values, based on Confucius's Five Relationships and cosmology, than the Taiwan Chinese patients did.

There is no doubt that cultural universality and diversity can explain the similarities and differences of the findings of these four models of Good/ Harmonious death. As 'each self is shaped according to a particular set of cultural and gender patterns' [60] and 'this context can be explained in term of individual culture and socialisation' (p.10). [3] Kellehear's [3] and Young and Cullen's studies [1] may represent studies of Western culture, while Chao's [27] and the present research may represent studies of Chinese culture. Based on the findings of these studies, Chinese people presented a stronger emphasis on moral-spiritual needs, with their views rooted in traditional Chinese thought, particularly, Confucian cosmology and the Five Relationships. For example, patients in all four studies asserted that dying in old age was an element of Good Death because of the 'good timing'. The Chinese patients would have better acceptance of the timing of death under other circumstances: completing social roles, accepting death as a natural part of life, and experiencing a meaningful life. These circumstances were moral-spiritual in nature.

Accordingly, there are obvious differences in the context of death awareness in Western and Chinese culture. For example, Cullen and Young claim that: 'Death is no longer a taboo... the resulting openness has made possible a new kind of good death for more people' (p.175). [1] However, in Taiwan and Hong Kong, death remains a social taboo. 'In Taiwan, there is a popular belief among lay people and health professionals that dying patients usually are not aware of their condition and should not be told the truth in order to keep hope' (p.178). [27] Therefore, not every member of health care team in these Chinese communities advocates open awareness.

Further, it is noted that differences in the findings of the studies may relate to clinical practice. For example, the Taiwan Chinese patients stayed in oncology wards, while my patients stayed in hospice units. The clinical practice and policy on 'truth-telling' could vary. On one hand, Chao [27] points out that 'the most significant factor of "settling all affairs" among the subjects, was knowing the reality of their dying status. If they did not realise that they were going to die, there was no way to accomplish unfinished wishes and business. Nineteen out of twenty subjects told [me] that they were aware of their disease outlook and they wanted to get the truth' (p.176). On the other hand, her patients' need for 'death awareness' appeared rather ambiguous. Chao has stressed that patients in Taiwan were always kept in closed awareness but she has not specified whether this practice applied to her patients. Also, she has not explained the meanings of 'disease outlook' and 'truth'.

In addition, the research design and purpose of these studies were different in nature; it is also possible that some of these differences are an artefact of these issues. Kellehear [3] uses a quantitative approach to test the five hypotheses of Good Death, while the other three studies use qualitative approaches to explore the meanings and perceptions of Good/Harmonious Death from the dying persons' perspective. Consequently, Kellehear's findings have a social focus and continue the interests of the study to the social dimension. This approach might overlook the holistic view of the dying experience. [27] The findings of Young and Cullen, [1] Chao [27] and the present research have a more existential outlook.

Summary

From the analysis of the hospice patients' view on Good Death, I identify seven elements to form the foundation of the theory of Harmonious Death. The Chinese social system is essentially relation-based, largely influenced by Chinese moral tradition with Confucianism as its core. Therefore, it is observed that the Chinese patients were concerned about their harmonious relationships with heaven, medical practitioners, and the family. Further exploration and discussion on how Chinese moral tradition has shaped the three relationships, has concluded that the theory of Harmonious Death has a strong moral-spiritual emphasis. The hospice patients rooted their views in Chinese moral tradition, particularly, Confucian cosmology, and the Five Relationships. Meanwhile, some traditional thoughts, Taoism, and Buddhism also contribute to patients' conceptions, but perhaps to a lesser extent.

On comparison, most previous studies on Good Death [1,3,27] have not emphasised the significance of moral-spiritual relationships (or the relationship with heaven) for the dying persons, as the findings of the present research did. Except for Kellehear's [3] research, the other studies mostly neglected socio-cultural influences on patients' view of Good Death. Chao's [27] and Young and Cullen's [1] studies provide inadequate discussions on the theoretical framework that supported their findings. Quill [61] argues that, 'The conceptual models ... of how death should be approached and what constitutes suffering are overly simplistic and woefully inadequate at the bedside' (p. 202). Dying persons' needs may remain unknown and unattended and they may die rather poorly despite the efforts made since the hospice movement began. On the other hand, an understanding of the contribution of Chinese moral tradition to the formation of the present theory of Harmonious Death will facilitate more effective and confident caring to meet the needs of Chinese dying persons. It also enables us to value the socio-cultural influences that have constantly affected people's views of life, death, and the afterlife.

12
Conclusion

Summary

A HARMONIOUS DEATH is one that maintains a harmonious relationship with heaven, medical practitioners, and family. Heaven refers to ancestors and heaven/gods. People may start with an awareness of dying. When people develop an awareness of dying, they often evaluate their relationships with their ancestors and heaven/gods who either grant them the Five Blessings or Six Sufferings as reward or punishment for their moral behaviour. They may further explore the meaning of life, death, and afterlife, which are closely related to their faiths, such as Taoism, Buddhism, or Confucianism. Meanwhile, people might seek hope for a cure or prolonged life.

Traditional Chinese medicine is a popular choice because it promotes health and longevity based on the philosophy of Taoism. The Taoist philosophy of health emphasises harmony of body-mind-spirit within each person.

People are also concerned about their relationships with medical practitioners. Medical practitioners have professional obligations to provide the dying individuals with comfort and treatment. People may also cling to some religions for spiritual comfort. For example, Buddhist teachings on suffering may enable them to accept their existing suffering better. Further, medical practitioners make most decisions for dying persons, including the place where they die. People most often respect the medical practitioner as the 'ruler' of their lives; therefore, they often play the passive and obedient role of the sick person. They may also believe that heaven controls their lives and death. Such belief is based on the teachings of Confucianism and Taoism. In this way, medical practitioners contribute primarily to the quality of the dying person's end stage of life.

Next, people need to maintain a harmonious relationship with their families. They hope to be loved, valued, and maintain family connectedness even after they die. Thus, they may make preparations for death and experience a sense of completion. The emphasis on harmonious relationships with heaven, medical practitioners, and their families reflects the importance placed on the Confucian values of the Five Relationships and cosmology. Family relationships are important in Chinese culture because three out of five human relationships occur within the family. Meanwhile, the patient's relationship with the medical practitioner resembles that of people and ruler.

I make several suggestions to translate these theoretical concepts into practical guidance in future policy and research directions, because one of my objectives in the present research is to identify some practical implications from the knowledge which derives from my theory. The goals of clinical implications of the theory include: 1) promoting truth-telling between Chinese hospice patients and health care professionals; 2) instilling and nurturing realistic hope for the patients; 3) providing patients with comfort from a holistic approach; 4) facilitating patients in maintaining connectedness with hospice staff and the family; 5) facilitating patients in maintaining their personal control if they wish; 6) facilitating patients in making preparations for death; and 7) facilitating patients in achieving better acceptance of the timing of their death as they wish. In order to help dying persons to achieve a Harmonious Death and make it the standard of care, further initiatives may need to be undertaken in the following areas: hospice philosophy, education, research, and health policy.

Implications of the study

Hospice philosophy

When Saunders[1] initiated the hospice movement, she distinguished hospice care from other streams of health care. She states that, 'Hospice care does not just enable the patient to die peacefully but to live fully until he or she dies.' While the meanings of 'peacefully' and 'fully' remain rather philosophical and abstract, it seems clear that the philosophy of hospice care is to assist patients to achieve a sense of spiritual integrity and peace of mind, which is beyond physical and psychosocial well being.

Based on the findings of this research, health care professionals cannot provide effective care unless they listen attentively to the dying and identify their needs. [2-3] The dying people needed to feel loved and valued, not just as patients, but as persons with different socio-cultural, moral-spiritual experiences and expectations. People needed to be cared for continuously with compassion and sensitivity, so that they did not feel they were a burden on their caregivers. As a consequence, they might be able to maintain their relationships with heaven, medical practitioners, and family in harmony, and experience a sense of completion and peace.

In order for patients to die a Good Death, several pioneer hospice leaders have emphasised the need to care for people with compassion. [4] Saunders [5-6] repeatedly cites the words of her dying patient, David Tasma, whom she came to know really well. He said, 'I only want what is in your mind and in your heart' (p.4). [6] Compassion has led people to explore 'the innate human capacity to experience the immaterial roots of self-awareness call it the level of self, soul or what you will — and so to receive the reassuring touch or what does not die, and with it the sense of a meaningful existence'. [7] Compassion is not a simple feeling-state but a complex emotional attitude toward another, characteristically involving imaginative dwelling on the condition of the other person'. [8] In Fromm's [9] words,

'Compassion or empathy implies that I experience in myself that which is experienced by the other person and hence that in this experience he and I are one. All knowledge of another person is real knowledge only if it is based on my experiencing in myself that which he experiences'.

'It (compassion) is also a sustained and practical determination to do whatever is possible and necessary to help alleviate their suffering'.[10] The death of Mother Theresa in 1997 has drawn people's attention once again to the essentiality of being a compassionate person. She claimed that the poor and dying people did not need people's sympathy and pity. They simply needed love and compassion. In practice, she picked up homeless dying persons and brought them back to her 'hospice home'. Someone would hold these people's hands and stay with them when they died. In sum, compassion comes from one's mind and heart. Compassion is a complex emotional attitude towards others, and a practical determination to help alleviate a person's suffering. Therefore, compassion will lead people to touch another person's soul and sense the meaning of (human) existence. In the end, the two persons' experiences and knowledge become one.

Compassion is the foundation of hospice philosophy and many hospice leaders repeatedly remind us of this. It is hoped that health care professionals will be willing to uphold such hospice philosophy and implement it in their clinical settings. Doyle [11] stresses that, 'We shall be judged by our willingness, indeed our eagerness, to share our facts and figures and sensitive insights about Man and how he reacts to suffering and loss with our students and colleagues in other disciplines and specialities because they care as much as I do' (p.2).

Education

Compassion and caring do not always come naturally. People may learn these skills and attitudes through their experiences and interactions with dying persons themselves. Accordingly, more work needs to be done through education.

Death education, which was started in Western countries in the 1960s, should be introduced to the formal education system at different levels of education in Asian countries: from primary to tertiary education. In Taiwan, for example, it has been documented that death education has been introduced in some tertiary settings. [12-13] Professional programmes on palliative care are important in both undergraduate and post-graduate programmes. Such programmes shall be evidence-based with an emphasis on skill acquisition. The academic levels of various programmes perhaps need more clarification and justifications, in order to meet the demands of clinical professional advancement. [14] Also, health care professionals' clinical competency in palliative care should be continuously and vigorously monitored.

Research

There are three major directions for future work in evaluating the findings of this research. These directions concern the replication, extension, and broadening of the present study.

Replication

Further replication of the study, using the same Grounded Theory method, may be applied to different ethnic groups. Such replication will test the validity of cross-cultural elements of dying a 'Harmonious Death' in different cultures. It is also important to identify the universality and diversity of Chinese culture. Therefore, replication of the present research can be made in other major Chinese communities such as mainland China, Taiwan, and overseas Chinese communities to justify the theoretical framework of the present research. From a methodological point of view, replication of the research can also be done in diverse populations, such as people in different socio-economic groups: the very poor and the wealthy; and people with different terminal illnesses, such as people with AIDS. This may rule out other factors affecting a Harmonious Death.

Extension

Another important part of future study is to extend and deepen the findings of this research to dying people in different clinical settings: independent hospices, hospital-based hospice units, nursing homes and their own homes. Attention to the quality of life of the terminally ill has too often been confined to hospice settings and has not been incorporated into other care settings. [15-16]

Broadening

The use of other qualitative research methods, such as longitudinal study or ethnography may broaden the findings of the present research. Another way to broaden the finding is to conduct studies to yield the viewpoints of relatives and hospice professionals. From previous literature, dying people, their primary caregivers, and the hospice professionals may have different attitudes towards death and dying. Therefore, it will be worthwhile to find out if this is also the case for their perceptions of what they mean to die a Harmonious Death.

Health policy

Hospice services continue to expand. In Hong Kong, hospice service aims to serve at least one-third of the people dying from cancer each year. This will require forty hospice care beds per million populations. [14] Based on the findings of the present research; there are two implications for health policy in the local community. First, hospice services need to include nursing homes in order to maintain the continuity of care. Second, community resources and support need to be increased so as to promote and increase home care services.

Inclusion of nursing homes for hospice services

Following the examples of other parts of the world, one way to expand hospice services is to include nursing homes. It has been reported that some nursing homes in China have started to provide hospice services. [17] In this way, the continuity of care can be maintained when people are transferred from the hospice setting to a nursing home. At present, the standards of care in nursing homes vary dramatically. For example, low staff numbers and a lack of training may have a negative effect on the quality of palliative care. [18] Therefore, it is essential for health care professionals who work in nursing homes to obtain a fundamental knowledge of hospice care through continuing education.

Increase community resources and support to promote home care services

Based on the findings of this research, it might be of value to people to stay at home as long as possible or to die at home. Therefore, people may require substantial nursing and personal care at home. [19] Family members, usually wives and other female relatives, are often the care providers. Consistent with some recent researches, [20] the findings of this research suggest that community resources and financial support should be increased in order to strengthen home-based hospice service. In this way, more dying persons and families may feel comfortable to die at home.

At a national level, China is still in its infancy in the provision of palliative care services. Some pioneer workers such as Zhou and Mi [21] have pointed out the need to develop a Chinese hospice model. Therefore, it is hoped that the findings of this research will be beneficial for health care professionals, in China and its neighbouring countries, in promoting and improving the quality of palliative care.

Conclusion

Interest in improving the care of dying people has developed from the concern of a few health care professionals to a widespread social concern over more than three decades. Despite such attention, a Good Death remains more a hope than standard health practice for all people. [21] This is partly due to the persistent cultural and social attitude that denies the existence of death. Birth is a cause for celebration but death remains a dreaded and unspeakable issue to be avoided by every possible means in some contemporary societies. The emphasis has been on avoiding problems and stopping unfavourable interventions rather than on a positive ideal of a Harmonious Death. As a result, people may die rather 'poorly'. It is anticipated that the theory of Harmonious Death will help to improve care for dying people in the following ways. First, the theory emphasises that dying is not just a medical experience and people's psychosocial, cultural, and moral-spiritual network can significantly influence their experiences. Thus, aspects of care expand considerations beyond physical and psychological comfort to include socio-cultural and moral-spiritual.

Second, the theory proposes potential interventions to implement and evaluate the concept of Harmonious Death. Health care professionals and institutions have a major responsibility to improve the care of dying patients in medical and non-medical aspects. This is important in improving the care for the dying. The operational perspective of Harmonious Death is not an impractical ideal, but a definite indication of how dying a Harmonious Death can become the criterion or dependent variables for good services and innovative studies. It also provides a conceptual base for hospice interventions.

This research contributes to the literature by developing a theory of how to die harmoniously and comparing its content to some of the previous work in Australia, the United Kingdom, and Taiwan. It is hoped that by clarifying some of the issues, health care professionals will be encouraged to initiate substantive research addressing the dynamics of dying a Harmonious Death and its implications in care for the dying.

Appendix

Interview Guide (In English)

Interview Questions

1. What is the nature of your current illness?

2. When was this diagnosis made (identify the stage of the disease)?

3. Who informed you of the diagnosis?

4. How was 'the bad news' announced?

5. What were your feelings on hearing your diagnosis?

6. What do you believe will be the outcome of your current illness?

7. Did you suspect that your illness might be terminal prior to diagnosis?

8. Has your prognosis been discussed with you?

9. When did you discover your prognosis?

10. When you felt ill, who were the first person(s) that you told about your illness?

11. What do you see as the causes of your illness?

12. Can you tell me how you are now?

13. What do you consider to be the main consequence of your current illness?

14. Can you tell me if there have been any positive changes since your illness?

15. What is your greatest concern?

16. Can you tell me of your difficult experiences in life?

17. What preparations are you making?

18. Who is closest to you?

19. Will you say farewell to your family or friends?

20. What are your plans for the future?

21. Can you describe what you feel about being here in hospice unit?

22. How can the health professionals in the hospice unit help?
    22.1 Where would you like to stay for the end phase of your life?
    22.2 What else would you like to accomplish?
    22.3 How would you like to go through your final day?
    22.4 Who would you like to stay with you?

23. Is there anything else you would like to tell me?

24. Do you have any questions or comments?
Thank you for giving me the information. Thank you very much.

References

Chapter one: Introduction

1 Glaser BG, Strauss AL. Awareness of dying. Chicago: Aldine Publishing Co.; 1965.
2 Kubler-Ross E. On death and dying. New York: Macmillan; 1969.
3 Weisman AD. Coping with cancer. New York: McGraw-Hill; 1979.
4 Pattison EM. The experience of death. Englewood Cliffs: Prentice-Hall Inc.; 1977.
5 Shneidman ES. Voices of death. New York: Harper Row; 1980.
6 Wahl CW. The fear of death. In: Feifel H, editor. The meaning of death. New York: Mc-Graw Hill; 1959. 25-26.
7 Kellehear A. Dying of cancer. The final year of life. Melbourne: Harwood Academic; 1990.
8 Young M, Cullen L. A Good Death. Conversations with East Londoners. London: Routledge; 1996.
9 Chao CSC. The meaning of good dying of Chinese terminally ill cancer patients in Taiwan. Unpublished PhD Thesis. Case Western Reserve University; 1993.
10 http://www.info.gov.hk/dh/useful/stat/tenlead_etxt.htm
11 Yeung WFE. The impact of hospice inpatient care on the quality of life of terminally ill cancer patients. Unpublished report. Hong Kong. Institute of Advanced Nursing Studies, Hospital Authority; 1997.
12 Mak MHJ. An investigation of the psychological responses towards dying and death of the terminally ill cancer patients in a Chinese community. Unpublished M.Sc. Thesis. Edinburgh: The University of Edinburgh; 1989.
13 Muzzin LJ. Anderson NJ. Figueredo AT. Gudelis SO. The experience of cancer. Social Science and Medicine.1994; 38(9): 1201-1208.
14 Clark D. History, gender and culture in the rise of palliative care. In: Payne S, Seymour J, Ingleton C editors. Palliative care nursing. Principles and evidence for practice. New York: Open University Press; 2004. 39-54.
15 Feifel H. Psychology and death. Meaningful rediscovery. American Psychologist.1990; 45 (4): 537-543.
16 Chung L. Setting up a nursing service in a new hospice: A Hong Kong experience. Asian Journal of Nursing Studies. Inaugural Issue.1993; 1(1): 46-51.
17 Hospital Authority. Annual Plan 1995-1996. Hong Kong: Hospital Authority; 1996.
18 Hwang TC. Introduction to death education. I. Taipei: Yip Keung Publishing Co. ; 1993. (in Chinese)

19 Qian Q. Preface. In: Tsui Y. Wang T.C. editors. Hospice care: Theory and practice. Beijing: Chinese Medical Press; 1992. 2.

20 Smith A, Zhu DZ. Hospice development in China: Like green shoots in the spring. In: Saunders C, Kastenbaum R, editors. Hospice care on the international scene. New York: Springer Publishing Co.; 1997. 193-205.

21 Aranda S. Changing Focus: Opportunities and challenges in palliative care delivery. In: Box M, Kellehear A, editors. Sink or swim –Palliative care in the mainstream. Proceedings of the Inaugural Victorian State Conference on Palliative care. La Trobe University. Melbourne. February 1999 Feb 10-12; Melbourne, Palliative Care Victoria Palliative Care Unit, La Trobe University.5-8.

22 Zhou Y, Mi J. Hospice care: A new problem of nursing study. Proceedings of the First East-West International Conference on Hospice Care. Tianjin: Tianjin Medical University; 1992.

23 Griffiths P. Progress in measuring nursing outcomes. Journal of Advanced Nursing.1995; 21: 1092-1100.

24 Kastenbaum R, Costa PT. Psychological perspectives on death. Annual Review of Psychology.1977; 28: 245-249.

25 Curtis AE, Fernsler JI. Quality of life of oncology hospice patients: A comparison of patient primary caregiver reports. Oncology Nursing Forum.1989; 16 (1): 49-53.

26 Payne SA. Langley-Evans A. Hillier R. Perceptions of a 'good' death: A comparative study of the views of hospice staff and patients. Palliative Medicine.1996; 10 (4): 307-312.

27 Benner P, Wrubel J. The primacy of caring: Stress and coping in health and illness. Menlo Park CA: Addison-Wesley Publishing Co.1989.

28 Leininger MM. Transcultural nursing: Concepts, theories and practices. New York: John Wiley & Sons; 1978.

29 Leininger MM. Care: The essence of nursing and health. Thorofare NJ: Slack Incorporated; 1984.

30 Leininger MM. Transcultural care: diversity and universality: A theory of nursing. Nursing Health Care.1985; 6 (4): 209-212.

31 Schultz R, Schlarb J. Two decades of research on dying: What do we know about the patient? Omega.1987-88; 18 (4): 299-317.

32 Field MJ, Cassel CK, editors. Approaching death: Improving care at the end of life. Committee on care at the end of life, Division of health care services, Institute of Medicine. Washington, D.C.: National Academy Press; 1997.

33 Beardsley T. A war not won. Scientific American.1994; 270 (1): 118-127.

34 Wang XS Yu S, Gu W and Xu G. China: Status of pain and palliative care. Journal of Pain and Symptom management.2002, 24(2): 177-179.

35 Clark D. History, gender and culture in the rise of palliative care. In: Payne S, Seymour J, Ingleton C. editors. Palliative care Nursing. Principles and evidence for practice. Berkshire: Open University Press, 2004. 51.

36 http://en.wikipedia.org/wiki/List_of_countries_by_population

37 http://www.deathreference.com/Bl-Ce/Causes-of-Death.html

38 Mak MHJ. 'Confucius' In Kastenbaum, R. et al. Editors. Macmillan Encyclopaedia of Death and Dying – e-Book version. New York: Thomson Gale Reference, 2003.

Chapter two: Literature review

1 Feifel H. Psychology and death. Meaningful rediscovery. American Psychologist. 1990; 45 (4): 537-543.

2 Feifel H. Psychology and death. Meaningful rediscovery. American Psychologist. 1990; 45 (4): 547.

3 Kastenbaum R, Costa PT. Psychological perspectives on death. Annual Review of Psychology. 1977; 28: 245-249.

4 Feifel H. The meaning of death. New York: McGraw-Hill; 1959.

5 Feifel H. New meanings of death. New York: McGraw-Hill; 1967.

6 Becker E. The denial of death. New York: Macmillan; 1973.

7 Kastenbaum R, Aisenberg R. The psychology of death. New York: Springer; 1972.

8 Farberow NL, Shneidman ES, editors. The cry for help. New York: McGraw Hill Book Co.; 1965.

9 Fulton RL. The clergyman and the funeral director: A study in role conflict. Social Forces. 1961; 39: 317-323.

10 Fulton RL, editor. Death identity. New York: John Wiley and Sons; 1965.

11 Fulton RL Death, grief and bereavement: A bibliography 1845-1975. New York: Arnold Press; 1977.

12 Glaser BG, Strauss AL. Awareness of dying. Chicago: Aldine Publishing Co.; 1965.

13 Glaser BG, Strauss AL. The discovery of Grounded Theory. Chicago: Aldine Publishing Co.; 1967.

14 Glaser BG, Strauss AL. Time for dying. Chicago: Aldine Publishing Co.; 1968.

15 Glaser BG, Strauss AL. Status passage. London: Routledge and Kewgan Paul; 1971.

16 Sudnow D. Passing on: The social organisation of dying. New Jersey, Eaglewood Cliffs: Prentice-Hall; 1967.

17 Sudnow D. Dying in a public hospital. In: Brim O, Freeman H, Levine S, Scotch N, editors. The dying patient. New York: Russell Sage Foundation; 1970. 91-208.

18 Benoliel JQ. The nurse and the dying patient. New York: Macmillan Company; 1967.

19 Benoliel JQ. Overview: care, cure and the challenge of choice. Earle A, et al. editors. The nurse as caretaker for the dying patient. New York: Columbia University Press. 1977. 6-18.

20 Benoliel JQ. Nurses and the human experience of dying. In: Feifel H, editor. New meanings of death. New York: McGraw-Hill. 1977. 124-141.

21 Hinton J. Dying. London: Penguin Books; 1967.

22 Kubler-Ross E. On death and dying. New York: Macmillan; 1969.

23 Parkes CM. Bereavement: Studies of grief in adult life. New York: International Universities Press; 1972.

24 Weisman AD. On dying and denying. A psychiatric study of terminality. New York: Behavioural sciences Press; 1972.

25 Choron J. Death and western thought. New York: Crowell-Collier; 1963.

26 Gorer G. Death, grief and mourning in contemporary Britain. London: Cresset Press; 1965.

27 Saunders C. The moment of truth: Care of the dying person. In: Person L. editor. Death and dying. London: The Press of Case Western Reserve University; 1969. 49-78.

28 Moody R. Life after life. Covington, GA: Mockingbird Books; 1975.

29 Moody R. The light beyond: The experience of almost dying. In: Bailey LW, Yates J, editors. The near death experience. New York: Routledge; 1996. 25-37.

30 Ring, K. (1996) Near death experiences: Implications for human evolution and planetary transformation. In Bailey, L.W. & Yates, J. (1996) The near death experience. A Reader. New York: Routledge. 179-197.

31 Kellehear A. Experiences near death: Beyond medicine religion. Melbourne: Oxford University Press; 1996.

32 Kastenbaum RJ. Avery D Weisman MD. An Omega interview. Omega. 1993; 27 (2): 103.

33 Kalish RA. Death, grief and caring relationship. Monterey: Brooks/Cole Publishing Company; 1981.

34 Veatch RM. Brain death. In: Shneidman ES, editor. Death: Current perspectives. 3rd ed. Palo Alto: Mayfield; 1984. 123-129.

35 Theodore de Bary et al., 1960. In: Chao CSC. The meaning of good dying of Chinese terminally ill cancer patients in Taiwan. Unpublished PhD Thesis. Case Western Reserve University; 1993. 164

36 Kellehear A. Dying of cancer. The final year of life. Melbourne: Harwood Academic; 1990.

37 Sweeting HN, Gilhooly MLM. Doctor, am I dead? A review of social death in modern societies. Omega. 1992; 24 (4): 251-269.

38 Knutson A. Cultural beliefs on life and death. In: Brim O, Freeman H, Levine S, Scotch N, editors. The dying patient. New York: Russell Sage Foundation; 1970. 42-64.

39 Kalish RA. Life and death — dividing the invisible. Social Science and Medicine. 1968; 2: 249-259.

40 Kastenbaum RJ. Death and bereavement in later life. In: Kntscher AH, editor. Death and bereavement. Charles C. Thomas: Springfield. 1969; I.L. 27-54.

41 Kastenbaum RJ. Death, society and human experience. New York: Macmillan; 1977.

42 Williamson JB, Shneidman ES. editors. Death: Current perspectives. 4th ed. Mountain View, Calif: Mayfield; 1995.

43 Bradbury M. Contemporary representations of 'good' and 'bad' death. In: Dickenson D, Johnson M, editors. Death, dying and bereavement. London: Sage. In association with The Open University. 1993; 68-71.

44 Wass H, Neimeyer RA, editors. Dying: Facing the facts. 3rd ed. Washington, D.C.: Taylor and Francis; 1995.

45 Li ZX. The knowledge of Shan Shu. Taipei: Tung Tai Book Co. Ltd.; 1994. (in Chinese).

46 Seale C. Caring for people who die: The experience of family and friends. Ageing and Society. 1990; 10: 413- 420.

47 Seale C. What happens in hospices: a review of research evidence. Social Science and Medicine. 1989; 28: 551-559.

48 Kastenbaum RJ. The psychology of death. 2nd ed. New York: Springer; 1992.

49 Jordan DK. Gods, ghosts and ancestors. The folk religions of a Taiwanese village.

Berkeley: University of California Press; 1972.

50 Baker H. Hong Kong images: People and animal. Hong Kong: Hong Kong University Press; 1990.

51 Yeung MK. To fight again. Hong Kong: Kan Sang Resource (Hong Kong). Ltd.; 1997. (in Chinese)

52 Blauner R. Death and social structure. Psychiatry. 1966; 29: 378-94.

53 Bok S. Lies to the sick and dying. In: Shneidman ES, editor. Death: Current perspectives. 3rd ed. Palo Alto: Mayfield; 1984. 171-186.

54 Nisbet R. Death. In: Shneidman ES, editor. Death: Current perspectives. 3rd ed. Palo Alto: Mayfield; 1984. 31-37.

55 His Royal Highness Charles Prince of Wales. Opening address. In: D.H.S.S. Proceedings of the Conference on care of the dying. London: H.M.S.O; 1985. 5-7.

56 Sontag S. Illness as metaphor. New York: Farrar, Straus, Giroux; 1978.

57 Sontag S. Illness as metaphor. In: Shneidman ES, editor. Death: Current perspective. 3rd ed. Palo Alto: Mayfield Publishing Co.; 1984. 97-113.

58 Epley RJ, McCaghy CH. The stigma of dying: Attitudes toward the terminally ill. Omega. 1977-8; 4: 379-393.

59 Aries P. The reversal of death: Changes in attitudes toward death in Western societies. In: Stannard DE, editor. Death in America. Philadelphia: University of Pennsylvania. 1975; 134-158.

60 So YP. Death. Be not proud. Hong Kong: Breakthrough Ltd.; 1981. (in Chinese)

61 Carnevali DL, Reiner AC. The cancer experience: Nursing diagnosis and management. Philadelphia: J.B. Lippincott; 1990.

62 Muzzin LJ. Anderson NJ. Figueredo AT. Gudelis SO. The experience of cancer. Social Science and Medicine. 1994; 38(9): 1201-1208.

63 Corner J. The impact of nurses' encounters with cancer on their attitudes towards the disease. Journal of Clinical Nursing; 1993; 2: 363-372.

64 Overmyer DT. Religions of China. New York: Harper Row; 1986.

65 Weisman AD. Coping with cancer. New York: McGraw-Hill; 1979.

66 http://www.info.gov.hk/dh/useful/stat/tenlead_etxt.htm

67 Kramer K. The sacred art of dying. How would religions understand death. New Jersey: Paulist Press; 1988.

68 Pattison EM. The experience of death. Englewood Cliffs: Prentice-Hall Inc.; 1977.

69 Shneidman ES. Voices of death. New York: Harper Row; 1980.

70 Kastenbaum RJ. Awareness of dying. In: Kastenbaum R, Kastenbaum B, editors. Encyclopaedia of death. Phoenix AZ: Oryx Press; 1989. 24-27.

71 Smith DC, Maher MF. Healthy Death. Counselling and Values. 1991; 36 (1): 42-48.

72 Lofland LH. The social shaping of emotion: The case of grief. Symbolic Interaction. 1985; 8: 171-90.

73 Antonff, S.R. and Spika, R. Patterning of facial expressions among terminal cancer patients. Omega. 1984-5; 15: 101-108.

74 Charmaz K. The social reality of death. Reading: Addison- Wesley; 1980.

75 Kastenbaum RJ. Death, society and human experience. 3rd ed. Columbus, Ohio: Charles, E. Merrill Publishing Co.; 1986.

76 Corr CA. Coping with dying: Lessons that we should not learn from the work of Elizabeth Kubler-Ross. Death Studies. 1993; 17: 69-83.

77 Kubler-Ross E. Death: The final stage of growth. Englewood Cliffs N.J.: Prentice-Hall; 1975.

78 Mak MHJ. Psychological responses to dying and death. Senior Nurse. 1992; 12 (3): 48-51.

79 Qvarnstrom U. Patients' reactions to impending death. International Nursing Review. 1979; 26(4): 117-119.

80 Cheng BY. Stress of bereavement. Social support and quality of life. A study on the bereaved spouse in Hong Kong. Unpublished Master of Social Science Thesis. Hong Kong: The Chinese University of Hong Kong; 1997.

81 Hinton J. The influence of previous personality on reactions to having terminal cancer. Omega. 1975; 6 (2): 95-111.

82 Bond S. Process of communication about cancer in a radiotherapy department. Unpublished Ph.D. Thesis. University of Edinburgh; 1978; 82-84.

83 Hinton J. Comparison of places and policies for terminal care. Lancet. 1979; 6 January, 29-32.

84 Knight M, Field D. Silent conspiracy: Coping with dying cancer patients on an acute surgical ward. Journal of Advanced Nursing. 1981; 6: 221-229.

85 Davis AJ, Slater P. The Good Death: Cross-cultural attitudes about euthanasia. Unpublished paper presented at International Conference on Medicine Law and Ethics, Sydney; 1986.

86 Wilson SA. The ethnography of death, dying and hospice care. Unpublished Ph.D. Thesis. University of Wisconsin – Milwaukee; 1989.

87 Samarel N. Caring for life and death. New York; Hemisphere Publishing Co.; 1991.

88 Taylor B. Hospice nurses tell their stories about a good death: the value of storytelling as a qualitative health research method. Annual Review of Health Social Sciences. 1993; 3: 97-108.

89 Aries P. The hour of our death. New York: Alfred A. Knopf; 1981.

90 McNamara B, Waddell C, Colvin M. The institutionalisation of the Good Death. Social Science and Medicine. 1994; 39 (11): 1501-8.

91 Hunt M. Scripts for dying at home — displayed in nurses, patients' and relatives' talk. Journal of Advanced Nursing. 1992; 17 (11): 1297-1302.

92 Wilkes LM. Nurses' descriptions of death scenes. Journal of Cancer Care. 1993; 2: 11-16.

93 White K. Ethical problems experienced by four palliative care nurses working in a hospice. Unpublished Master of Nursing Thesis, Australian Catholic University; 1994.

94 McNamara B, Waddell C, and Colvin M. Threats to the Good Death: The cultural context of stress and coping among hospice nurses. Sociology of Health and illness. 1995; 17 (2): 222-244.

95 McNamara B. Nursing concerns in hospice care organisations. Cancer Forum. 1996; 20(1): 19-29.

96 Taylor B. Promoting a good death: Nurses' practice insights. In: Gray G, Pratt R, editors. Issues in Australian nursing 5: The nurse as clinician. Melbourne: Churchill Livingstone; 1995. 209-220.

97 Shneidman ES. An appropriate death. In: Shneidman ES, editor. Deaths of man.

Bath: Pitman Press; 1973. 25-32.

98 Weisman AD. Appropriate death and the hospice program. The Hospice Journal. 1988; 4 (1): 65-77.

99 Kastenbaum RJ. Health dying: A paradoxical guest continues. Journal of Social Issues. 1979; 35 (1): 185-206.

100 Smith DC, Maher MF. Achieving a healthy death: The dying person's attitudinal contributions. The Hospice Journal. 1993; 9 (1): 21-32.

101 Berger PL, Luckmann T. The social construction of reality. Harmondsworth: Penguin; 1975.

102 Corless IB. Dying well: Symptom control within hospice care. Annual Review of Nursing Research. New York: Springer Publishing Co.; 1994. 125-147.

103 Henderson V, Nite G. Principles and practice of nursing. 6th ed. New York: Macmillan Publishing Co.; 1997.

104 Wotton M. A peaceful death. Nursing Praxis in New Zealand. 1993; 8 (1): 47-49.

105 Callahan D. Pursuing a peaceful death. Hastings Center Report. 1993; 23 (4): 33-38.

106 Loxterkamp, D. (1993). Reflections in family practice. A Good Death is hard to find: Preliminary reports of a hospice doctor. JABFP. 1993; 6 (4): 415-418.

107 Reigle J. Commentary on pursuing a peaceful death. AACN Nursing Scan in Critical Care. 1994; 4(1): 22

108 Butler RN, Burt R, Foley KM, Morris J, Morrison RS. A peaceful death: how to manage pain and provide quality care. A round table discussion: Part 2. Geriatrics. 1996; 51(6): 32-5, 39-40, 42.

109 Jennings B. Individual rights and the human good in hospice co-published simultaneously in ethics and in hospice care: Challenges to hospice values in a changing health care environment. The Hospice Journal. 1997; 12 (2): 1-7.

110 Byock I. Dying well: The prospect for growth at the end of life. New York: Riverhead Books; 1997.

111 Reoch R. Dying well: A holistic guide for dying their carers. London: Gaia Books Ltd.; 1997.

112 Maslow A. The Editorial. Abe Maslow 1908-1970. Psychology Today. 1970; 4 (3):16.

113 Davis AJ, Slater P. US. and Australian nurses' attitudes and beliefs about the Good Death. Image: Journal of Nursing Scholarship. 1989; 21(1): 34-39.

114 Alizade AM. One will die: Ethical aspects of death and clinical implications. Revista de Psicoanalisis. 1988; 45 (4): 859-870.

115 Kearl MC. Endings. A sociology of death and dying. New York: Oxford University Press; 1989.

116 Mak MHJ. An investigation of the psychological responses towards dying and death of the terminally ill cancer patients in a Chinese community. Unpublished M.Sc. Thesis. Edinburgh: The University of Edinburgh; 1989.

117 World Health Organisation. Cancer pain relief and palliative care: Report of a WHO expert committee. Geneva: World Health Organisation; 1993, 52.

118 Richman J. From despair to integrity: An Eriksonian approach to psychotherapy for the terminally ill. Psychotherapy. 1995; 32 (2): 317-322.

119 Saunders DE. Jr. A good and peaceful death: A personal statement. Journal of South Carolina Medical Association. 1996; 92 (2): 44-7.

120 Payne SA, Langley-Evans A, Hillier R. Perceptions of a 'good' death: A comparative study of the views of hospice staff and patients. Palliative Medicine. 1996; 10 (4): 307-312.

121 Low JTS, Payne S. Palliative care. The good and bad death perceptions of health professionals working in palliative care. European Journal of Cancer Care. 1996; 5(4): 237-241.

122 Young M, Cullen L. A Good Death. Conversations with East Londoners. London: Routledge; 1996.

123 Justice C. Dying the Good Death: The pilgrimage to die in India's Holy city. Albany: State University of New York Press; 1997.

124 Wilkes LM. Reflection on the Good Death and the nurse in palliative care. In: Parkers J, Aranda S, editors. Palliative care: Explorations and challenges. Sydney: Maclennan and Petty Pty. Ltd.; 1998. 115.

125 Webb M. The Good Death: The new American search to reshape the end of life. New York: Bantam Books. 1997.

126 Nimocks MJA, Webb L. Connell J. Communication and the terminally ill: A theoretical model. Death Studies. 1987; 11: 323-344.

127 Illich I. Limits to medicine. Medical nemesis: The expropriation of health. London: Marion Boyars; 1976. 127.

128 McDonald RT, Carroll JD. Appropriate death: College students' preferences Vs. actuarial projections. Journal of Clinical Psychology. 1981; 37(1): 28-31.

129 Sweeting HN, Gilhooly MLM. Dementia and the phenomenon of social death. Sociology of Health and Illness. 1997; 19 (1): 93-117.

130 Rodin J. Health, control and ageing. In: Baltes M.M. Baltes P.B. editors. The psychology of control and ageing. Hillsdale, New York: Eribaum. 1986. 139-167.

131 Johnston M, Tookman A, Honeybun J. The impact of a death on fellow hospice patients. British Journal of Medical Psychology. 1992; 65: 67-72.

132 D'Angelo B. Death with dignity: Supporting a patient's decision. American Nephrology Nurses' Association Journal. 1986; 13(6): 330-333.

133 Madan TN. Dying with dignity. Social Science and Medicine. 1992. 35(4): 425-432.

134 Sogyal Rinpoche. The Tibetan book of living and dying. London: Rider; 1992.

135 Kelner MJ, Bourgeault IV. Patient control over dying: Responses of health care professionals. Social Science and Medicine. 1993; 36 (6): 757-765.

136 Travellbee J. Interpersonal aspects of nursing. 2nd ed. Philadelphia: F.A. Davis; 1971.

137 Anderson H. After the diagnosis: An operational theology for the terminally ill. Journal of Pastoral Care. 1989; 43 (2): 141-150.

138 Hull MM. A family experience: Hospice supported home care of a dying relative. Unpublished PhD. Thesis. University of Rochester; 1989. 3.

139 Lipman A, Marden PW. Preparation for death in old age. Journal of Gerontology. 1996; 21: 426-431.

140 Kalish RA, Reynold DK. Death and Ethnicity: A psychocultural study. Los Angeles: University of Southern California Press; 1976.

141 Riley Jr JW. What people think about death.death? In: Brim OG, Freeman HE, Levine S, Scotch N.A. The dying patient. New York: Sage; 1970. 30-41.

142 Weisman AD, Hackett TP. Predilection to death. Psychosomatic Medicine.

1961; 23: 232-256.

143 Metcalf P, Hungtington R. Celebrations of death: The anthropology of mortuary ritual. 2nd ed. Cambridge: Cambridge University Press; 1991.

144 King A, Lee R. Social life developmentlife development in Hong Kong. Hong Kong: Chinese University Press; 1981.

145 Ho MW. The development of a quality of life scale for patients with life threatening illness in a chronic context. Unpublished Ph.D. Thesis. Hong Kong: The Chinese University of Hong Kong; 1991.

146 Gall TL, editor. Worldmark encyclopaedia of cultures and daily life. Vol. 3 Asia Oceania. London: Gale; 1997.

147 Henderson H, Thompson SE, Holidays, festivals and celebrations of the World Dictionary. 2nd ed. Detroit: Omnigraphics Inc.; 1997.

148 Fu WF. Respect of death and respect of life. Taipei: Chung Ching Publishing Co.; 1993. (in Chinese)

149 Analects 11: 11, In: Soothhill WE. The Analects. London: Oxford University Press; 1937.

150 Cheng HK. Chinese wisdom on death. Taipei: Tung Tai Publishing Co.; 1994. (in Chinese)

151 Fu PW. Religions behind Confucian view of death and dying. Philosophy and Culture. 1994; 21 (7): 600-607. (in Chinese)

152 Overmyer DT. China. In: Holck F.H. editor. Death and Eastern thought. Nashville Tennessee: Abingdon Press; 1974. 198-222.

153 Watson B. (Translator). The complete work of Chuang Tzu. New York: Columbia University Press; 1968. 235.

154 Watson B. (Translator). Chuang Tzu. New York: Columbia University Press; 1964.

155 Hwang TC. Introduction to death education. II. Taipei: Yip Keung Publishing Co.; 1993. (in Chinese)

156 Berling JA. A pilgrim in Chinese culture. Negotiating religious diversity. Maryknoll NY: Orbis Books; 1997.

157 Hsu FLK. Americans and Chinese. Passages to difference. 3rd. ed. Honolulu: The University Press of Hawaii; 1981.

158 Watson JL. Rawski ES. Death ritual in late imperial modern China. Berkeley: University of California Press; 1988.

159 Saunders C. Foreword. In: Dunlop R. Cancer: Palliative care. New York: Springer; 1998. vii.

160 Nuland SB. How we die. London: Chatto Windus; 1993.

161 Peck MS. Further along the road less travelled: The unending journey toward spiritual growth. New York: Simon and Schuster; 1993.

162 Cella DF, Tross S. Psychological adjustment to survival from Hodgkin's disease. Journal of Consulting and Clinical Psychology. 1986; 54: 616-622.

163 Houts PS, Yasko JM, Kahn SB, Schlezel GW, Marconi KM. Unmet psychological, social and economic needs of persons with cancer in Pennsylvania. Cancer. 1986; 58: 2355-2361.

164 Cohen SR, Mount BM, Bruera E, Provost M, Rowe J, Tong K. Validity of the McGill quality of life questionnaire in the palliative care setting: A multi-centre Canadian study demonstrating the importance of the existential domain. Palliative Medicine. 1997; 11: 3-20.

165 Yeung WFE. The impact of hospice inpatient care on the quality of life of terminally ill cancer patients. Unpublished report. Hong Kong. Institute of Advanced Nursing Studies, Hospital Authority; 1997.

166 Choy YSC. An exploratory study on anticipatory grieving - case studies of spouses of terminally ill patients. Unpublished Master of Social Work Thesis. Hong Kong: The University of Hong Kong; 1987.

167 Ng LN. An exploratory study on an interventive approach to work with the spouse of patients with terminal illness. Unpublished Master of Social Work Thesis. The University of Hong Kong; 1987.

168 Tsang WH. Attitudes towards 'life' and 'death' in Chinese bereaved widows: Implications for bereavement work in Hong Kong. Unpublished M.S.W. Dissertation Department of Social Work and Social Administration. The University of Hong Kong; 1996.

169 Wong LC. A study of hospice care: Communication between the health care professionals and the patients. Unpublished Master of Social Science Thesis. Hong Kong: The University of Hong Kong; 1992.

170 Schultz R, Schlarb J. Two decades of research on dying: What do we know about the patient? Omega. 1987-88; 18 (4): 299-317.

171 Hwang TC. A cross cultural study of attitudes towards death and dying between Chinese and American college students. Unpublished Ed.D. Thesis. Drake University; 1988.

172 Ahlner-Elmqvist M et al. Place of death: hospital – based advanced home care versus conventional care. Palliative Medicine. 2004; 18: 585-593.

173 Strauss AL, Glaser BG. Social organisation of medical work. Chicago: Chicago University Press; 1985.

174 Shneidman ES. Autopsy of a suicidal mind. New York: Oxford University Press, 2004.

175 Zerwekh JV. Nursing care at the end of life. Palliative care for patients and families. Philadelphia: F.A. Davis, 2006.

176 Kubler-Ross E. Kessler D. Life lessons. New York: Touchstone Publishing, 2000.

177 Chen KY. (Translator) Lao Tzu: Text notes comments. Chinese Material Centre. 1961. XLII

Chapter three: Methodology

1 Siegel K. Research issues in psychosocial oncology. Journal of Psychosocial Oncology. 1983; 1 (1): 101-104.

2 Berg BL. Qualitative research method for the social sciences. Boston: Allyn Bacon; 1989. 2-3.

3 Manning SS. Ethical decisions: A grounded theory approach to the experience of social work administrators. Unpublished Ph.D. Thesis. University of Denver; 1990.

4 Denzin NK, Lincoln YS, editors. Handbook of qualitative research. London: Sage; 1994.

5 Glaser BG. Emerging Vs forcing: Basics of Grounded Theory analysis. CA: Mill Valley: The Sociology Press; 1992. 12.

6 Leininger MM. Transcultural care: diversity and universality: A theory of nursing. Nursing and Health Care. 1985; 6 (4): 209-212.

7 Minichiello V, Aroni R, Timewell E, Alexander L. In-depth interviewing: Research people. Melbourne: Longman Cheshire; 1990.

8 Chao CSC. The meaning of good dying of Chinese terminally ill cancer patients in Taiwan. Unpublished PhD Thesis. Case Western Reserve University; 1993.

9 Mak MHJ. Moral education. Asian Culture. 1990; 18 (3): 62-71.

10 Seale C. Caring for people who die: The experience of family and friends. Ageing Society. 1990; 10: 413- 420.

11 Feifel H. Psychology and death. Meaningful rediscovery. American Psychologist. 1990; 45 (4): 537-543.

12 Corr CA. A task-based approach to coping with dying. Omega. 1992; 24(2): 81-94.

13 Seale C. Qualitative interviewing. In: Seale C, editor. Researching society and culture. London: Sage; 1998. 202-216.

14 Merton RK. On theoretical sociology. New York: Free Press; 1967. 39.

15 Maxwell JA. Qualitative research design: An interpretive approach. Thousand Oaks, CA: Sage; 1976. 29, 31.

16 Fawcett J. Analysis and evaluation of nursing theories. Philadelphia: FA. Davis; 1993.

17 Strauss AL. Qualitative analysis for social scientists. Cambridge: Cambridge University Press; 1987.

18 Glaser BG, Strauss AL. Awareness of dying. Chicago: Aldine Publishing Co.; 1965. 79.

19 Strauss AL, Corbin J. Grounded theory methodology. An overview. In: Denzin NK. Lincoln YS, editors. Handbook of qualitative research. London: Sage; 1994. 273-285.

20 Lincoln Y, Guba E. Naturalistic inquiry. Newbury park, CA: Sage Publications; 1985.

21 Glaser BG, Strauss AL. The discovery of Grounded Theory. Chicago: Aldine Publishing Co.; 1967.

22 Morse JM. Field PA. Nursing research: The application of qualitative approaches. 2nd ed. New York: Chapman Hall; 1996.

23 Mak MHJ. Sham M. A preliminary study of affective states of dying patients in a hospice in Hong Kong. Abstracts. 2nd EORTC International Hong Kong Symposium On Current Trend in Cancer Care. 1995 Feb. 13-15.

24 Davison BJ, Degner LF. Promoting patient decision-making in life-death situations. Seminars in Oncology Nursing. 1998; 14 (2): 129-136.

25 Kellehear A. Dying of cancer. The final year of life. Melbourne: Harwood Academic; 1990.

26 Morse JM. editor. Critical Issues in Qualitative Research Methods. London: Sage; 1994.

27 Yeung WFE. The impact of hospice inpatient care on the quality of life of terminally ill cancer patients. Unpublished report. Hong Kong. Institute of Advanced Nursing Studies, Hospital Authority; 1997.

28 Hospital Authority. Cancer incidence and mortality in Hong Kong 1992. Hong Kong: Hong Kong Cancer Registry; 1992.

29 Sandelowski M. Focus on qualitative methods. Sample size in qualitative

research. Research in Nursing and Health. 1995; 18: 179-183.

30 Morse JM. editor. Critical Issues in Qualitative Research Methods. London: Sage; 1994.

31 West HG. Having cancer. Unpublished PhD Thesis. University of California; 1991.

32 Lofland J. Analysing social settings. Belmont California: Wadsworth; 1971.

33 Bryant A, Payne S. Difficulties inherent in research with cancer patients. Journal of Cancer Care. 1993; 2: 143-6.

34 Robbins M. Evaluating palliative care. Establishing the evidence base. Oxford: Oxford University Press; 1998.

35 Charmaz K. Identity dilemmas of chronically ill men. In: Strauss A. Corbin JM, editors. Grounded Theory in practice. London: Sage. 1997. 35-62.

36 Jones S. In-depth interviewing. In: Walker R, editor. Applied Qualitative Research. Aldershor: Gower. 48-49.

37 Seale C, Kelly M. Coding and analysing data. In: Seale C, editor. Researching society and culture. London: Sage; 1998. 146-163.

38 Glaser BG. Theoretical sensitivity. Advances in the methodology of Grounded Theory. Mill Valley: Sociology Press; 1978.

39 Hutchinson SA. Grounded Theory: The method. In: Munchall PL, Oiler CJ, editors. Nursing research: A qualitative perspective. Norwalk, CT: Appleton-Century Crofts; 1986. 118.

40 Morse JM. Qualitative and quantitative methods: Issues in sampling. In: Chinn P.L. editor. Nursing Research Methodology. Rockville MD: Aspen; 1986; 181-191.

41 Morse JM. editor. Completing a qualitative project. London: Sage; 1997.

42 Davies B, Reimer JC, Brown P, Martens N. Challenges of conducting research in palliative care. Omega. 1995; 31 (4): 263-273.

Chapter four: Being aware of dying

1 Seale C, Kelly M. Coding and analysing data. In: Seale C, editor. Researching society and culture. London: Sage; 1998. 146-163.

2 Kellehear A. Dying of cancer. The final year of life. Melbourne: Harwood Academic; 1990.

3 Hwang TC. Introduction to death education. I and II. Taipei: Yip Keung Publishing Co.; 1993. (in Chinese).

4 Glaser BG, Strauss AL. Awareness of dying. Chicago: Aldine Publishing Co.; 1965.

5 Weisman AD. On dying and denying. A psychiatric study of terminality. New York: Behavioural sciences Press; 1972.

6 Young M, Cullen L. A Good Death. Conversations with East Londoners. London: Routledge; 1996.

7 Cheng BY. Stress of bereavement. Social support and quality of life. A study on the bereaved spouse in Hong Kong. Unpublished Master of Social Science Thesis. Hong Kong: The Chinese University of Hong Kong; 1997.

8 Galanti GA. Caring for patients from different cultures: Case studies from American hospitals. Philadelphia: University of Pennsylvania Press; 1997.

9 Lederburg P, Latimer E. Psychosocial ethical issues in the care of cancer patients. In: DeVita VT, Hellman S, Rosenberg SA, editors. Cancer: Principles and Practice of Oncology. 4th ed. Philadelphia: J.B. Lippincott; 1989.

10 Kubler-Ross E. On death and dying. New York: Macmillan; 1969.

11 Weisman AD. Coping with cancer. New York: McGraw-Hill; 1979.

12 Pattison EM. The experience of death. Englewood Cliffs: Prentice-Hall Inc.; 1977.

13 Peck MS. The road less travelled: A new psychology of love, traditional values and spiritual growth. New York: Simon and Schuster; 1978.

14 Lack S, Lamerton R, editors. The hour of our death. A record of the Conference on the care of the dying held in London. London: Geoffrey Chapman; 1974.

15 Miyaji NT. The power of compassion: Truth-telling among American doctors in the care of dying patients. Social Science and Medicine. 1993; 36 (3): 249-264.

16 Kleinman A. The illness narratives. New York: Basic Books; 1988. 16-17.

17 Chao CSC. The meaning of good dying of Chinese terminally ill cancer patients in Taiwan. Unpublished PhD Thesis. Case Western Reserve University; 1993.

18 Fielding R. Clinical communication skills. Hong Kong: Hong Kong University Press; 1995.

19 Fielding R, Ko L, Wong LSW. Inconsistencies between belief and practice: Assessment of Chinese cancer patients' knowledge of their disease. Journal of Cancer Care. 1995; 4: 11-15.

20 Arathuzik MD. The appraisal of pain coping in cancer patients. Western Journal of Nursing Research. 1991; 13: 714-731.

21 Frank-Stromborg M, Wright PS, Segalla M, Dielmann J. Psychosocial impact of the cancer diagnosis. Oncology Nursing Forum. 1984; 11 (3): 16-22.

22 Glaser BG, Strauss AL. The discovery of Grounded Theory. Chicago: Aldine Publishing Co.; 1967.

23 Glaser BG, Strauss AL. Time for dying. Chicago: Aldine Publishing Co.; 1968.

24 Glaser BG, Strauss AL. Status passage. London: Routledge and Kewgan Paul; 1971.

25 Weisman AD. Appropriate death and the hospice program. The Hospice Journal. 1988; 4 (1): 65-77.

26 Saunders C. Foreword. In: Dunlop R. Cancer: Palliative care. New York: Springer; 1998. vii.

27 Tsim KF, Lui PY. Report on seminar of the hospice film: Love until next life, care of the care receivers and care givers. China Hospice Foundation Newsletter. 1995; 12: 69-71. (in Chinese).

28 McIntosh J. Communication and awareness in a cancer ward. London: Croom Helm; 1977. 94.

29 Timmermans S. Dying of awareness: The theory of awareness contexts revisited. Sociology of Health and Illness. 1994; 16 (3): 322-339

30 Seale C. Communication awareness about death: a study of a random sample of dying people. Social Science and Medicine. 1991; 32 (8): 943-952.

31 Brewin TB, Sparshott M. Relating to the relatives. Breaking bad news communication and support. Oxford: Radcliffe Medical Press; 1996.

32 Cartwright A. Changes in life. Care in the year before death 1969-1987. Public

Health Review. 1991; 13: 81-87.

33 Wass H, Neimeyer RA, editors. Dying: Facing the facts. 3rd ed. Washington, D.C.: Taylor and Francis; 1995.

34 Field MJ, Cassel CK, editors. Approaching death: Improving care at the end of life. Committee on care at the end of life, Division of health care services, Institute of Medicine. Washington, D.C.: National Academy Press; 1997.

35 Kellehear A. Health promoting palliative care. Melbourne: Oxford University Press; 1999

36 Lee SK, Tsim KF, Lui PY. Report of seminar on hospice film: The moment of life death — from hospice care to the meanings of life for the terminally ill cancer patients. China Hospice Foundation Newsletter. 1995; 12: 65-68. (in Chinese).

37 Li ZX. The knowledge of Shan Shu. Taipei: Tung Tai Book Co. Ltd.; 1994. (in Chinese).

38 Mak MHJ. Cultural responses to death and dying: The experience in Hong Kong. Abstracts. The Social Context of Death, Dying and Disposal. 3rd International Conference. The University of Cardiff, UK. 1997 April, 4-6.

39 Lip E. Chinese numbers: Significance, symbolism and traditions. Singapore: Times Book International; 1992.

40 Cooper JC. An illustrated encyclopaedia of traditional symbols. London: Thames Hudson Ltd.; 1992.

41 Mauk J. Communication at the end of life. In: Forman WB, Kitzes JA, Anderson RP, Sheehan DK. Hospice and Palliative Care. Concepts and Practice. 2nd ed. Boston: Jones and Bartlett Publisher. 2003; 67-85.

42 Pollard A. Cairns J. Rosenthal M. Transitions in living and dying: defining palliative care. In: Aranda S. O'Connor M. editors. Palliative care nursing: A guide to practice. Melbourne: Ausmed Publications; 1999. 5-20.

43 Zerwekh JV. Nursing care at the end of life. Palliative care for patients and families. Philadelphia: F.A. Davis, 2006.

Resources
Education for physicians on end-of-life care (EPEC)
The EPEC Project (www.epec.net)

Chapter five: Maintaining hope

1 Moto JA. Hope, suicide, and medical practice. Journal of the American Medical Association. 1975; 234: 1168-1169.

2 Nathan J. What to do when they say 'It's cancer'. A survivor's guide. Sydney: Allen Unwin; 1998.

3 Hall BA. The struggle of the diagnosed terminally ill person to maintain hope. Nursing Science Quarterly. 1990; 3: 177-184.

4 Kessler D. The rights of the dying. A companion for life's final moments. New York: Harper Collins; 1997.

5 Wilkes LM. Nurses' descriptions of death scenes. Journal of Cancer Care. 1993; 2: 11-16.

6 Wilkes LM. Reflection on the Good Death and the nurse in palliative care.

In: Parkers J, Aranda S, editors. Palliative care: Explorations and challenges. Sydney: Maclennan and Petty Pty. Ltd.; 1998. 115-125.

7 White K. Ethical problems experienced by four palliative care nurses working in a hospice. Unpublished Master of Nursing Thesis, Australian Catholic University; 1994.

8 Hinton J. Dying. London: Penguin Books; 1967.

9 Miller JF. Hope-inspiring strategies of the critically ill. Applied Nursing Research. 1989; 2: 23-29.

10 Fromm E. The revolution of hope. Toward a humanised technology. New York: Harper and Row; 1968.

11 Flemming K. The meaning of hope to palliative cancer patients. International Journal of Palliative Nursing. 1997; 3 (1): 14-18.

12 Hunt M. Scripts for dying at home — displayed in nurses, patients' and relatives' talk. Journal of Advanced Nursing. 1992; 17 (11): 1297-1302.

13 Speck P. Spiritual issues in palliative care. In: Doyle D, Hanks G, MacDonald N, editors. Oxford textbook of palliative medicine. 2nd ed. Oxford: Oxford University Press; 1998. 805-814.

14 Anderson H. After the diagnosis: An operational theology for the terminally ill. Journal of Pastoral Care. 1989; 43 (2): 141-150.

15 Corr CA. A task-based approach to coping with dying. Omega. 1992; 24(2): 81-94.

16 Overmyer DT. Religions of China. New York: Harper Row; 1986.

17 The Holy Bible, New International version. Michigan: Zondervan Bible Publishers; 1978. Roman, 5: 2-5.

18 Smith DC, Maher MF. Achieving a healthy death: The dying person's attitudinal contributions. The Hospice Journal. 1993; 9 (1): 21-32.

19 Bradbury M. Contemporary representations of 'good' and 'bad' death. In: Dickenson D, Johnson M, editors. Death, dying and bereavement. London: Sage. In association with The Open University. 1993; 68-71.

20 Nuland SB. How we die. London: Chatto Windus; 1993; 223.

21 Cattell E. Nurse practitioners' role in complementary and alternative medicine: Active or passive? Nursing Forum. 1999; 34 (3): 14-23.

22 Chan KS, Lam Z, Chun R, Dai D, Leung A. Chinese patients with terminal cancer. In: Doyle D, Hanks G, MacDonald N, editors. Oxford textbook of palliative medicine. 2nd ed. Oxford: Oxford University Press; 1998. 793-795.

23 Smaje C, Field D. Absent minorities? Ethnicity and the use of palliative care services. In: Field D, Hockey J, Small N, editors. Death, gender and ethnicity. London: Routledge; 1997. 142-165.

24 Wong CW. The seeking of Chinese medical advice by the patients. A preliminary report on the survey. Medical Policy Research Group, Hong Kong Social Welfare Society. Hong Kong; 1998. (in Chinese).

25 Cassileth B. The alternative medicine handbook. The complete reference guide to alternative and complementary therapies. New York: W.W. Norton; 1998.

26 Ahern EM. Chinese-style and Western-style doctors in northern Taiwan. In: Kleinman A, et al. editors. Culture and healing in Asian societies. Cambridge MA: Schenkman. 1978; 101-110.

27 Bullock M, Pheley A, Kiresuk T, Lenz S, Culliton P. Characteristics complaints of patients seeking therapy at a hospital-based alternative medicine clinic. The

Journal of Alternative and Complementary Medicine. 1997; 3: 31-37.

28 Alspach G. Alternative and complementary therapies: Treading tentatively out of the mainstream. Critical Care Nurse. 1998; 18 (5): 13-16.

29 Cheng BY. Stress of bereavement. Social support and quality of life. A study on the bereaved spouse in Hong Kong. Unpublished Master of Social Science Thesis. Hong Kong: The Chinese University of Hong Kong; 1997.

30 Chao CSC. The meaning of good dying of Chinese terminally ill cancer patients in Taiwan. Unpublished PhD Thesis. Case Western Reserve University; 1993.

31 Yeung WFE. The impact of hospice inpatient care on the quality of life of terminally ill cancer patients. Unpublished report. Hong Kong. Institute of Advanced Nursing Studies, Hospital Authority; 1997.

32 Glaser BG, Strauss AL. Awareness of dying. Chicago: Aldine Publishing Co.; 1965.

33 Erikson EH. Childhood and society. 2nd ed. New York: Norton; 1963.

34 Young M, Cullen L. A Good Death. Conversations with East Londoners. London: Routledge; 1996.

35 Festinger L. A theory of social comparison processes. Human Relations. 1954; 7: 117-140.

36 Elizabeth Kubler-Ross. Death Studies. 1993; 17: 69-83.

37 Weisman AD. On dying and denying. A psychiatric study of terminality. New York: Behavioural sciences Press; 1972.

38 Morse JM. Doberneck B. Delineating the concept of hope. Image: Journal of Nursing Scholarship. 1995; 27(4): 277-285.

39 Doyle D, Hanks G, MacDonald N, editors. Oxford textbook of palliative medicine. 3rd ed. Oxford: Oxford University Press; 2004.

40 Cousins N. The physician as communicator. Journal of the American Medical Association. 1982; 248 (5): 587-589.

41 Wong-Wylie G, Jevne RF. Patient hope: Exploring the interactions between physicians and HIV seropositive individuals. Qualitative Health Research. 1997; 7(1): 32-56.

42 Zerwekh JV. Nursing care at the end of life. Palliative care for patients and families. Philadelphia: F.A. Davis Co., 2006

Chapter six: Being free from pain and suffering

1 Saunders C. Hospices world-wide: A mission statement. In: Saunders C. Kastenbaum R. editors. Hospice care on the international scene. New York: Springer Publishing Co.; 1997. 3-12.

2 International Association of Study of Pain. Subcommittee on taxonomy. Pain terms: A list with definitions and notes on usage. Pain. 1980; 8: 249-252.

3 Melzack R. The puzzle of pain. Harmondsworth: Penguin; 1973.

4 Cupples SA. Pain as hurtful experience: A philosophical analysis and implications for holistic nursing care. Nursing Forum. 1992; 27(1): 5-11.

5 Kellehear A. Dying of cancer. The final year of life. Melbourne: Harwood Academic; 1990.

6 Ahles TA, Martin JB. Cancer pain: A multi-dimensional perspective. In: Turk DC, Feldman CS, editors. Non-invasive approaches to pain management in the

terminally ill. New York: The Haworth Press; 1992. 25-48.

7 Chao CSC. The meaning of good dying of Chinese terminally ill cancer patients in Taiwan. Unpublished PhD Thesis. Case Western Reserve University; 1993.

8 World Health Organisation. Cancer pain relief and palliative care: Report of a WHO expert committee. Geneva: World Health Organisation; 1993.

9 Mak MHJ. Sham M. A preliminary study of affective states of dying patients in a hospice in Hong Kong. Abstracts. 2nd EORTC International Hong Kong Symposium On Current Trend in Cancer Care. 1995 Feb. 13-15.

10 Yeung WFE. The impact of hospice inpatient care on the quality of life of terminally ill cancer patients. Unpublished report. Hong Kong. Institute of Advanced Nursing Studies, Hospital Authority; 1997.

11 Kwan C. Problems and concerns of terminal cancer patients' families identified by nurses during hospitalisation in a hospice unit. Poster presented at 5th Hong Kong International Cancer Congress. 1998 Nov. 8-11 Hong Kong.

12 Sze FKH, Chung TK, Wong E, Lam KK, Lo R, Woo J. Pain in Chinese cancer patients under palliative care. Palliative Medicine. 1998; 12: 271-277.

13 McNamara B, Waddell C, and Colvin M. Threats to the Good Death: The cultural context of stress and coping among hospice nurses. Sociology of Health and illness. 1995; 17 (2): 222-244.

14 Zimmerman L, Story KT, Gaston-Johansson F, Rowles JR. Psychological variables, cancer pain. Cancer Nursing. 1996; 19(1): 44 -53.

15 Fielding R. Clinical communication skills. Hong Kong: Hong Kong University Press; 1995.

16 Saunders C. Caring for the dying. In: Lack S. Lamerton R. The hour of our death. A record of the Conference on the care of the dying held in London. London: Geoffrey Chapman; 1975. 18-27.

17 Brenneis JM. Spirituality and suffering. In: Parris WCV, editor. Cancer pain management. Principles and practice. Boston: Butterworth Heinemann; 1997. 507-515.

18 Edwards RB. Pain and the ethics of pain management. Social Sciences and Medicine. 1984; 18: 512-523.

19 Saunders C. The management of terminal illness. London: Hospital Medical Publishing. 1967.

20 Saunders C. Foreword. In: Dunlop R. Cancer: Palliative care. New York: Springer; 1998. vii.

21 Lam CYJ, Chung TK, Chiu WC. A preliminary study on patient-related barriers to cancer pain management in Hong Kong. Unpublished report for Special Course on oncology nursing. Hong Kong: The Chinese University of Hong Kong; 1995.

22 Wills BSH, Wootton SY. Concerns and misconceptions about pain among Hong Kong Chinese cancer patients. Paper presented at 5th Hong Kong International Cancer Congress. 1998 Nov. 8-11. Hong Kong.

23 Galanti GA. Caring for patients from different cultures: Case studies from American hospitals. Philadelphia: University of Pennsylvania Press; 1997.

24 Ahles TA, Blanchard EB, Ruckdeschel JC. The multidimensional nature of cancer - related pain. Pain. 1983; 17: 272-288.

25 Ferrell BR. Humanising the experience of pain and illness. In: Ferrell BR, editor. Suffering. London: Jones and Bartlett Publisher; 1996. 211-222.

26 Foley KM. Pain assessment and cancer pain syndromes. In: Doyle D, Hanks GW, MacDonald N, editors. Oxford textbook of palliative medicine. 2nd ed. Oxford: Oxford University Press; 1998. 11-33.

27 Rimer BK, Kediera P, Levy MH. The role of patient education in cancer pain control. In: Turk DC, Feldman C.S. editors. Non-invasive approaches to pain management in the terminally ill. New York: The Harworth Press; 1992. 171-192.

28 Wujcik D, Utley S. The nurse' role. In: Parris WCV, editor. Cancer pain management. Principles and practice. Boston: Butterworth-Heinemann; 1997. 429-442.

29 Turk DC, Feldman CS. Facilitating the use of non-invasive pain management strategies with the terminally ill. In: Turk DC, Feldman CS, editors. Non-invasive approaches to pain management in the terminally ill. New York: The Howarth Press; 1992. 193-214.

30 Sloan PA, Donnelly MB, Schwartz RW. Sloan DA. Residents' management of the symptoms associated with terminal cancer. The Hospice Journal. 1997; 12 (3): 5-15.

31 Foley KM. Pain assessment and cancer syndrome. In: Doyle D, Hanks G, MacDonald N, editors. Oxford textbook of palliative medicine. Oxford: Oxford University Press; 1993. 148-165.

32 Dunlop R. Cancer: Palliative care. London: Springer-Verlag; 1998.

33 Jaffe C, Ehrlich CH. All kinds of love: Experiencing hospice. Amitylle N.Y.: Baywood Publication; 1997.

34 Benner P, Wrubel J. The primacy of caring: Stress and coping in health and illness. Menlo Park CA: Addison-Wesley Publishing Co. 1989. 1.

35 Cassell E. The nature of suffering and the goals of medicine. New England Journal of Medicine. 1982; 306: 640

36 Brallier LW. The suffering of terminal illness: cancer. In: Starck PL. McGovern JP, editors. The hidden dimension of illness: Human suffering. New York: National League of Nursing; 1992. 203-225.

37 Benoliel JQ. Foreword. In: Ferrell BR, editor. Suffering. London: Jones Bartlett Publisher; 1996. vii-x.

38 Morris JN. Sherwood S. Wright SM. Gutkin CE. The last weeks of life: Does hospice care make a difference? In: Mor V. Greer DS. Kastenbaum R, editors. The hospice experiment. Baltimore: John Hopkins University Press; 1988. 109-132.

39 Seale C, Cartwright A. The year before death. Aldershot: Ashgate; 1994.

40 Portenoy RK, Thaler HT, Kornblith AB. et al. Symptom prevalence, characteristics and distress in a cancer population. Quality Life Research. 1994; 3: 183-189.

41 Cohen SR, Mount BM, Strobel MG, Bui F. The McGill quality of life questionnaire: A measure of quality of life appropriate for people with advanced disease. A preliminary study of validity and acceptability. Palliative Medicine. 1995; 9: 207-219.

42 Maes JL. Suffering: A caregiver' guide. Nashville, TN: Abingdon Press; 1990.

43 Seale C, Addington HJ. Euthanasia: Why people want to die earlier. Social Science and Medicine. 1994; 39 (5): 647-654.

44 Yuen R, Mak Y, Wong J, Leung C, Cheng D, Yip C. A pilot study on cancer

patients' requests for euthanasia. Poster presented at 5th International Cancer Congress. 1998 Nov. 8-11. Hong Kong.

45 Goh CR. A palliative care curriculum for Asia. Paper presented at 14th Asia Pacific Cancer Conference/4th Hong Kong International Cancer Congress. 1997 Nov. 16-19.

46 Seale C, Addington HJ. Euthanasia: the role of good care. Social Science and Medicine. 1995; 40 (5): 581-587.

47 Glaser BG, Strauss AL. Awareness of dying. Chicago: Aldine Publishing Co.; 1965.

48 Quill TE. Death and dignity. New York: Norton; 1993.

49 Cheng BY. Stress of bereavement. Social support and quality of life. A study on the bereaved spouse in Hong Kong. Unpublished Master of Social Science Thesis. Hong Kong: The Chinese University of Hong Kong; 1997.

50 Cartwright A, Hockey L, Anderson JL. Life before death. London: Routledge Kegan Paul; 1973.

51 Shneidman ES. An appropriate death. In: Shneidman ES, editor. Deaths of man. Bath: Pitman Press; 1973. 25-32.

52 Portenoy RK, Thaler HT, Kornblith AB. et al. The Memorial symptom assessment scale: An instrument for the evaluation of symptom prevalence, characteristics and distress. European Journal of Cancer. 1994; 30: 1326-36.

53 Morse JM, Bottorff JL, Hutchison S. The paradox of comfort. Nursing Research. 1995; 44: 14-19.

54 Arruda EN, Larson PJ, Meleis AI. Comfort: immigrant Hispanic cancer patients' views. Cancer Nursing. 1992; 15 (6): 387-394.

55 Bottorff JL, Gogag M, Engelberg-Lotzkar M. Comforting: exploring the work of cancer nurses. Journal of Advanced Nursing. 1995; 22 (6): 1077-1084.

56 Breitbart W, Bruera E, Chochinov H, Lynch M. Neuro-psychiatric syndromes and psychological symptoms in patients with advanced cancer. Journal of Pain Symptom Management. 1995; 10: 131-141.

57 Becker R, & Gamlin R. Fundamental aspects of palliative care nursing. Salisbury: Quay Books; 2004.

58 Zerwekh JV. Nursing care at the end of life. Palliative care for patients and families. Philadelphia: F.A. Davis, 2006.

Resources
American Society of Pain Management Nurses: (http://www.aspmn.org)
American Academy of Pain Management: (http://www.aapainmanage.org)
Wisconsin Cancer Pain Initiative Cancer Society: (http://cis.nci.nih.gov)

Chapter seven: Maintaining social relations

1 Halldorsdottir S. Five basic modes of being with another. In: Gaut DA, Leininger MM, editors. Caring: The compassionate healer. New York: National League for Nursing. 1991; 37-48.

2 Krause K. Coping with cancer. Western Journal of Nursing Research. 1993; 15: 31-43.

3 Schubert PE. Lionberger HJ. Mutual connectedness. Journal of Holistic

Nursing. 1995; 13 (2): 102-116.

4 Walton J. Spiritual relationships. A concept analysis. Journal of Holistic Nursing. 1996; 14 (3): 237-250.

5 Flemming K. The meaning of hope to palliative cancer patients. International Journal of Palliative Nursing. 1997; 3 (1): 14-18.

6 Speck P. Spiritual issues in palliative care. In: Doyle D, Hanks G, MacDonald N, editors. Oxford textbook of palliative medicine. 2nd ed. Oxford: Oxford University Press; 1998. 805-814.

7 Benoliel JQ. ForwardForeword. In: Ferrell BR, editor. Suffering. London: Jones Bartlett Publisher; 1996. vii-x.

8 May R. Man's search for himself. New York: Norton Company; 1953. 88.

9 Patterson JG. Zderad LT. Humanistic nursing. New York: National League for Nursing; 1988.

10 Ma JLC. The adjustment process of patients suffering from neoplasm of nasopharynx throughout the course of illness: A panel study in Hong Kong. Hong Kong: The University of Hong Kong; 1995.

11 Sudnow D. Passing on: The social organisation of dying. New Jersey, Eaglewood Cliffs: Prentice-Hall; 1967.

12 Yeung WFE. The impact of hospice inpatient care on the quality of life of terminally ill cancer patients. Unpublished report. Hong Kong. Institute of Advanced Nursing Studies, Hospital Authority; 1997.

13 Becker E. The denial of death. New York: Macmillan; 1973.

14 Carr B, Mahalingam I, editors. Companion Encyclopaedia of Asian philosophy. London: Routledge; 1997.

15 Chan KS, Lam Z, Chun R, Dai D, Leung A. Chinese patients with terminal cancer. In: Doyle D, Hanks G, MacDonald N,. editors. Oxford textbook of palliative medicine. 2nd ed. Oxford: Oxford University Press; 1998. 793-795.

16 Bolande HA. The rebirth of the traditional funeral. Eastern Express. 1996 Jan 4. 16 Feature.

17 Glaser BG, Strauss AL. Awareness of dying. Chicago: Aldine Publishing Co.; 1965.

18 Dunlop R. Cancer: Palliative care. London: Springer-Verlag; 1998.

19 Brallier LW. The suffering of terminal illness: cancer. In: Starck PL. McGovern JP, editors. The hidden dimension of illness: Human suffering. New York: National League of Nursing; 1992. 203-225.

20 Kwan C. Problems and concerns of terminal cancer patients' families identified by nurses during hospitalisation in a hospice unit. Poster presented at 5th Hong Kong International Cancer Congress. Hong Kong, 1998 Nov. 8-11 Hong Kong.

21 Cheng HL, editor. New essays in Chinese philosophy. New York: Peter Lang; 1997.

22 Ferrell BR. The family. In: Doyle D, Hanks G, MacDonald N, editors. Oxford textbook of palliative medicine. 2nd ed. Oxford: Oxford University Press; 1998. 908-929.

23 Leung WT. Towards a model of cities in radical transition. Unpublished Ph.D. Thesis. Regent University; 1994.

24 Shum M. The first year of an independent hospice in Hong Kong. Annuals of Academy of Medicine. Hong Kong; 1994.

25 Koo L. Concept of disease causation, treatment prevention among Hong Kong Chinese. Social Science and Medicine. 1987; 25 (4): 405-417.

26 Lee RPL, Cheung YW. Health and health care. In: Lau SK, Lee MK, Wan PS, Wong SL, editors. Indicators of social development. Hong Kong: The Chinese University Press; 1993. 59-112.

27 Ferrell BR, Ferrell BA, Rhiner M, Grant MM. Family factors influencing cancer pain management. Post Graduate Medical Journal. 1991; 67 (Supplement 2): S64-9.

28 Wee B. Palliative care in Hong Kong. European Journal of Palliative Care. 1997; 4 (6): 216-218.

29 Yeung MK. To fight again. Hong Kong: Kan Sang Resource (Hong Kong). Ltd.; 1997. (in Chinese)

30 Yang TC. Philosophy of death. Taipei: Hung Yip Publisher. ; 1994. (in Chinese)

31 Bryce D, editor. Philosophy and religion in China by Leon Wieger. Felinfach Lampeter. Dyfed: Llanerch Enterprises; 1988. 31-32.

32 Ho YFD. Filial piety and its psychological consequences. In: Bond M, editor. The handbook of Chinese psychology. Hong Kong: Oxford University Press; 1996. 155-167

33 Doyle D. Upon reflection. A farewell address. Paper delivered at Geneva: Switzerland. 1999 Sept. 25.

34 Field D, Hockey J, Small N. Making sense of difference: gender and ethnicity in modern Britain. In: Field D, Hockey J, Small N, editors. Death, gender and ethnicity. London: Routledge; 1997. 1-28.

35 Davis-Friedmann D. Long lives: Chinese elderly and the Communist resolution. Expanded edition. Stanford: Stanford University Press; 1991.

36 Webb M. The Good Death: The new American search to reshape the end of life. New York: Bantam Books. 1997. 401.

37 Wu SC. Chinese funeral and Feng Shui. The world after death. Taipei: Mo Ling Publishing Co.; 1984. (in Chinese)

38 Travellbee J. Interpersonal aspects of nursing. 2nd ed. Philadelphia: F.A. Davis; 1971.

39 Overmyer DT. China. In: Holck F.H. editor. Death and Eastern thought. Nashville Tennessee: Abingdon Press; 1974. 198-222.

40 Conco D. Christian patient's views of spiritual care. Western Journal of Nursing Research. 1995; 17 (3): 266-276.

41 Cheng BY. Stress of bereavement. Social support and quality of life. A study on the bereaved spouse in Hong Kong. Unpublished Master of Social Science Thesis. Hong Kong: The Chinese University of Hong Kong; 1997.

42 Cohen SR, Mount BM, Strobel MG, Bui F. The McGill quality of life questionnaire: A measure of quality of life appropriate for people with advanced disease. A preliminary study of validity and acceptability. Palliative Medicine. 1995; 9: 207-219.

43 Kellehear A. Health promoting palliative care. Melbourne: Oxford University Press; 1999.

44 Robbins M. Evaluating palliative care. Establishing the evidence base. Oxford: Oxford University Press; 1998.

45 Jaffe C, Ehrlich CH. All kinds of love: Experiencing hospice. Amitylle N.Y.:

Baywood Publication; 1997.

46 Wong-Wylie G, Jevne RF. Patient hope: Exploring the interactions between physicians and HIV seropositive individuals. Qualitative Health Research. 1997; 7(1): 32-56.

47 Zerwekh JV. Nursing care at the end of life. Palliative care for patients and families. Philadelphia: F.A. Davis Co., 2006

Chapter eight: Experiencing personal control

1 McLean GL. Facing death. Conversations with cancer patients. London: Churchill Livingstone; 1993.

2 Zimmerman L, Story KT, Gaston-Johansson F, Rowles JR. Psychological variables, cancer pain. Cancer Nursing. 1996; 19(1): 44-53.

3 Rodin J. Health, control and ageing. In: Baltes MM, Baltes PB editors. The psychology of control and ageing. Hillsdale, New York: Eribaum. 1986. 141.

4 Mesler MA. The philosophy and practice of patient control in hospice: The dynamics of autonomy versus paternalism. Omega. 1994-5; 30 (3): 173-189.

5 Smith DC, Maher MF. Achieving a healthy death: The dying person's attitudinal contributions. The Hospice Journal. 1993; 9 (1): 21-32.

6 Taylor B. Promoting a good death: Nurses' practice insights. In: Gray G, Pratt R, editors. Issues in Australian nursing 5: The nurse as clinician. Melbourne: Churchill Livingstone; 1995. 209-220.

7 McNamara B, Waddell C, Colvin M. The institutionalisation of the Good Death. Social Science and Medicine. 1994; 39 (11): 1501-8.

8 McNamara B, Waddell C, and Colvin M. Threats to the Good Death: The cultural context of stress and coping among hospice nurses. Sociology of Health and illness. 1995; 17 (2): 222-244.

9 Weisman AD. On dying and denying. A psychiatric study of terminality. New York: Behavioural sciences Press; 1972.

10 Weisman AD. Appropriate death and the hospice program. The Hospice Journal. 1988; 4 (1): 65-77.

11 Kalish RA. Death, grief and caring relationship. Monterey: Brooks/Cole Publishing Company; 1981.

12 D'Angelo B. Death with dignity: Supporting a patient's decision. American Nephrology Nurses' Association Journal. 1986; 13(6): 330-333.

13 Madan TN. Dying with dignity. Social Science and Medicine. 1992. 35(4): 425-432.

14 Chao CSC. The meaning of good dying of Chinese terminally ill cancer patients in Taiwan. Unpublished PhD Thesis. Case Western Reserve University; 1993.

15 Young M, Cullen L. A Good Death. Conversations with East Londoners. London: Routledge; 1996.

16 Kahn DL, Steeves RH. An understanding of suffering. In: Ferrell BR, editor. Suffering. London: Jones Bartlett Publisher. 1996. 4-27.

17 Justice C. Dying the Good Death: The pilgrimage to die in India's Holy city. Albany: State University of New York Press; 1997.

18 Chan KS, Lam Z, Chun R, Dai D, Leung A. Chinese patients with terminal cancer. In: Doyle D, Hanks G, MacDonald N, editors. Oxford textbook of

palliative medicine. 2nd ed. Oxford: Oxford University Press; 1998. 793-795.

19 Kessler D. The rights of the dying. A companion for life's final moments. New York: Harper Collins; 1997.

20 Yeung WFE. The impact of hospice inpatient care on the quality of life of terminally ill cancer patients. Unpublished report. Hong Kong. Institute of Advanced Nursing Studies, Hospital Authority; 1997.

21 Emanuel EJ, Fairclough D, Slutsman J, Omundsen E, Emanuel LL. Predictors outcomes of significant care giving needs and economic burdens among terminally ill oncology patients: Results from the Commonwealth- Cummings Project. Journal of Clinical Oncology. 1998; 17: 1628.

22 Strauss AL, Glaser BG. Social organisation of medical work. Chicago: Chicago University Press; 1985.

23 Davis AJ, Slater P. US. and Australian nurses' attitudes beliefs about the Good Death. Image: Journal of Nursing Scholarship. 1989; 21(1): 34-39.

24 Johnston M, Tookman A, Honeybun J. The impact of a death on fellow hospice patients. British Journal of Medical Psychology. 1992; 65: 67-72.

25 Dunlop R. Cancer: Palliative care. London: Springer-Verlag; 1998.

26 Byock I. Dying well: The prospect for growth at the end of life. New York: Riverhead Books; 1997.

27 Catalan-Fernandez JG, Pons-Sureda O, Recober-Martinez A, Avella-Mestre A, Carbonero-Malberti JM, Benito-Oliver E, Garau-Llinas I. Dying of cancer. The place of death and family circumstances. Medical Care. 1991; 29 (9): 841-851.

28 Callahan M, Kelly P. Final gifts. Understanding the special awareness, needs and communications of the dying. New York: Poseidon Press; 1992.

29 Quill TE. A midwife through the dying process: Stories of healing and hard choices at the end of life. Baltimore: John Hopkins Press; 1996

30 Wass H, Neimeyer RA, editors. Dying: Facing the facts. 3rd ed. Washington, D.C.: Taylor and Francis; 1995.

31 Glaser BG, Strauss AL. Awareness of dying. Chicago: Aldine Publishing Co.; 1965.

32 Samarel N. Caring for life and death. New York: Hemisphere Publishing Co.; 1991. 72.

33 Benner P, Wrubel J. The primacy of caring: Stress and coping in health and illness. Menlo Park CA: Addison-Wesley Publishing Co. 1989.

34 Cassidy S. The loneliest journey. London: Darton, Longman and Todd; 1995.

35 De Raeve L. Dignity and integrity at the end of life. International Journal of Palliative Nursing. 1996; 2(2): 71-76.

36 Grealish L. Beyond Hypocrites: Ethics in palliative care. International Journal of Palliative Nursing. 1997; 3 (3): 151-155.

37 Kastenbaum RJ. The psychology of death. 2nd ed. New York: Springer; 1992.

38 Davison BJ, Degner LF. Promoting patient decision-making in life--death situations. Seminars in Oncology Nursing. 1998; 14 (2): 129-136.

39 Yeung MK. To fight again. Hong Kong: Kan Sang Resource (Hong Kong). Ltd.; 1997. 37. (in Chinese).

40 Sogyal Rinpoche. The Tibetan book of living and dying. London: Rider; 1992. 93.

41 Fu WF. Respect of death and respect of life. Taipei: Chung Ching Publishing Co.; 1993. (in Chinese).

42 Bryce D, editor. Philosophy and religion in China by Leon Wieger. Felinfach Lampeter. Dyfed: Llanerch Enterprises; 1988. 106.

43 Wing RL. The Tao of power. A translation of the Tao Te Ching by Lao Tsu. New York: A Dolphin Book Doubleday; 1986.

44 Palsson M. Norberg A. Breast cancer patients' experiences of nursing care with the focuses on emotional support: The implementation of a nursing intervention. Journal of Advanced Nursing. 1995; 21: 227-285.

45 Jaffe C, Ehrlich CH. All kinds of love: Experiencing hospice. Amitylle N.Y.: Baywood Publication; 1997.

46 Eutsler EN. Community resources for hospice/ palliative care patients. In: Forman WB, Kitzes JA, Anderson RP, Sheehan DK. Hospice and Palliative Care. Concepts and Practice. 2nd ed. Boston: Jones and Bartlett Publisher. 2003; 261-267.

47 Kung H, Jens W. A dignified dying. London: SCM Press Ltd.; 1995.

48 Sigrist D. Journey's end. A guide to understanding the dying process. 2nd ed. New York: Genesee Region Home Care; 1996.

49 Glaser BG, Strauss AL. Time for dying. Chicago: Aldine Publishing Co.; 1968.

50 Kramer K. The sacred art of dying. How would religions understand death? New Jersey: Paulist Press; 1988. 91.

51 Zerwekh JV. Nursing care at the end of life. Palliative care for patients and families. Philadelphia: F.A. Davis Co., 2006.

Chapter nine: Preparing to depart and bidding farewells

1 Smith DC, Maher MF. Healthy Death. Counselling and Values. 1991; 36 (1): 42-48.

2 Kellehear A. Dying of cancer. The final year of life. Melbourne: Harwood Academic; 1990.

3 White K. Ethical problems experienced by four palliative care nurses working in a hospice. Unpublished Master of Nursing Thesis, Australian Catholic University; 1994.

4 Taylor B. Promoting a good death: Nurses' practice insights. In: Gray G, Pratt R, editors. Issues in Australian nursing 5: The nurse as clinician. Melbourne: Churchill Livingstone; 1995. 209-220.

5 Chao CSC. The meaning of good dying of Chinese terminally ill cancer patients in Taiwan. Unpublished PhD Thesis. Case Western Reserve University; 1993.

6 Mak MHJ. Moral education. Asian Culture. 1990; 18 (3): 62-71.

7 Hirst PH. Moral education in a secular society. London: University of London Press [for the] National Children's Home; 1974.

8 Sih KT. Will Confucian thought survive in the modern age? Chinese Culture. 1976. 17 (2): 27-30.

9 Goh CR. Problems of pain and quality of life assessment in a multi-cultural context. Paper presented at the 2nd International Conference on Cancer pain in the Pacific Basin, Perth: Western Australia; 1995.

10 Braun KL, Nichols R. Death and dying in four Asian American cultures: A descriptive research. Death Studies. 1997; 21(4): 327-359.

11 Waddell C, McNamara B. The stereotypical fallacy: A comparison of Anglo and Chinese Australians' thoughts about facing death. Mortality; 1997; 2(2): 149-161.

12 Cooper JC. An illustrated encyclopaedia of traditional symbols. London: Thames Hudson Ltd.; 1992.

13 Li ZD. Chinese traditional auspicious patterns. Shanghai: Shanghai Popular Science Press, 1989. (in English and Chinese).

14 Nuland SB. The doctor's role in death. In: Spiro H.M. McCrea Curnen M.G. Wandel L.P. editors. Facing death: Where culture, religion and medicine meet. New Heaven: C.T. Yale V. Press; 1996. 41.

15 Wu SC. Chinese funeral and Feng Shui. The world after death. Taipei: Mo Ling Publishing Co., 1984. (in Chinese).

16 Young M, Cullen L. A Good Death. Conversations with East Londoners. London: Routledge; 1996.

17 Dunn M. The good death guide. Oxford: How to Book Ltd.; 2000.

18 Lipman A, Marden PW. Preparation for death in old age. Journal of Gerontology. 1996; 21: 426-431.

19 Glaser BG, Strauss AL. Time for dying. Chicago: Aldine Publishing Co.; 1968.

20 Kalish RA, Reynold DK. Death and Ethnicity: A psychocultural research. Los Angeles: University of Southern California Press; 1976.

21 Riley Jr JW. What people think about death. In: Brim O.G. Freeman H.E. Levine S. Scotch N.A. The dying patient. New York: Russel Sage; 1970. 30-41.

22 McDonald RT, Carroll JD. Appropriate death: College students' preferences Vs. actuarial projections. Journal of Clinical Psychology. 1981; 37(1): 28-31.

23 Bolande HA. The rebirth of the traditional funeral. Eastern Express. 1996 Jan 4. 16 Feature.

24 Jaffe C, Ehrlich CH. All kinds of love: Experiencing hospice. Amitylle N.Y.: Baywood Publication; 1997.

25 Davis-Friedmann D. Long lives: Chinese elderly and the Communist resolution. Expanded edition. Stanford: Stanford University Press; 1991.

26 Bryce D, editor. Philosophy and religion in China by Leon Wieger. Felinfach Lampeter. Dyfed: Llanerch Enterprises; 1988. 32-33.

27 Overmyer DT. China. In: Holck F.H. editor. Death and Eastern thought. Nashville Tennessee: Abingdon Press; 1974. 198-222.

28 Cheng HK. Chinese wisdom on death. Taipei: Tung Tai Publishing Co.; 1994. (in Chinese).

29 Wong CW. The seeking of Chinese medical advice by the patients. A preliminary report on the survey. Medical Policy Research Group, Hong Kong Social Welfare Society. Hong Kong; 1998. (in Chinese).

30 Li ZX. The knowledge of Shan Shu. Taipei: Tung Tai Book Co. Ltd.; 1994. (in Chinese).

31 Hsu FLK. Americans and Chinese. Passages to difference. 3rd. ed. Honolulu: The University Press of Hawaii; 1981.

32 Webb M. The Good Death: The new American search to reshape the end of life. New York: Bantam Books. 1997.

33 Mak MHJ. Cultural care — Isn't it needed in the basic nursing curriculum in Hong Kong? Hong Kong Nursing Journal. 1991; 56: 40-44.

34 Kessler D. The rights of the dying. A companion for life's final moments. New York: Harper Collins; 1997.

35 Emanuel LL, Emanuel EJ. The medical directive: A new comprehensive advance care document. Journal of the American Medical Association. 1991; 325: 3288-3293

Chapter ten: Accepting the timing of one's death

1 Hunt M. Scripts for dying at home — displayed in nurses, patients' and relatives' talk. Journal of Advanced Nursing. 1992; 17 (11): 1297-1302.

2 Wilkes LM. Nurses' descriptions of death scenes. Journal of Cancer Care. 1993; 2: 11-16.

3 White K. Ethical problems experienced by four palliative care nurses working in a hospice. Unpublished Master of Nursing Thesis, Australian Catholic University; 1994.

4 Taylor B. Promoting a good death: Nurses' practice insights. In: Gray G, Pratt R, editors. Issues in Australian nursing 5: The nurse as clinician. Melbourne: Churchill Livingstone; 1995. 209-220.

5 Weisman AD. Coping with cancer. New York: McGraw-Hill; 1979.

6 Wilson SA. The ethnography of death, dying and hospice care. Unpublished Ph.D. Thesis. University of Wisconsin – Milwaukee; 1989.

7 Kearl MC. Endings. A sociology of death and dying. New York: Oxford University Press; 1989.

8 Shneidman ES. An appropriate death. In: Shneidman ES, editor. Deaths of man. Bath: Pitman Press; 1973. 29.

9 Hinton J. Dying. London: Penguin Books; 1967. 43.

10 McDonald RT, Carroll JD. Appropriate death: College students' preferences Vs. actuarial projections. Journal of Clinical Psychology. 1981; 37(1): 28-31.

11 Nimocks M.J.A. Webb L. Connell J.R. Communication and the terminally ill: A theoretical model. Death Studies. 1987; 11: 323-344.

12 Weisman AD. On dying and denying. A psychiatric study of terminality. New York: Behavioural sciences Press; 1972.

13 Tsim KF, Lui PY. Report on seminar of the hospice film: Love until next life, care of the care receivers and care givers. China Hospice Foundation Newsletter. 1995; 12: 69-71. (in Chinese).

14 Glaser BG, Strauss AL. Time for dying. Chicago: Aldine Publishing Co.; 1968.

15 Kastenbaum RJ. The psychology of death. 2nd ed. New York: Springer; 1992.

16 Young M, Cullen L. A Good Death. Conversations with East Londoners. London: Routledge; 1996.

17 McNamara B, Waddell C, and Colvin M. Threats to the Good Death: The cultural context of stress and coping among hospice nurses. Sociology of Health and illness. 1995; 17 (2): 222-244.

18 Maslow A. The Editorial. Abe Maslow 1908-1970. Psychology Today. 1970; 4 (3):16.

19 Sih KT. Will Confucian thought survive in the modern age? Chinese Culture. 1976. 17 (2): 27-30.

20 Chan KS, Lam Z, Chun R, Dai D, Leung A. Chinese patients with terminal cancer. In: Doyle D, Hanks G, MacDonald N, editors. Oxford textbook of palliative medicine. 2nd ed. Oxford: Oxford University Press; 1998. 793-795.

21 Ho YFD. Filial piety and its psychological consequences. In: Bond M, editor. The handbook of Chinese psychology. Hong Kong: Oxford University Press; 1996. 155-167.

22 Braun KL, Nichols R. Death and dying in four Asian American cultures: A descriptive study. Death Studies. 1997; 21(4): 327-359.

23 Sweeting HN, Gilhooly MLM. Dementia and the phenomenon of social death. Sociology of Health and Illness. 1997; 19 (1): 93-117.

24 Li ZX. The knowledge of Shan Shu. Taipei: Tung Tai Book Co. Ltd.; 1994. (in Chinese).

25 Justice C. Dying the Good Death: The pilgrimage to die in India's Holy city. Albany: State University of New York Press; 1997.

26 Wass H, Neimeyer RA, editors. Dying: Facing the facts. 3rd ed. Washington, D.C.: Taylor and Francis; 1995.

27 Doka KJ, Morgan JD, editors. Death and spirituality. Amityville N.Y.: Baywood Publishing Co.; 1993.

28 Zerwekh JV. A family care giving model for hospice nursing. The Hospice Journal. 1995; 10 (1): 27-44.

29 Klass, 1993 cited by Jaffe C, Ehrlich CH. All kinds of love: Experiencing hospice. Amitylle N.Y.: Baywood Publication; 1997. 234–235.

30 Fu PW. Religions behind Confucian view of death and dying. Philosophy and Culture. 1994; 21 (7): 600-607. (in Chinese).

31 Overmyer DT. China. In: Holck F.H. editor. Death and Eastern thought. Nashville Tennessee: Abingdon Press; 1974. 198-222.

32 Yeung MK. To fight again. Hong Kong: Kan Sang Resource (Hong Kong). Ltd.; 1997. (in Chinese).

33 Kleinman A. The illness narratives. New York: Basic Books; 1988. 148.

34 Erikson EH. Childhood and society. 2nd ed. New York: Norton; 1963.

35 Fromm E. The revolution of hope. Toward a humanised technology. New York: Harper and Row; 1968. 84.

36 Neuberger J. Caring for dying people of different faiths. 2nd ed. London: Mosby; 1994.

37 Corr CA. Coping with dying: Lessons that we should not learn from the work of Elizabeth Kubler-Ross. Death Studies. 1993; 17: 69-83.

38 Kastenbaum RJ. Avery D Weisman MD. An Omega interview. Omega. 1993; 27 (2): 97-103.

39 Shelly JA. Spiritual care, planting seeds of hope. Critical Care Update. 1982 Dec. 9-14.

40 Cohen SR, Mount BM, Strobel MG, Bui F. The McGill quality of life questionnaire: A measure of quality of life appropriate for people with advanced disease. A preliminary study of validity and acceptability. Palliative Medicine. 1995; 9: 207-219.

41 Cohen SR, Mount BM, Tomas J, Mount L. Existential well being is an important determinant of quality of life: Evidence from the McGill quality of life questionnaire. Cancer. 1996; 77: 576-586.

42 Cohen SR, Mount BM, Bruera E, Provost M, Rowe J, Tong K. Validity of the

McGill quality of life questionnaire in the palliative care setting: A multi-centre Canadian study demonstrating the importance of the existential domain. Palliative Medicine. 1997; 11: 3-20.

43 Kessler D. The rights of the dying. A companion for life's final moments. New York: Harper Collins; 1997. 85.

44 Quill TE. A midwife through the dying process: Stories of healing and hard choices at the end of life. Baltimore: John Hopkins Press; 1996.

45 Brallier LW. The suffering of terminal illness: cancer. In: Starck PL. McGovern JP, editors. The hidden dimension of illness: Human suffering. New York: National League of Nursing; 1992. 203-225.

46 Sogyal Rinpoche. The Tibetan book of living and dying. London: Rider; 1992. 183.

47 Cohen S, Boston P, Mount B, Porterfield P. Changes in quality of life following admission to palliative care units. Palliative Medicine. 2001; 15 (5): 363-371.

48 Zhoc J, Li K, Yeo W, Johnson P, Mak Y, Lee J Cross-cultural validation of the McGill Quality of life questionnaire in Hong Kong Chinese. Palliative Medicine. 2001; 15(5): 387-397

Chapter eleven: A Harmonious Death

1 Young M, Cullen L. A Good Death. Conversations with East Londoners. London: Routledge; 1996.

2 Tu WM, editor. The living tree. The changing meaning of being Chinese today. Stanford: Stanford University Press; 1994.

3 Kellehear A. Dying of cancer. The final year of life. Melbourne: Harwood Academic; 1990.

4 Brallier LW. The suffering of terminal illness: cancer. In: Starck PL. McGovern JP, editors. The hidden dimension of illness: Human suffering. New York: National League of Nursing; 1992. 203-225.

5 Benoliel JQ. Forward. In: Ferrell BR, editor. Suffering. London: Jones Bartlett Publisher; 1996. vii-x.

6 King AYC. Kuan-Hsi and network building: A sociological interpretation. In: Tu WM, editor. The living tree. The changing meaning of being Chinese today. Stanford: Stanford University Press; 1994. 109-126.

7 Chang H. Confucian cosmological myth and Neo-Confucian transcendence. In: Smith RJ, Kwok DWY, editors. Cosmology ontology human efficacy. Essays in Chinese thought. Honolulu: University of Hawaii Press; 1993; 14-32.

8 King A, Lee R. Social life and development in Hong Kong. Hong Kong: Chinese University Press; 1981.

9 Henderson H, Thompson SE, Holidays, festivals and celebrations of the World Dictionary. 2nd ed. Detroit: Omnigraphics Inc.; 1997.

10 Weisman AD. On dying and denying. A psychiatric study of terminality. New York: Behavioural sciences Press; 1972.

11 Lederburg P, Latimer E. Psychosocial and ethical issues in the care of cancer patients. In: DeVita VT, Hellman S, Rosenberg SA, editors. Cancer: Principles and Practice of Oncology. 4th ed. Philadelphia: J.B. Lippincott; 1989.

12 Gaudry E, Spielberger CD. Personal power. Use, misuse and abuse. Victoria:

Harper Collins; 1995.

13 Li ZX. The knowledge of Shan Shu. Taipei: Tung Tai Book Co. Ltd.; 1994. (in Chinese).

14 Littleton CS, editor. The sacred East. Melbourne: Cardigan Street Publishers; 1996.

15 Li SP. Ching cosmology popular precepts. In: Smith RJ, Kwok DWY, editors. Cosmology, ontology, and human efficacy. Essays in Chinese thought. Honolulu: University of Hawaii Press. 1993. 113-137.

16 Neuberger J. Caring for dying people of different faiths. 2nd ed. London: Mosby; 1994.

17 Fu WF. Respect of death and respect of life. Taipei: Chung Ching Publishing Co.; 1993. (in Chinese).

18 Speck P. Spiritual issues in palliative care. In: Doyle D, Hanks G, MacDonald N, editors. Oxford textbook of palliative medicine. 2nd ed. Oxford: Oxford University Press; 1998. 805-814.

19 Martin JP. Eastern spirituality and health care. In: Carson VB, editor. Spirituality dimensions of nursing practice. Philadelphia: W.B. Saunders. Co. 1989. 114-131.

20 Wong CW. The seeking of Chinese medical advice by the patients. A preliminary report on the survey. Medical Policy Research Group, Hong Kong Social Welfare Society. Hong Kong. 1998. (in Chinese).

21 Dow TI. Yin-Yang dialectical monism. In: Cheng HL, editor. New essays in Chinese philosophy. New York: Peter Lang. 1997; 175-194.

22 Blauner R. Death and social structure. Psychiatry. 1966; 29: 378-94.

23 Bok S. Lies to the sick and dying. In: Shneidman ES, editor. Death: Current perspectives. 3rd ed. Palo Alto: Mayfield; 1984. 171-186.

24 Yeung MK. To fight again. Hong Kong: Kan Sang Resource (Hong Kong). Ltd. 1997. (in Chinese).

25 Galanti GA. Caring for patients from different cultures: Case studies from American hospitals. Philadelphia: University of Pennsylvania Press; 1997.

26 Miyaji NT. The power of compassion: Truth-telling among American doctors in the care of dying patients. Social Science and Medicine. 1993; 36 (3): 249-264.

27 Chao CSC. The meaning of good dying of Chinese terminally ill cancer patients in Taiwan. Unpublished PhD Thesis. Case Western Reserve University; 1993.

28 Cousins N. The physician as communicator. Journal of the American Medical Association. 1982; 248 (5): 587-589.

29 Dunlop R. Cancer: Palliative care. London: Springer-Verlag; 1998.

30 Foley KM. Pain assessment and cancer syndrome. In: Doyle D, Hanks G, MacDonald N, editors. Oxford textbook of palliative medicine. Oxford: Oxford University Press; 1993. 148-165.

31 Lam CYJ, Chung TK, Chiu WC. A preliminary study on patient-related barriers to cancer pain management in Hong Kong. Unpublished report for Special Course on oncology nursing. Hong Kong: The Chinese University of Hong Kong; 1995.

32 Wills BSH, Wootton SY. Concerns and misconceptions about pain among Hong Kong Chinese cancer patients. Paper presented at 5th Hong Kong International Cancer Congress. 1998 Nov. 8-11. Hong Kong.

33 Overmyer DT. Religions of China. New York: Harper and Row; 1986.

34 Cheng HK. Chinese wisdom on death. Taipei: Tung Tai Publishing Co.; 1994. (in Chinese).

35 Glaser BG, Strauss AL. Awareness of dying. Chicago: Aldine Publishing Co.; 1965

36 Cheng BY. Stress of bereavement. Social support and quality of life. A study on the bereaved spouse in Hong Kong. Unpublished Master of Social Science Thesis. Hong Kong: The Chinese University of Hong Kong; 1997.

37 Doyle D. Upon reflection. A farewell address. Paper delivered at Geneva: Switzerland. 1999 Sept. 25.

38 Mesler MA. The philosophy and practice of patient control in hospice: The dynamics of autonomy versus paternalism. Omega. 1994-5; 30 (3): 173-189.

39 Chan KS, Lam Z, Chun R, Dai D, Leung A. Chinese patients with terminal cancer. In: Doyle D, Hanks G, MacDonald N, editors. Oxford textbook of palliative medicine. 2nd ed. Oxford: Oxford University Press; 1998. 793-795.

40 Slote WH. Psychocultural dynamics within the Confucian family. In: Slote WH, DeVos GA, editors. Confucianism and the family. Albany: State University of New York Press; 1998. 37-52.

41 Bryce D, editor. Philosophy and religion in China by Leon Wieger. Felinfach, Lampeter, Dyfed: Llanerch Enterprises; 1988. 106.

42 Sih KT. Will Confucian thought survive in the modern age? Chinese Culture. 1976. 17 (2): 27-30.

43 So YP. Death. Be not proud. Hong Kong: Breakthrough Ltd.; 1981. (in Chinese).

44 Kuo ECY. Confucianism and the Chinese family in Singapore: continuities and changes. In: Slote WH, DeVos GA, editors. Confucianism and the family. Albany: State University of New York Press; 1998. 231-148.

45 Conco D. Christian patient's views of spiritual care. Western Journal of Nursing Research. 1995; 17 (3): 266-276.

46 Bolande HA. The rebirth of the traditional funeral. Eastern Express. 1996 Jan 4. 16 Feature.

47 Duan D. Philosophy of death. Hunan: Hunan People's Press; 1996. (in Chinese).

48 Moore TW. Philosophy of education. London: Rutledge and Kegan Paul; 1982.

49 Hirst PH. Moral education in a secular society. London: University of London Press [for the] National Children's Home; 1974.

50 Toong J, editor. Seminar on East Asian man – Modern Asian Man. IEAP News. 1987; 8: 2-3.

51 Slote WH, DeVos GA, editors. Confucianism and the family. Albany: State University of New York Press; 1998.

52 Mak MHJ. Moral education. Asian Culture. 1990; 18 (3): 62-71.

53 Wing RL. The Tao of power. A translation of the Tao Te Ching by Lao Tsu. New York: A Dolphin Book Doubleday; 1986.

54 Tu WM. Confucius and Confucianism. In: Slote WH, DeVos GA, editors. Confucianism and the family. Albany: State University of New York Press; 1998. 3-36.

55 Choy HL, Lai B, Har YW. Analects of Confucius. Beijing: Sinolingua; 1994. 4.

(in Chinese and English).

56 Kubler-Ross E. On death and dying. New York: Macmillan; 1969.

57 Pattison EM. The experience of death. Englewood Cliffs: Prentice-Hall Inc.; 1977.

58 Lee E. A Good Death. A guide for patients and carers facing terminal illness at home. London: Rosendale Press; 1995.

59 Byock I. Dying well: The prospect for growth at the end of life. New York: Riverhead Books; 1997.

60 Mackie F. The ethnic self. In: Kellehear A. editor. Social self, global culture – An introduction to sociological ideas. Melbourne: Oxford University Press; 1996. 34-44.

61 Quill TE. A midwife through the dying process: Stories of healing and hard choices at the end of life. Baltimore: John Hopkins Press; 1996.

Chapter twelve: Conclusion

1 Saunders C. The moment of truth: Care of the dying person. In: Person L. editor. Death and dying. London: The Press of Case Western Reserve University; 1969. 49-78.

2 Corr CA. Coping with dying: Lessons that we should not learn from the work of Elizabeth Kubler-Ross. Death Studies. 1993; 17: 69-83.

3 Callahan M, Kelly P. Final gifts. Understanding the special awareness, needs and communications of the dying. New York: Poseidon Press; 1992.

4 Brykczynska G, editor. Caring. The compassion and wisdom of caring. London: Arnold; 1997.

5 Saunders C. Caring for the dying. In: Lack S. Lamerton R. The hour of our death. A record of the Conference on the care of the dying held in London. London: Geoffrey Chapman; 1975. 18-27.

6 Saunders C. Kastenbaum R. editors. Hospice care on the international scene. New York: Springer Publishing Co.; 1997.

7 Kearney M. Mortally wounded. Stories of soul pain, death and healing. Dublin: Marino Books; 1996. 179.

8 Blum, 1980 cited by Finn WF. Patients' wants and needs: The Physicians' responses. In: DeBellis Marcus RE, Kutscher AH, Torres CS, Barrett V, Siegel ME, editors. Suffering. Psychological and social aspects in loss, grief and care. London: The Haworth Press; 1986. 11.

9 Fromm E. The revolution of hope. Toward a humanised technology. New York: Harper and Row; 1968. 79.

10 Sogyal Rinpoche. The Tibetan book of living and dying. London: Rider; 1992. 187.

11 Doyle D. Upon reflection. A farewell address. Paper delivered at Geneva: Switzerland. 1999 Sept. 25.

12 Chao CSC. The meaning of good dying of Chinese terminally ill cancer patients in Taiwan. Unpublished PhD Thesis. Case Western Reserve University; 1993.

13 Hwang TC. A cross cultural study of attitudes towards death and dying between Chinese and American college students. Unpublished Ed.D. Thesis. Drake University; 1988.

14 Mak MHJ. Cultural responses to death and dying: The experience in Hong Kong. Abstracts. The Social Context of Death, Dying and Disposal. 3rd International Conference. The University of Cardiff, UK. 1997 Apr. 4-6.

15 Ferrell BR. To know suffering. Oncology Nursing Forum. 1993; 20(10): 1471-1477.

16 Abu-Saad HH. Evidence-based Palliative care across the life span. Oxford: Blackwell; 2001.

17 Smith A, Zhu DZ. Hospice development in China: Like green shoots in the spring. In: Saunders C, Kastenbaum R, editors. Hospice care on the international scene. New York: Springer Publishing Co.; 1997. 193-205.

18 Mor et al., cited by Dunlop R. Cancer: Palliative care. London: Springer-Verlag; 1998.

19 Young M, Cullen L. A Good Death. Conversations with East Londoners. London: Routledge; 1996.

20 Emanuel EJ, Fairclough D, Slutsman J, Omundsen E, Emanuel LL. Predictors outcomes of significant care giving needs and economic burdens among terminally ill oncology patients: Results from the Commonwealth- Cummings Project. Journal of Clinical Oncology. 1998; 17: 1628.

21 Zhou Y, Mi J. Hospice care: A new problem of nursing study. Proceedings of the First East-West International Conference on Hospice Care. Tianjin: Tianjin Medical University; 1992.

Bibliography

Beauchamp TLY. and Veatch RM. Editors. *Ethical issues in death and dying.* 2nd ed. New Jersey: Prentice Hall, 1996.

Benoliel JQ. Institutional dying: A convergence of cultural values, technology, and social organization. In Wass H. Berardo FM. and Neimeyer RA. editors. *Dying: facing the facts.* 2nd ed. Washington, DC: Hemisphere Publishing, 1988, 185-200.

Beresford P. Adshead L. and Croft S. *Palliative care, social work and service users: making life possible.* Philadelphia: Jessica Kingsley Publishers, 2007.

Berger AM. Shuster JL. and Von Roenn JH. Editors. *Principles and practice of palliative care and supportive oncology.* Philadelphia: Lippincott Williams and Wilkins, 2007.

Booth S. editor *Palliative care consultations in advanced breast cancer.* New York: Oxford University Press, 2006.

Burns N. Measuring Cancer Attitudes. In Frank-Stromborg M. *Instruments for Clinical Nursing Research.* Sudbury, MA: Jones & Bartlett Publishers, 1992, 297-309.

Chan HYL. and Pang SMC. Quality of life concerns and end-of-life care preferences of aged persons in long-term care facilities. *Journal of Clinical Nursing.* 2007, 16(11): 2158-2166.

Charmaz K. Discovering chronic illness: using grounded theory. *Social Science and Medicine.* 1990, 30: 1161-1172.

Cheng HK. *Beyond of death.* Taipei: Ching Chung Publishing Co., 1999. (in Chinese)

Chiarella M. *Policy in end-of-life care: education, ethics, practice and research.* London: Quay Books Division, MA Healthcare, 2006.

Clark SE. and Marley J. Good grief. *The Medical Journal of Australia.* 1993, 158: 834-841.

Corr CA. Nabe CM. and Corr DM. *Death and dying, life and living.* Belmont CA: Wadsworth, 2006.

Davies E. and Higginson IJ. *Better palliative care for older people.* Copenhagen: WHO Regional Office for Europe, 2004.

De Raeve L. Ethical issues in palliative care research. *Palliative Medicine.* 1994, 8: 298-305.

Dobratz MC. Causal influences of psychological adaptation in dying. *Western Journal of Nursing Research*. 1993, 15(6): 708-729.

Dority B. In the hands of the people: recent victories of the death with dignity movement. *The Humanist*. 1996, 56: 6-8.

Emanuel LL. and Librach SL. Editors. *Palliative care: core skills and clinical competencies*. Philadelphia, PA: Saunders/Elsevier, 2007.

Faull C. and Woof R. *Palliative care*. Oxford: Oxford University Press, 2002.

Filmer P. Jenks C. Seale C. and Walsh D. Developments in social theory. In C. Seale, Editor. *Researching society and culture*. London: Sage, 1998, 23-36.

Fu WF. *The wisdom of life*. Taipei: San Chee Publishing, 1997. (in Chinese)

Gates MF. Transcultural comparison of hospital and hospice as caring environments for dying patients. *Journal of Transcultural nursing*. 1991, 2(2): 3-15.

George R. and Houghton P. *Healthy dying*. Bristol PA: Jessica Kingsley, 1997.

Glaser BG. *Emergency vs. forcing: basics of grounded theory analysis*. Mill Valley, CA: The Sociology Press, 1992.

Goddard NC. Spirituality as integrative energy: A philosophical analysis as requisite precursor to holistic nursing practice. *Journal of Advanced Nursing*. 1995, 222: 808-815.

Goldman A. Hain R. and Liben S. *Oxford textbook of palliative care for children*. New York: Oxford University Press, 2006.

Greisinger AJ. Lorimor RJ. Aday LA. Winn RJ. and Baile WF. Terminally ill cancer patients: their most important concerns. *Cancer Practice*. 1997, 5(3): 147-54.

Grey A. The spiritual component of palliative care. *Palliative Medicine*. 1994, 8: 215-221.

Halldorsdottir S. and Hamrin E. Experiencing existential changes: the lived experience of having cancer. *Cancer Nursing*. 1996, 19(1): 29-36.

Harrison J. and Burnard P. *Spirituality and Nursing Practice*. Aldershot: Ashgate, 1994.

Higginson I. *Quality standards, organizational, and clinical audit for hospice and palliative care services*. London: National Council for Hospice and Specialist Palliative Care Services, 1992.

Ho SMY. and Shiu WCT. Death anxiety and coping mechanism of Chinese cancer patients. *Omega*. 1995, 31(1): 59-65.

Krause K. Coping with Cancer. *Western Journal of Nursing Research*. 1993: 15(1): 31-43.

Lai Y. Continuing hospice care of cancer: a three year experience. *Journal of Formosa Medical Association*. 1994, 93: 98-102.

Lars S. *A good death: on the value of death and dying*. Maidenhead: Open University Press, 2005.

Lau BWK. Feng Shui: an example of sense of coherence in Chinese geomancy? *Asian Culture Quarterly*. 1996, 24(4): 55-61.

Lee E. *A good death: a guide for patients and carers facing terminal illness at home*. London: Rosendale, 1995.

Ling J. and O'Síoráin L. *Palliative care in Ireland*. New York: Open University Press, 2005.

Loewe M. *Chinese ideas of life and death*. London: George Allen & Unwin: 1982.

Mak MHJ. Death awareness: An experience of Chinese patients with terminal cancer. *Omega*. 2001, 43(3): 259-279.

Mak MHJ. Accepting one's death: An experience of Chinese hospice patients. *Omega*. 2002, 45(3): 227-244.

Mak MHJ, 'Confucius' In Kastenbaum, R. et al. (Eds.) *Macmillan Encyclopaedia of Death and Dying* – eBook version. New York: Thomson Gale Reference, 2003.

Mak MHJ, 'Qin Shih Huang's Tomb' In Kastenbaum, R. et al. (Eds.) *Macmillan Encyclopaedia of Death and Dying* – eBook version. New York: Thomson Gale Reference, 2003.

Mays N. and Pope C. editor. *Qualitative research in health care*. London: BMJ Publishing Group: 1996.

McDonald M. Reflections on Ming, Fate and Destiny. *Asian Culture Quarterly*. 1993, 21(3): 9-28.

Melia K. Rediscovering Glaser. *Qualitative Health Research*. 1996, 6(3) 368-378.

Miller G. and Dingall R. editors. *Context and method in qualitative research*. London: Sage. 1997.

Morse JM. *Qualitative health research*. London: Sage. 1992.

Morton A. Translator. Chien M. The characteristics of Chinese culture. *Asian Culture Quarterly*. 1994, 22(1): 1-36.

Mount BM. et al., Ethical issues in palliative care research revisited. *Palliative Medicine*. 1995, 9: 165-170.

Murray JA. and Murray MH. Benchmarking: A tool for excellence in palliative care. *Journal of Palliative Care*. 1992, 8(4): 41-45.

Oppenheim AN. *Questionnaire design, interviewing and attitude measurement*. London: Pinter Publishers. 1992.

Orne RM. The meaning of survival: The early aftermath of a near-death experience. *Research in Nursing and Health*. 1995, 18(3): 239-247.

Palmer E. and Howarth J. *Palliative care for the primary care team*. London: Quay Books, 2005.

Parkes CM. Terminal care: home, hospital or hospice? *Lancet*. 1985, 1: 155-7.

Payne S. Seymour J. and Ingleton C. editors. *Palliative care nursing: principles and evidence for practice*. Maidenhead: Open University Press, 2004.

Petrinovich LF. *Living and dying well*. New York: Plenum Press. 1996.

Rinpoche S. *Glimpse after glimpse. daily reflections on living and dying*. New York: Harper Collins, 1995.

Ross LA. Teaching spiritual care to nurses. *Nurse Education Today*. 1996, 16: 38-43.

Royal College of Nursing. *Palliative Nursing Group Standards of Care for palliative nursing*. RCN Dynamic Quality Improvement Programme. Middlesex: Royal college of nursing. 1993.

Samarel N. The experience of receiving therapeutic touch. *Journal of Advanced Nursing*. 1992, 17, 651-657.

Seale C. Dying at the best time. *Social Science and Medicine*. 1995, 40(3): 589-595.

Searle L and Nyatanga B *Work-based learning in cancer and palliative care*. London: Quay Books, 2006.

Shen SM. On quality of life in Hong Kong. In Lau SK. Wan PS., Lee MK. Wong SL. *The development of social indicators research in Chinese societies*. Hong Kong: The Chinese University of Hong Kong. 1992, 129-146.

Strauss AL. and Glaser BG. Anguish. *A case history of a dying trajectory*. London:

Martin Robinson, 1977.

Sweeting HN. and Gilhooly MLM. Anticipatory grief: A review. *Social Science and Medicine*. 1990, 30: 1073-1080.

Taylor EJ. Amenta M. and Highfield M. Spiritual care practices of oncology nurses. *Oncology Nursing Forum*. 1995, 22(1): 31-39.

The West Midlands Paediatric Macmillan Team. *Palliative care for the child with malignant disease*. New York: Springer, 2006.

Vachon MLS. Caring for the caregiver in oncology and palliative care. *Seminars in Oncology Nursing*. 1998, 14(2): 152-157.

Vallerand AH. Measurement issues in the comprehensive assessment of cancer pain. *Seminars in Oncology Nursing*. 1997, 13(1): 16-24.

Yeung M. Editor. *If death is near you*. Taipei: Little Lion, 1996.(in Chinese)

Zerwekh J. The truth-tellers: how hospice nurses help patients confront death. *American Journal of Nursing*. 1994, 94: 30-34

Index

Printed in the United Kingdom
by Lightning Source UK Ltd.
128882UK00002B/43-45/P